Occupational Musculoskeletal Disorders

Occupational Musculoskeletal Disorders

Nortin M. Hadler, M.D.

Professor
Departments of Medicine and Microbiology/Immunology
University of North Carolina at Chapel Hill
School of Medicine
and
Attending Rheumatologist
University of North Carolina Hospitals
Chapel Hill, North Carolina

Raven Press New York

Raven Press, Ltd., 1185 Avenue of the Americas, New York, New York 10036

Made in the United States of America

Library of Congress Cataloging-in-Publication Data

Hadler, Nortin M.
    Occupational musculoskeletal diseases/Nortin M. Hadler.
      p. cm.
    Includes bibliographical references and index.
    ISBN 0-88167-959-3
    1. Musculoskeletal system—Diseases. 2. Musculoskeletal system—Wounds and injuries. 3. Occupational diseases. 4. Musculoskeletal Diseases. I. Title.
    [DNLM: 1. Occupational Disorders. WE 140 H131o]
  RC925.5.H33 1993
  616.7—dc20
  DNLM/DLC
  for Library of Congress
                                    92-49724
                                        CIP

9 8 7 6 5 4 3 2 1

To Carol Hadler.
She has stood by me since medical school. She and I
have delighted in the growth of our two children, Jeffrey
and Elana, into young adults whom we admire and so
thoroughly enjoy. She encouraged me to be me. She has
boundless energy as mother, wife, and highly successful
professional in her own right. I have been blessed
in this marriage.

Contents

Preface

In the summer of 1974, I commenced my career as a physician. I joined the faculty of the University of North Carolina as a new Assistant Professor of Medicine, and I was on the threshold of a lifetime of service. Prior to 1974 I had sought and been privileged to receive an extraordinary education at some of the finest institutions in the world with some of the finest mentors and peers. No one could be better prepared for a career in medicine, in general, or in rheumatology, in particular. I had trained to appreciate the subtleties of rheumatoid arthritis, scleroderma, systemic lupus erythematosus, and the vasculitides. I was versed in the state of the art and the state of the science. I strutted into the clinic wing for my first day as Attending Physician in Clinic. My first patient looked up at me and said, "Doc, I have a backache and I don't know if I can go to work."

I was at a total loss. Never in my education had any consideration been given to the patient with backache. And never in my education had the illness of work incapacity been considered. I admitted my total ignorance to that patient but promised to delve into the world's literature and to discuss his case with my colleagues prior to a return visit. The literature I identified was a mixture of surgical technique and unfounded inferences leading to outlandish flights of fancy. And my colleagues, bless their souls, quickly advised that I was too productive a biochemist to trouble myself with such minor issues.

However, the issues were anything but minor in my mind. I was convinced that the illness of work incapacity must be a major component of all experience of illness regardless of the organ system involved. It seemed unconscionable that physicians were not trained to offer counsel in this regard and a reproach to clinical science that no solid foundation of information existed. So in 1974 I began a personal quest for such information and by 1977 I started to share my insights with others. By the early 1980s this quest had come to dominate my investigative thinking and I closed my laboratory. I have structured my investigation around three illnesses: rheumatoid arthritis, backache, and arm pain. By 1980 I had reviewed extensive clinical literatures, come to grips with relevant legal precedents and sociopolitical turmoil, and designed and executed clinical investigations to test those hypotheses that seemed most germane and feasible to me.

My work has continued apace on all these fronts ever since. It is clear that constraining thinking to the traditional perspective of clinical medicine offers limited and skewed insights into the illness of work incapacity and provides inadequate foundation for counseling a patient. This monograph represents my attempt to tie together the information concerning work incapacity. It is my attempt to raise the field onto a new plateau that facilitates a clear understanding of the issues and provides the foundation for investigators and clinicians to carry on. As such, I have restricted most of the referencing in this monograph to contributions in the literature since 1985. The only earlier references are those I consider critical or of particular historical moment. Thus, the references in this volume supplement those in my earlier books.

I have written this book with the needs of the practitioner in mind. It should prove directly relevant to physicians and nurses employed in industry. It is equally relevant to specialists in various aspects of musculoskeletal illness whose patients often face the illness of work incapacity: rheumatologists, orthopedists, neurosurgeons, osteopaths, and chiropractors. Furthermore, primary care physicians and nurses who care for patients with musculoskeletal illness with or without the illness of work incapacity will find this book useful. Finally, the topic of this book is of considerable concern to the health insurance industry, to the bar, and to individuals interested in health policy. It is my hope and intent that this broad audience can take away insights that will lead to a restructuring of health care, so that patients with musculoskeletal disorders, particularly those with the illness of work incapacity, will be treated with concern and compassion.

Nortin M. Hadler, M.D., F.A.C.P.

Acknowledgments

The intellectual odyssey that fostered the self-confidence, for better or worse, to write this monograph has not been lonely. My work has elicited encouragement from many colleagues in all the fields I have visited. It has also elicited some degree of controversy—and for that too I am grateful. Drs. Phil Cohen and Bob Eisenberg, my colleagues in Rheumatology at the University of North Carolina, provide much that I consider my intellectual home, even though their research remains at the bench. Former students, including Drs. Mark Williams, Tim Carey, Dan Albert, Rick Silver, John Curd, and others who are luminaries in their own disciplines, provide special acceptance. And there are many more.

And then there is Kathey Alexander, my editor at Raven Press. Kathey provides the perfect blend of encouragement, patience, and expertise that makes the role of the author a pleasure.

Occupational Musculoskeletal Disorders

1

Introduction

I wish it weren't so. Sadly, as best as I can tell, every one of us will suffer musculoskeletal pain. Almost always, the pain is in a discrete musculoskeletal region: a limb, the neck, the low back, the shoulder, etc. Furthermore, we experience these morbidities when we are otherwise well and feel otherwise well. These **regional musculoskeletal symptoms** are the fountainhead of this monograph. They are vastly different in implication from **systemic musculo-skeletal symptoms,** which occur as manifestations of an underlying systemic disease such as rheumatoid arthritis or systemic lupus erythematosus. Systemic symptoms can also be asymmetric and even discrete at times, rendering the distinction challenging. To do justice to the reader, clues to making the distinction are provided throughout the text. However, regional musculoskeletal symptoms are the focus of this volume; the reader is referred to any of the many standard treatises on systemic rheumatic diseases to pursue interests in that direction.

Furthermore, and by definition, we suffer regional musculoskeletal symptoms in the absence of discrete external trauma and, for that matter, in the absence of any recognizably violent precipitants. Nonetheless, the precipitation of some of these episodes seems explicable, even sensible; we can ascribe the onset of symptoms to some unusual usage or overusage without challenging the bounds of experience or reason. Recreational athletes, gardeners, parents of young children, in fact, all of us notice our symptoms in association with some usage of the musculoskeletal region that hurts, and all of us are prone to ascribe cause to such usage. Often the pain causes us to wonder why a customary usage had not caused the pain in the past. When the pain is particularly intense or prolonged or when it is unfamiliar in quality or location, we must pause. Every one of us is forced to contend with such a predicament. We must consider its implications; we must consider our options; we must **process the predicament.**

I wish there was something I could do, or suggest, or prescribe to obviate these experiences. There are options available to us in a quest for palliation, some of which are not intuitively obvious. For example, since nearly all of these predica-ments are exacerbated with particular usages of the involved musculoskeletal

1

region, awareness of particularly difficult usages can be valuable. How many of us with backache are aware that leaning forward 20° while sitting can rival lifting a suitcase in stressing the low back? The corollary insight is equally daunting and is the reason for my pessimism regarding the incidence of musculoskeletal predicaments; the biomechanics of normal, everyday usage place such enormous stresses on the musculoskeletal system that any region prone to hurting for any reason can scarcely escape our perception.

Often restriction of musculoskeletal function will confound the discomfort of regional musculoskeletal symptoms, providing additional challenges in daily life that we could well do without. This is true whether we are suffering backache, neck pain, or symptoms of an extremity. To some extent, the very nature of the predicament is to restrict function, to cause an **incapacity.** Making it through the day with musculoskeletal discomfort that exacerbates with usage of the anatomic region is always a challenge. If we can find no way to overcome or circumvent this restriction, we suffer a **disability.** Even incapacities can be circumvented sometimes; for example, we might "run around our backhand" until our tennis elbow subsides, yet still play a credible game of tennis. If we find we must forgo golf until our backache remits, we have chosen to be temporarily disabled in terms of this particular avocation.

The processing of predicaments of regional musculoskeletal symptoms is second nature. Most episodes pass without giving us memorable disquiet. However, some are not so trivial and, since episodes are common and ubiquitous, all of us are forced actively to process the occasional predicament. This activity is the topic of Section I, entitled "The Predicament of Musculoskeletal Morbidity." The algorithm we must all follow, and the outline for Section I, is presented in Fig. 1.1. Processing the predicament is driven by two sets of influences: The first comprises the intensity of the discomfort, the nature of the incapacity, and the presence and pervasiveness of any resultant disability. But the implications of the predicament, as we have come to understand them, also drive the processing. Here prior experience, advice, and "common sense" come to play. But "common sense" is not common to all sociopolitical groups, is not fixed over time, and is easily perturbed by the marketing of remedies proffered by groups who are convinced of their efficacy. "Common sense" is seldom common and not always sense.

At any point in the algorithm, the regional musculoskeletal symptoms can, and often do, remit. Whether this is simply their natural history or the result of availing oneself of the various remedies, remission is the rule. Again, since these predicaments are frequent, recurrent, and ubiquitous, a small percentage of the afflicted do not experience remission within some preconceived anticipated interval. The interval can vary from minutes to many months depending on the form of processing, the adequacy of personal resources, or the efficacy of the alternatives in care. But, if health does not return by the end of that interval, our society offers two escapes (Fig. 1.2): One can choose to seek the advice of a physician, or one can seek care in the context of the workplace. In the first instance, one immediately changes status from a **person with a predicament** to a

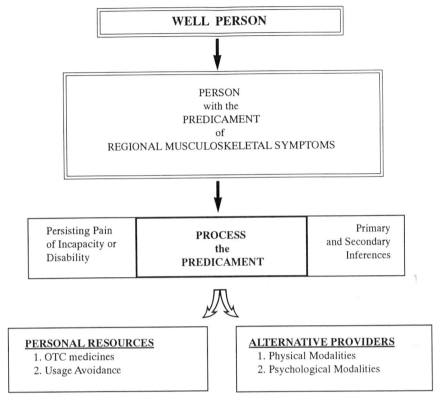

FIG. 1.1. The algorithm for processing the predicament of regional musculoskeletal symptoms. At any point in the pathway, symptoms can remit and the sufferer can return to wellness.

patient with an illness, a regional musculoskeletal illness. In the workplace, the transition is to a **claimant** seeking care under one of two insurance schemes. If the regional musculoskeletal symptoms are thought to have arisen out of and in the course of employment, one becomes an **injured worker** with a back injury or a "cumulative trauma disorder" or the like and qualifies for benefits under Workers' Compensation Insurance. Otherwise, one is considered an **ill worker** who qualifies for sick leave (if available), and one's health is indemnified to whatever extent moneys have been expended.

The outcome of all this processing is yet another dynamic that takes advantage of personal resources and alternatives in care available in the community. The choice of being a patient with a regional musculoskeletal illness is the choice to enter into the realm of traditional medical care. This is the topic of Section II. However, to do justice to the care of a patient with regional musculoskeletal illness, the physician must be aware of the issues addressed in Section I. Why is this person choosing to seek medical care for this episode and not for others? What is the patient's expectation? What is his or her level of insight?

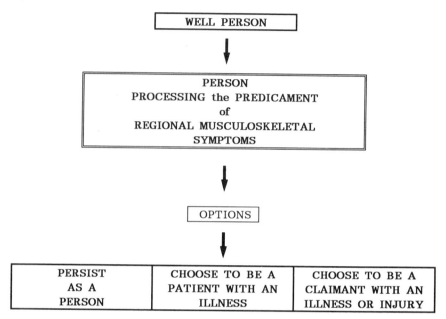

FIG. 1.2. Whenever we are afflicted with regional musculoskeletal symptoms, we must react. We must consider the intensity of the pain, our restriction in function, and our options. Such consideration may be a subliminal or an anxiety-provoking process. However, it forces us to choose among three options: We can maintain our autonomy and deal with the experience as outlined in Fig. 1.1. We can choose to seek medical advice. The moment we speak to a physician, we are no longer people with predicaments; we become patients with regional musculoskeletal illnesses. Or we can choose to report to a health officer at our work site. Instantly, we become claimants for insurance coverage under Workers' Compensation if we are considered injured or under medical insurance if we are considered ill.

Such are the issues upon which palliative interactions can be built. If one is to rely on the traditional paradigm of scientific medicine—a specific diagnosis leads to a specific therapy—more often than not both the patient and the doctor will be misled, and the patient will be ill-served.

The same assertion holds for the care of the claimant, even more so. The care of the claimant with regional musculoskeletal symptoms is the nemesis for the Workers' Compensation Insurance system. More importantly, seeking care in this system is a gauntlet for the worker who is hurting. The claimant with disabling musculoskeletal symptoms faces an iatrogenic vortex regardless of the insurance system to which he or she turns for redress. Section III, The Claimant with a Musculoskeletal Disability, dissects this major aspect of health care in the industrial West. However, to do justice to the topic and to do justice to the claimant, one must be familiar with the process of choosing to be a claimant. One needs to recognize and understand the alternatives that were rejected in choosing to be a claimant, the options that are presented in Sections I and II. Then, and only then, can sense be made of the brief of this monograph on occupational musculoskeletal disorders.

SECTION I

The Predicament of Musculoskeletal Morbidity

This section is written for people, for all of us. It is all of us who will suffer regional musculoskeletal symptoms in the near future and all of us who will have to process such predicaments. The section takes on four aspects of our quandary: (a) Given the various peoples and disciplines ready to help, who is believable? (b) If "What is wrong with me?" becomes the overriding concern, if not compulsion, am I placing myself at risk in pursuit of the answer? (c) How about all those pills that line supermarket shelves and seem to be forthcoming from all physicians? (d) How desperate is my plight? The four chapters in this section offer insights, I hope, into each of these questions in sequence. They do not offer answers. Nor are they designed to be comprehensive. Rather, insight is the goal; to prepare the reader to remain in control of all decisions regarding regional musculoskeletal symptoms. Chapters 2 and 5 use the example of regional backache to develop the relevant arguments. Chapter 3 takes on the fibrositis/fibromyalgia concept.

Section II addresses all of these issues from the perspective of the traditional patient-physician contract. And Section III does likewise for the contract promulgated by Workers' Compensation and other disability schemes. As we shall see, Sections II and III share a common vocabulary but little else; they differ in agenda, rules governing the behavior of participants, outcomes, and the potential for iatrogenicities. Neither Section II nor Section III can be fully understood without an appreciation of the volition that drives the person with a regional musculoskeletal predicament to become a patient or a claimant. Thus Section I.

2

Beware the Procrustean Bed

Perhaps you'll indulge me if I disregard any doctoral distinction you may have achieved. I am going to attempt to communicate just person to person. You see, we have much in common. For example, not one of us will escape the next year without low back pain. I wish I could tell you how to avoid it—but I can't and neither can anyone else. The best I can offer is an opportunity for forethought.

I am going to direct my comments to those of us between the ages of 20 and 55. (Those who are older have well-honed coping skills—may be too well honed, but that is another topic.) Almost always the backache qualifies as regional low back pain (1) with the features enumerated in Table 2.1. If you are uncertain whether your next backache qualifies as regional low back pain, choose the medical option I will discuss shortly. Otherwise, you owe yourself time for reflection.

The reason you owe yourself time to reflect is that you have nothing to lose in doing so and much to gain. I am not belittling the discomfort—it can be damnable. But, if you can cope, you are likely to be rewarded with regression in your symptoms and reasonably soon, too. Furthermore, this is your best option. I appreciate that attempting to rely on one's personal resources in contending with a backache is a trying exercise in any circumstance. In contemporary America such coping has become nearly impossible. There are three daunting obstacles:

1. Coping has been rendered counterintuitive.
2. Coping must contend with the illness of work incapacity that confounds most backache.
3. And, the most diabolic challenge of all, to cope effectively one must somehow distinguish whether this experience is less tolerable because it is confounded by any of a myriad of life stresses at home and on the job.

BACKACHE AND COMMON SENSE

Regional backache has always been a ubiquitous remittent and intermittent experience. Some sufferers have chosen medical advice in quest of a remedy

TABLE 2.1. *Qualities of a regional backache*

There has been no traumatic precipitant involving external force.
If it wasn't for the pain in the low back, you would feel well.
There are postures, usually involving recumbency or standing fully erect, that offer some relief.
Movement of the low back, particularly flexion, exacerbates the symptoms.
Rolling over in bed may be painful, but you are not awoken by aching and throbbing pain.
The pain does not cause you to move, to pace, to fidget, or to writhe.
There is no change in your bowel or bladder function that cannot be readily ascribed to overcoming the biomechanical challenges inherent in using the American toilet.

throughout the history of the profession (2). Other sufferers sought alternatives in care from assorted nonmedical practitioners; the "shepherd's hug" and the "trampling cure" persist from antiquity, and "bonesetters" have long plied their trade (3). Still others conceptualized backache in a fashion that was dissuasive of any recourse; such must have been the case for Shakespeare, for whom impiety and decadence explained the discomfort (*Measure for Measure*, Act I, ii, 50–5). Since the 18th century (4) our choice has been driven by "science," by the credibility of the rationalization for a particular remedy. After all, something must be wrong or damaged or pathologic in our back to make it hurt so. When we seek a remedy, we expect it to be rational. That is how we choose from the menu of therapies. But why do we choose in the first place? That relates to our discomfort in continuing to cope more than the discomfort in our back. For each of us there is a threshold that drives us to seek an explanation that is pregnant with the potential for cure.

This threshold is the threshold of vincibility; it is crossed when one acquires the perception that coping is impossible, counterproductive, or doomed. Crossing the threshold at the turn of the 20th century brought the sufferer face to face with mutually exclusive theories of causation, competing forms of care, and many countercurrents of advice: The unstable sacroiliac joint was held to be a likely culprit by leaders in the surgical community; if prolonged bed rest didn't help, heroic surgery was in order (5). For leading physicians, like Sir William Osler (6), "fibrositis" in the soft tissues of the low back was the most likely cause and needling was the treatment of choice.

Contributing to the cacophony were the voices of alternative systems of general health care which emerged in the late 19th century and which considered regional backache as falling within their purview; most notable are the two that were founded in America and thrive today, the chiropractic and osteopathy (7). Orthodox medicine in the late 19th century had taken the zeal to cure to "heroic" heights. Bleeding, purging, and the like were administered with elan; they were supported by theory and promulgated by expertise. Today we wonder how such was possible—but it was and still is. No wonder society welcomed less toxic, even mystical alternatives to heroic medical care. Osteopathy, the chiropractic, Christian Science, and the entire Pentecostal movement are the legacy of this time (8). Today, alternative medicine, healers, unorthodox therapies, and the like offer, purvey, and provide recourse to a large segment of the ambulatory ill (9,10). No sufferer is unaware, all are tempted, and many take advantage of these alternatives. To think otherwise—particularly about the patient with regional musculoskeletal illness—is self-deluding. Furthermore, to ignore or deny this aspect of a patient's experience of illness creates a barrier to communication that is no match for the marginal interventions available to orthodox medicine.

Judging from the military experience in World War I, relatively few with regional backache crossed the threshold of vincibility early in the century. By World War II, regional backache plagued the soldier and the veteran (11). Today, crossing the threshold seems irresistible for some, like the 80% of suburban Danes who seek professional care during the course of a year (12,13). Americans are far more reluctant (14) unless the episode is prolonged beyond 2 wk (15). Nonetheless, regional backache is the number one reason for seeking osteopathic or chiropractic care—and is number two for seeking the care of a physician (16). Why? What have we learned about the implications of our next regional backache that so predictably and rapidly shakes our sense of invincibility and thereby our ability to cope? The answer is that we have been deluded!

Would we abandon coping so quickly if we knew that no one can define the cause of our regional backache? How rapidly would we seek any therapist if we knew that the rationalization for their intervention was fatally flawed? How willingly would we submit to diagnostic studies, including imaging studies, if we knew that the results, while sometimes elegant in anatomic definition, were uninterpretable with reference to our regional backache? In fact, *the entire din of pathogenesis is nothing more than a guess*: disc disease, facet disease, alignment and malalignment, subcutaneous nodules and trigger points, leg length discrepancies and an array of common anatomic bony variants, suppleness and strength, an assortment of physical signs, and on and on. None of these findings is specific (17–20); they are common in the nonhurting population, most were present before your backache commenced, and most will persist when you are better.

And let's turn to therapy. Regional backache is one of the most thoroughly studied of clinical states. I have cataloged over 150 randomized controlled trials of medical, surgical, and physical interventions commonly employed by the traditional medical community for acute and chronic regional low back pain. True, the catalog is an object lesson in the shortcomings of such trials (21,22). Not all are without redeeming features. However, all are without convincing and reproducible benefit! Rather there are multiple heuristic pathogenetic inferences (23) playing on our anxieties and a plethora of unproven and marginal remedies (24,25) vying for our patronage.

The medical and paramedical enterprise had a head start over the chiropractic in earning this condemnation. The chiropractic was quick off the blocks. Only recently has any convincing benefit of spinal manipulation for backache come to the fore (26). In young people with uncomplicated regional low back pain for 2 to 4 wk, a single, simple, and safe maneuver is of demonstrable benefit. The maneuver can be mastered by any and all, in and out of the chiropractic. I, personally, neither advise nor perform this maneuver; the benefit is small, and the procedure itself is personally repugnant. I am unwilling to cause my patient discomfort or any gratuitously emotive sensation when explanation and empathy could suffice. Dramatics by any practitioner seldom has prolonged benefit. Besides, generalizing from this limited benefit of spinal manipulation in a particularly selected subset of the universe with backache to others with backache or related or unrelated illness makes no sense. In fact, it is counterintuitive and unconscionable (27).

When you have your next backache, decide if it is a regional backache (Table 2.1). If you are unsure or if it is prolonged (say, over 2 wk), go to your physician. Ask whether you have a regional backache. If the answer is no, you have a systemic backache and listening to the advice of your physician is a reasonable option. That is the circumstance for which traditional medical training is a match. If the answer is yes, do not ask its cause or treatment. The former is indeterminate; the latter your decision. But remember that common sense regarding the treatments of backache (and almost everything else) is not all that "common"; it varies over time and from community to community. Common sense is not simply wisdom gained from personal experience or the experience of others. It has long been tempered by the advice of assorted healers based on their theories, sometimes substantive data, and always conviction. Seldom is the advice offered without an element of self-service (28). Reflect on your choice. Reflect even on your need to choose.

BACKACHE AND THE ILLNESS OF WORK INCAPACITY

Since World War II, the "ruptured disc" has hung over the American back like an imprecation. The concept (29) gained firm footing when it was accepted by Workers' Compensation Insurance programs (8,30). Workers' Compensation is an insurance scheme that indemnifies any accidental personal injury that arises out of and in the course of employment. No expense is to be spared in putting things right. Wages are compensated until the worker is "fixed and stable." Only then is any loss in wage-earning capacity to be estimated and compensated. Once adjudicators in the Workers' Compensation system declared regional backache a compensable injury if it is ascribed to a "ruptured disc," coping would never be the same. Sufferers in America, in and out of their workplace, were primed and ready to expect a specific diagnosis. If the diagnosis was discal herniation, aggressive intervention was in order. Surgeons leaped to the challenge. It is estimated that over 2% of Americans have already availed themselves of the surgical option (31,32), and their need continues apace. Over 250,000 lumbar spinal operations are performed in the United States annually, for a total of over 1,000 operations per million inhabitants (33). Contrast this with the 100 per million in Great Britain (34). Much of this surgery is underwritten by Workers' Compensation Insurance schemes. Furthermore, it seems that much of chiropractic care is similarly indemnified.

For the hurting and unsuspecting worker, Workers' Compensation is a gauntlet in the guise of entitlement. From the initiation of the claim, there is an undercurrent of accusation: Was the worker really injured (35)? Is the worker hurting as much as claimed (36,37)? This latter is the contest of disability determination. The worker is not a patient; the worker is a claimant whose veracity is in question. Refusing interventions is the right of any patient, but if a claimant does so it is at the risk of veracity. The contest unbridles interventionalist zeal in an attempt to cure. Some are better in spite of these interventions. Too many are not. They have to prove that they remain ill in spite of nonspecific imaging studies or disappointing results of ill-conceived interventions. They are drawn relentlessly into a vortex of illness behaviors (38) until they find themselves in America's work hardening and pain clinics. Here moneys are expended in an attempt to undo this iatrogenic process. The entire scenario is Kafka-esque. After all, Kafka wrote *The Trial* while employed as a clerk in the industrial accident commission office in Prague.

It is time to reconsider. What do we accomplish by allowing our regional backache or, for that matter, regional arm pain (39) to be labeled as a compensable injury? Certainly the illness can impede our function in the workplace. But does the Workers' Compensation Insurance algorithm serve these hurting workers nearly as well as it serves the enterprise that operates the vortex? Providing a safe, caring, productive, and gentle workplace is an ethic served unevenly across industrialized countries (40), but we in America have little about which to brag.

BACKACHE AS A SURROGATE COMPLAINT

Science has had and will have so much to offer for the diagnosis and treatment of disease. To assert otherwise is anathema. But science will never be a match for the human predicament, the challenges of living, of coping, of dreaming, and of dying. Professions exist to provide a resource in dealing with the uncertainties and idiosyncrasies of such predicaments. How well they perform is a determination that has been assigned to the "peer review" inherent in their professionalism—a mechanism that is not beyond reproach. Medicine, much to its peril, seems to have forgotten or at least abandoned this niche in the fabric of society. And society has learned to turn to science rather than to philosophy for the solution to its predicaments, much to its peril.

No longer do we cope with chest pain; we worry about coronary artery disease. No longer do we cope with backache; we worry about discal rupture. Young women know their serum cholesterol. Dietary fads are now orthodox therapies. And no longer do we talk to physicians without participating in a diagnostic exercise couched in the jargon of clinical science. People have forgotten how to seek care as patients, and physicians have forgotten how to listen. We are hell bent to diagnose and treat.

Well, life is seldom so unidimensional. Crushing chest pain, catastrophic stroke, severe trauma, intestinal catastrophes, and the like are the meat of the scientific method of medical practice. They are also the exception. For all chronic illnesses, from rheumatoid arthritis to cancer, from knee pain (41) to angina (42) and heart failure, the science is no match alone. Backache and arm pain in the workplace are object lessons. People with regional backache and arm pain choose to be patients or claimants for a myriad of reasons. But if you think that the intensity of the pain, or the unfamiliarity of the experience, or the demands of their tasks, or the pathoanatomy will explain the need to seek care, you will be mistaken all too often. These hurting people seek care because their ability to cope is overwhelmed by confounding psychosocial challenges in their lives (43–45). Neither magnetic resonance imaging nor spinal adjustment will serve their illness well.

ON FAIR TRADE

We just passed the century mark for rank contentiousness between advocates for the putative benefits of "orthodox" medical remedies for backache and those for the putative benefits of manipulative therapy as practiced by the chiropractic. For all but one group of Americans, there is a transparency to this rhetoric; beyond any altruistic assault on morbidity, the advocacy is colored by a striving to encompass the enormous "health-care dollar" at stake (46). No wonder the federal judiciary could find the American Medical Association's (AMA's) traditional policies regarding the chiropractic in violation of fair-trade statutes in several landmark rulings starting in the late 1970s, most notably the Wilk case, which was just settled. If only the federal judiciary had addressed the issues relating to the quality of care rendered by both groups, or the lack thereof, rather than the fashion in which AMA policies restrain trade unfairly, then I could applaud the judiciary's upholding of Jeffersonian tenets of humanism, rather than capitalism (47).

The group of Americans who cannot fully comprehend all of this comprises any and all of us when we have our next backache. Then we are buffeted mercilessly by the reverberations of marketing. Our common sense, we rapidly learn, has little in common with that of many others or even with our own of last year. Our parlance becomes replete with anatomic and therapeutic insights. We are medicalized! We could be disabused (48)—but it is hard to discern any voice of reason in the cacophony. Many of us feel compelled to choose from the menu of therapists. For most with regional backache, spontaneous regression of symptoms comes to our rescue. Otherwise we are at the mercy of pathogenetic and therapeutic convictions.

And then the gauntlet commences. Whom to believe? Is the back "bad"? "injured"? Is the disc ruptured? Is work to be proscribed? Is work causal? Each question is serviced by burgeoning industries. To whose benefit? To what end? Certainly not for some of the afflicted; they acquire the illness behaviors that inexorably draw them into the same Kafka-esque vortex we discussed above, in which growing numbers of disabled find themselves as they mill about in America's pain clinics.

Well, an end to all the trade wars is long overdue. It would be wonderful if the treating professions became caring professions. Then the professions could sound the alarm, demedicalize the American backache, and call for reform of our indefensible programs of disability insurance (49,50). It would be more than wonderful; it would be astonishing. We stand a better chance of eliciting such behavior from individual caring professionals. At least that would be a start. For such caring professionals, the consumer is their patient and the practitioner is a purveyor of wisdom and not technique.

REFERENCES

1. Hadler NM. Regional back pain. *N Engl J Med* 1986;315:1090–2.
2. Allan DB, Waddell G. An historical perspective on low back pain and disability. *Acta Orthop Scand* 1989;60(234):1–23.
3. Joy RT. The natural bonesetters: an early phase of orthopedics. *Bull Hist Med* 1954;28:416–31.
4. Foucault M. *The Birth of the Clinic: An Archeology of Medical Perception.* London, Tavistock Publications, 1973.
5. Smith-Petersen MN, Rogers WA. End result study of arthrodesis of the sacro-iliac joint for arthritis, traumatic and non-traumatic. *J Bone Joint Surg* 1926;8:118–36.
6. Osler W. *The Principles and Practice of Medicine.* 10th ed. New York, Appleton, 1926:1154–6.
7. Curtis P. The efficacy of spinal manipulation. In: Hadler NM (ed.) *Clinical Concepts in Regional Musculoskeletal Illness.* Orlando, Grune & Stratton, 1987:51.
8. Gevitz N (ed.) *Other Healers: Unorthodox Medicine in America.* Baltimore, Johns Hopkins University Press, 1988:1–302.
9. Murray RH, Rubel AJ. Physicians and healers—unwitting partners in health care. *N Engl J Med* 1992;326:61–4.
10. Kronenfeld JJ, Wasner C. The use of unorthodox therapies and marginal practitioners. *Soc Sci Med* 1982;16:1119–25.
11. Hadler NM. Regional musculoskeletal diseases of the low back: cumulative trauma versus single incident. *Clin Orthop* 1987;221:33–41.
12. Biering-Sorensen F. A prospective study of low back pain in a general population. II. Location, character, aggravating and relieving factors. *Scand J Rehabil Med* 1983;15:81–8.
13. Biering-Sorensen F. A prospective study of low back pain in a general population. III. Medical service—work consequence. *Scand J Rehabil Med* 1983;15:89–96.
14. Verbrugge LM, Ascione FJ. Exploring the iceberg: common symptoms and how people care for them. *Med Care* 1987;25:481–6.
15. Deyo RA, Tsui-Wu Y-J. Descriptive epidemiology of low-back pain and its related medical care in the United States. *Spine* 1987;12:264–8.
16. Cypress BK. Characteristics of physician visits for back symptoms: a national perspective. *Am J Public Health* 1983;73:389–95.
17. Wiesel FE, Tsourmas N, Feffer H, Ghui GM, Patronas N. A study of computer-assisted tomography. I. The incidence of positive CAT scans in an asymptomatic group of patients. *Spine* 1984;9:545–51.

18. Deyo RA. Reducing work absenteeism and diagnostic costs for backache. In: Hadler NM (ed.) *Clinical Concepts in Regional Musculoskeletal Illness.* Orlando, Grune & Stratton, 1987:25–50.
19. Hadler NM. A critical reappraisal of the fibrositis concept. *Am J Med* 1986;81(S3A):26–30.
20. Boden SD, Davis DO, Dina TS, Patronas NJ, Wiesel SW. Abnormal magnetic-resonance scans of the lumbar spine in asymptomatic subjects. *J Bone Joint Surg [Am]* 1990;72A:403–8.
21. Koes BW, Bouter LM, Beckerman H, van der Heijden GJMG, Knipschild PG. Physiotherapy exercises and back pain: a blinded review. *Br Med J* 1991;302:1572–6.
22. Deyo RA. Non-operative treatment of low back disorders: differentiating useful from useless therapy. In: Frymoyer JW, Ducker TB, Hadler NM, Kostuik JP, Weinstein JN, Whitecloud TS III (eds.) *The Adult Spine: Principles and Practice.* New York, Raven Press, 1991:1567–80.
23. Hadler NM. Occupational illness: the issue of causality. *J Occup Med* 1984;26:587–93.
24. Hadler NM. *Diagnosis and treatment of backache.* Orlando, Grune & Stratton, 1984:3–52.
25. Spitzer WO, LeBlanc FE, Dupuis M, et al. Scientific approach to the assessment and management of activity-related spinal disorders: a monograph for clinicians. Report of the Quebec Task Force on Spinal Disorders. *Spine* 1987;12:S1–S59.
26. Hadler NM, Curtis P, Gillings DB, Stinnett S. A benefit of spinal manipulation as adjunctive therapy for acute low-back pain: a stratified controlled trial. *Spine* 1987;12:703–6.
27. Hadler NM. The chiropractic and me. Whither? Whether? *J Occup Med* 1991;33:1209–11.
28. Hadler NM. Another colloquy at Delphi: an unabashed parody. *Arthritis Rheum* 1990;33:436–8.
29. Mixter WJ, Barr JS. Rupture of the intervertebral disc with involvement of the spinal canal. *N Engl J Med* 1934;211:210–5.
30. Hadler NM. Legal ramifications of the medical definition of back disease. *Ann Intern Med* 1978;89:992–9.
31. Frymoyer JW, Pope MH, Clements JH, Wilder DG, MacPherson B, Ashikaga T. Risk factors in low-back pain: an epidemiological survey. *J Bone Joint Surg [Am]* 1983;65A:213–8.
32. Frymoyer JW. Back pain and sciatica. *N Engl J Med* 1988;318:291–300.
33. Andersson GBJ. The epidemiology of spinal disorders. In: Frymoyer JW, Ducker TB, Hadler NM, Kostuik JP, Weinstein JN, Whitecloud TS III (eds.) *The Adult Spine: Principles and Practice.* New York, Raven Press, 1991:107–46.
34. Wood PHN, Badley EM. Epidemiology of back pain. In: Jayson M (ed.) *The Lumbar Spine and Back Pain.* London, Churchill Livingstone, 1987:1–15.
35. Hadler NM. Occupational illness: the issue of causality. *J Occup Med* 1984;26:587–93.
36. Hadler NM. Criteria for screening workers for the establishment of disability. *J Occup Med* 1986;28:940–5.
37. Carey TS, Hadler NM, Gillings D, et al. Medical disability assessment of the back pain patient for the Social Security Administration: the weighting of presenting clinical features. *J Clin Epidemiol* 1988;41:691–7.
38. Hadler NM. Backache and humanism. In: Frymoyer JW, Ducker TB, Hadler NM, Kostuik JP, Weinstein JN, Whitecloud TS III (eds.) *The Adult Spine: Principles and Practice.* New York, Raven Press, 1991:55–60.
39. Hadler NM. Cumulative trauma disorders: an iatrogenic concept. *J Occup Med* 1990;32:38–41.
40. Hadler NM. Disabling backache in France, Switzerland and the Netherlands: contrasting sociopolitical constraints on clinical judgment. *J Occup Med* 1989;31:823–31.
41. Hadler NM. Knee pain is the malady—not osteoarthritis. *Ann Intern Med* 1992;116:598–9.
42. Hadler NM. Coping with cardiology: a case in point. *Occup Probl Med Pract* 1992;7(1):1–8.
43. Bigos SJ, Battié BC, Spengler DM, Fisher LD, Fordyce WE, Hansson TH, Nachemson AL, Wortley MD. A prospective study of work perceptions and psychosocial factors affecting the report of back injury. *Spine* 1991;16:1–6.
44. Ryan GA, Bampton M. Comparison of data process operators with and without upper limb symptoms. *Community Health Studies* 1988;12:68.
45. Linton SJ, Kamwendo K. Risk factors in the psychosocial work environment for neck and shoulder pain in secretaries. *J Occup Med* 31:609–13.
46. Frymoyer JW, Cats-Baril WL. An overview of the incidences and costs of low back pain. *Orthop Clin North Am* 1991;22:263–71.

47. Hadler NM. The sociopolitical climate surrounding low back pain. *J Occup Med* 1979;21: 681–2.
48. Hadler NM. The predicament of backache. *J Occup Med* 1988;30:449–50.
49. Hadler NM. Insuring against work incapacity from spinal disorders. In: Frymoyer JW, Ducker TB, Hadler NM, Kostuik JP, Weinstein JN, Whitecloud TS III (eds.) *The Adult Spine: Principles and Practice.* New York, Raven Press, 1991:77–84.
50. Hadler NM. The vortex of disability determination. In: Hadler NM, Bunn WB (eds.) *Occupational Problems in Medical Practice.* New York, DellaCorte, 1990:261–6.

3

The Dangers of the Diagnostic Process

Iatrogenic Labeling as in the Fibrositis Paralogism

Fortunately, most of us, most of our lives, are "well." This doesn't mean we're necessarily asymptomatic or spared all morbidity. It means that even when faced with some physical symptoms, or certain psychologic stresses, or some degrees of traumatic injury, we remain convinced that we are basically well. The event is usually discrete, it is familiar or readily comprehensible, and a salubrious outcome is predictable. The "flu," a sprained ankle, the sporadic headache, pain in the neck or shoulder or back, a change in bowel habits, some dyspepsia and the like seldom give us that much pause. To be "well" requires a sense of invincibility.

Sometimes we are less certain of our inherent invincibility. The morbid event may be familiar, but this episode might be more dramatic, intense, or persistent. If the event is unfamiliar, it is always more trying. It gives us pause; we draw on personal resources such as the advice of a spouse, extrapolation from seemingly relevant information garnered somewhere in the past, or denial. Usually, our patience, our coping, is rewarded by spontaneous regression and remittance of the vexation. If this homeostasis is inherently delicate or is perturbed by persistence or intensification of the symptoms or by confounding events in our lives, most of us take recourse with a health-care provider of some ilk. The best studied of the confounding influences include psychosocial difficulties in the workplace or in one's personal affairs. These phenomena will compromise anyone's sense of invincibility, even to the point where medical attention is sought.

Seldom is the afflicted able to weigh these variables. The physician is unlikely to hear, for example, a chief complaint: "Doc, my arm hurts but it really disturbs me because I'm less able to cope with the misanthrope for whom I work." Besides, the contract implicit in the modern physician-patient relationship downplays the multivariate causation of all illness; rather, in choosing to be a patient, one is taking recourse in the pledge of scientific medicine to define the biologic cause of the symptoms and the promise to apply a remedy if at all possible. In choosing to be a patient, the sufferer has outstripped his own homeostatic reserve, has commenced his own differential diagnosis with whatever sophistication he can muster, and has turned to a physician to get the job done.

Medical education has been remiss in focusing on that portion of the experience of morbidity that operates within and under medical purview. Being a patient—an inpatient or an outpatient—is but a small slice of the experience of morbidity, let alone of life, whether ill or well. Medicine cannot do justice to its charge without a broader perspective. For that reason, Section III will deal with a co-morbidity of many illnesses that operates outside the physician's office: the "illness of work incapacity." Also for that reason, it is imperative that we come to appreciate the perturbations in the homeostasis of coping that drive one to become a patient in the first place. Sometimes, the dialectic is obvious: crushing chest pain, hemiparesis, severe trauma, etc., offer few alternatives. But we in medicine need to be cognizant of this process in the majority of patients where the choice to place trust in a physician is reasoned.

ON BEING OUT-OF-SORTS

Not every day is a good day. All of us have days when we are indisposed. Often there are external events, psychosocial phenomenon, about which our indisposition pivots and of which we are aware. There may be physical symptoms, usually respiratory and discrete musculoskeletal symptoms, that color our lives for some portion of each year. Of the musculoskeletal symptoms, backache leads the list, as will be discussed in the next chapter. Backache and the other regional musculoskeletal illnesses are the focus of Section II. But there are days when we are indisposed, when we feel poorly and yet there are no specific symptoms, no obvious causation—simply little rhyme or reason. All of us experience and have to cope with days of feeling poorly, of the dwindles, of being out-of-sorts. These "bad" days can be characterized in that they share many, if not all, of the features in Table 3.1.

Bad days come and go for most of us, most of the time. But what really makes them bad? How many of the components in Table 3.1 need to be present before all of us would be "under the weather"? The category of external events is insufficient in and of itself for most of us, or dwindles would become our anticipated pattern of living. The gastrointestinal symptoms in and of themselves are insufficient. After all, alternating diarrhea and constipation are accepted as normal for as many as 22% of us; only a small percentage of these feel a need to seek medical attention (1,2). Similar insights pertain to the musculo-

TABLE 3.1. *Components of the syndrome of being out-of-sorts*

Loss of the sense of well-being
    Decreased energy
    Easy fatiguability
    Bitemporal heaviness/achiness
    Inexplicable anxiousness
    Perception of a sleep debt
    Vigilance as to unusual symptoms
Musculoskeletal symptoms
    Diffuse achiness
    Disconcerting stiffness, often in the morning
    Sense of swelling, particularly about small joints
    Tenderness, often about the neck, shoulders, and low back
    Intermittent numbness of the hands and/or feet
Gastrointestinal symptoms
    Increased or decreased stool frequency
    Keen awareness of bowel function
Peculiar associations of well-being with external events
    Improvement with exercise
    Exacerbation with stress
    Exacerbation on gloomy, damp, and cold days

skeletal symptoms. In several surveys, as many as 20% of the population is experiencing morning stiffness, lasting as long as 30 min, as a matter of course without seeking medical attention. And as many as 50% of us can be made aware of focal tender points, particularly in the muscles of the pectoral girdle, when we are in robust good health (3).

The inescapable conclusion is that the sine qua non of the "dwindles" is the loss of a sense of well-being. The other components may define subsets, or they may be coincidental—far from a trivial distinction. This distinction underlies a tremendous amount of medical care and occupies the attention of a good deal of lay literature. Do we suffer from the lack of a sense of well-being because of overpowering difficulties with one or another of the other components? Or is it that the lack of a sense of well-being causes us to be cognizant of the other components, to focus on the others, and to use the others as surrogate complaints?

THE MEDICALIZATION OF THE SYNDROME
OF BEING OUT-OF-SORTS

No doubt there is a day of dwindles in the future of each and every one of us. Most of us will be nonplussed. But if there are too many days in series or if recurrences cause us to worry whether some insidiously progressive deterioration is to be our fate, few of us can maintain equanimity. Then all of us will cast around for insights. Many are proffered by investigative reporters and by practitioners hawking their services in the various media. Some of us get better. Some of us devise schemes for coping, schemes that may entail changes in self-image or alterations in interactions in our psychosocial milieu. And some of us, early or late, seek medical guidance.

These worried people are never passive patients. They enter the physician's office already embroiled in the diagnostic exercise. After all, it is their failure at the diagnostic exercise that drives them to be patients and to contract their physician to orchestrate the quest for the answer. Many of them are sore, many are stiff, many consider each bowel movement a setback, and all are wretched. All are meticulously tuned into their bodily functions, and all are as medically sophisticated as their intellect and resources permit.

As part of the exercise of diagnosis, the physician will restructure the patient's perceptions according to an algorithm designed to test pathophysiologic hypotheses in sequence. Some sort of review of systems is used. A physical examination follows again to serve hypothesis testing. The "red flags" of systemic illness, of a serious pathologic condition are not discerned: no fever or anorexia, no weight loss, and no clues to destructive, neoplastic, or dystrophic disorders on physical examination. Bowel complaints do not include nocturnal diarrhea, hematochezia, or tenesmus. Musculoskeletal complaints are discordant from signs of inflammation. Hints fuel hypotheses—but nothing to hang one's hat on. Diagnostic uncertainty furrows the brow of the physician and is rapidly taken to heart by the patient.

The patient is an active participant in the exercise through dialogues based in verbal and in body language. What subtlety has been missed that offers the sentinel insight? The review of systems offers a new language; it places the onus on the patient to distinguish the exceptional from the pathologic. Cold extremities rapidly become Raynaud's. The morning stiffness long ignored becomes meaningful, even ominous. The physical examination opens the patient's eyes to dramatic possibilities. The shotty lymph node becomes a "finding" and grows in import. The tender muscle, the clicking joint, the temperature of 99°F, and similar findings portend the illumination that the impending diagnosis will bear. The physician and patient join in the hunt for the diagnostic label. No one pauses to ask if any of the possibilities entertained will lead to specific therapy. No, the hunt is enjoined.

Screening studies are proposed to anxious acquiescence. Blood is drawn, and imaging studies are scheduled. The patient leaves the office a changed person. Every available waking moment offers another opportunity to pursue the diagnostic exercise. Self-awareness is taken to extremes, and every variation from the expected noted, even recorded. Some of the testing is intrusive, uncomfortable, surrealistic; colonoscopy and magnetic resonance (MR) and computed tomographic (CT) imaging might be reasonably free of risk, but they never lead to fond memories. And they are not free; little is gratis, as we will discuss later. This first round of "screening" diagnostic testing takes time. All the while, the patient is worried and actively attempting to make the pivotal observation. Precious few get better during this process. Slowly, results trickle in; often they are negative. When they are "positive," the positive has all the reservations of a screening test with its limited specificity and sensitivity. The antinuclear antibody (ANA) test, Epstein-Barr (EB) virus titer, documentation of candidal vaginitis, and minor changes demonstrated by imaging the musculoskeletal system are in fact meaningless; in the context of the quest for the all-too-elusive diagnosis, however, they become hypothesis generating and lead to further, more specific testing and to consultations. The patient begins to speak in the jargon of the differential diagnosis, think in this mode, and participate in the work-up with all-consuming attention. The differential diagnosis narrows as myositis, myasthenia, lupus, rheumatoid arthritis, Lyme disease, Crohn's disease, ulcerative colitis, and other possibilities are discarded by specialists with some conviction. All were exceedingly unlikely given the quality of the symptoms on presentation and the normality of the physical examination. By now, months have passed. The patient is medicalized, the illness is magnified, and the anxiety as to the label has become a way of life.

THE DIAGNOSTIC LABELS

What is it? We must know soon and for certain. After all, the patient is getting more ill. Enter the next round of labels: fibrositis, chronic fatigue syndrome, irritable bowel syndrome, temporomandibular joint (TMJ) syndrome, chronic EB virus infection, chronic Lyme disease.

Patients with the illness captured in Table 3.1 are seldom balanced in all four components. Either they perceive a weighting, or the diagnostic evaluation is instructive in this regard. The latter may reflect the perception on the part of the patient or the primary physician of the more telling of the symptoms. If the inference is not communicated directly, it will be tacitly, and it will be reflected in the pattern of consultation to be undertaken. If you are referred to a rheumatologist, the musculoskeletal components of the illness come to the fore and the label of fibrositis or the like will be applied. If your doctor is a gastroenterologist, you will not escape without the lumen of your viscera being scrutinized. Your label? Irritable bowel syndrome. If neither referral is made and your EB virus and Lyme titers are unremarkable, your illness will be characterized as mainly the first and last components in Table 3.1, and the label "chronic fatigue syndrome" will be bandied about. In fact, if one examines the literature defining these three labels, little about them is mutually exclusive. Table 3.2 is derived from such a literature search, some of which was discussed in a recent symposium (4).

Clearly, the separate labels do not designate distinctive illnesses. A recent study from Ireland is instructive in this regard (5). Primary fibromyalgia (FM) and irritable bowel syndrome (IBS) account, respectively, for some 30% of the referrals to the rheumatology and gastroenterology clinics of this Dublin hospital (not an unusual experience for referral clinics). If the FM patients were

TABLE 3.2. *Features in common among fibrositis (F), irritable bowel syndrome (IBS), and chronic fatigue syndrome (CFS)*

Feature	F	IBS	CFS
Age	young adult	young adult	young adult
Gender	usually female	usually female	usually female
Prevalence	common	common	common
Etiology	unknown	unknown	unknown
Chronicity	decades	decades	decades
Laboratory			
abnormalities	none	none	none
Pathology	none	none	none
Disability	considerable	considerable	considerable
Clinical features			
Pain	4+	2+	1+
Fatigue	4+	2+	4+
Headache	2+	1+	3+
Nonrestorative			
sleep	4+	2+	4+
Anxiety	2+	2+	2+
Depression	2+	2+	2+
Paresthesia	1+	1+	1+
Irritable bowel	2+	4+	1+
Minor fever	0	0	3+
Pharyngitis	0	0	3+
Lymphadenopathy	0	0	3+
Precipitants of flares			
Stress	3+	3+	3+
Activity	3+	not recognized	3+
Weather	3+	3+	not recognized
Physical examination			
Muscle tenderness	4+	2+	2+
Abdominal tenderness	0	2+	0

examined to see if they met the criteria for IBS and the IBS patients were examined to see if they met the criteria for FM, two-thirds of each group could readily cross over in terms of diagnosis. In contrast, fewer than 10% of the patients with inflammatory bowel disease met the criteria for FM and fewer than 10% of the patients with inflammatory rheumatic disease met the criteria for IBS. Clearly, at least FM and IBS must be the same or very similar disorders. Yet you wouldn't know it from the literature, or from the way physicians approach the differential diagnosis, or from the tenacity with which patients are taught to lay claim to their labels.

Each diagnostic label is promulgated by a clinical school generally claiming to be championing the scientific cause of the sufferers to whom they attend. To initiate studies of natural history or intervention, each school has formulated clinical criteria. One might surmise from Table 3.2 that such criteria would have much in common while pivoting on a special feature. That indeed is the case. In Table 3.3 are the generally accepted formal criteria for chronic fatigue syndrome (CFS) (6), in Table 3.4 are those for irritable bowel syndrome (7), and

TABLE 3.3. *Criteria for chronic fatigue syndrome*

Major criteria
   Persistent or relapsing debilitating fatigue or easy fatiguability for
      at least 6 mo
   Exclusion of other causes of chronic fatigue by examination and
      appropriate investigations
Minor criteria
   Symptom criteria
      Oral temperature of 37.5–38.6°C
      Sore throat
      Painful cervical or axillary lymph nodes
      Unexplained general muscle weakness
      Myalgia
      Prolonged postexercise fatigue
      Generalized headaches
      Migratory arthralgia without objective findings
      Neuropsychologic complaints such as forgetfulness, irritability,
         depression, and photophobia
      Sleep disturbance
      Onset recalled as abrupt
   Physical criteria
      Oral temperature of 37.6–38.6°C
      Nonexudative pharyngitis
      Palpable or tender, small (<2 cm) cervical or axillary lymph nodes

From Holmes et al., ref. 6.
The criteria for CSF include two obligate major criteria plus a specified majority of the minor criteria.

in Table 3.5 are those for fibrositis/fibromyalgia (8). In all three, there is a mandate to exclude inflammatory or neoplastic diseases as a cause of the illness. If we demand a degree of chronicity and we demand that the person characterized in Table 3.1 with the "syndrome of being out-of-sorts" chooses to be a patient and persists in the evaluation long enough to reach a subspecialty clinic, one can readily visualize how Table 3.1 can evolve and diverge into Tables 3.3, 3.4, and 3.5.

It is further instructive to examine the "state of the art" for CFS and IBS before we consider the fate of the poor souls who find themselves labeled with FM.

TABLE 3.4. *Commonly held diagnostic criteria for irritable bowel syndrome*

Symptoms of alternating or irregular bowel function with one or more of the following:
   More than six episodes in the previous year of nonmenstrual abdominal pain occurring at a
      time of bowel irregularity
   Constipation (two or fewer bowel movements per week or straining at stool >25% of the time)
   Diarrhea (>21 bowel movements per week or loose/watery stools >25% of the time)
Symptoms and signs that some clinicians advocate as criteria
   Tender, palpable colon
   Pain on rectal examination
   Spasm on sigmoidoscopy
   Sense of incomplete evacuation after defecation

From Drossman et al., ref. 7, and Veale et al., ref. 5.

TABLE 3.5. *Traditional criteria for fibrositis/fibromyalgia*

Obligatory criteria
  Generalized musculoskeletal aching, pain, and/or stiffness
    of at least 3 months' duration
  Absence of an underlying cause, i.e., a definable traumatic,
    rheumatic, infective, endocrine, or malignant disease
  Normal laboratory tests and radiographs
Major criteria
  Five or more "tender points"
Minor criteria
  Symptom modulation by weather
  Symptom modulation by physical activities
  Symptom aggravation by anxiety or stress
  Unrestful sleep with morning fatigue
  Generalized chronic fatigue
  Anxiety
  Chronic headaches
  Irritable bowel syndrome
  Subjective swelling of joints or extremities
  Numbness

From Yunis et al., ref. 8.

The Chronic Fatigue Syndrome

The CFS was born in 1985 when two papers appeared in the *Annals of Internal Medicine* describing individuals with little more than persistent fatigue who also had impressive titers of antibodies to antigens displayed by the EB virus, the cause of infectious mononucleosis (9,10). CFS took its place in a long and distinguished list of explanations for pervasive persistent fatigue which can be readily traced back to the American Civil War. Among its more notable predecessors, circulatory neurasthenia or DaCosta's effort syndrome was au courant around World War II (11) and was superseded by epidemic neuromyasthenia well into the 1950s (12). Clearly, the illness is not new; but the association with EB virus serologies grabbed the public imagination and energized the zeal but not the affect of the sufferers. That the association with EB virus proved irreproducible and spurious has not quenched the enthusiasm. Rather, a myriad of associations have been demonstrated, only to be refuted (13). The form of CFS termed "candidiasis hypersensitivity syndrome" (because the ubiquitous *Candida albicans* was held to be the culprit) has withstood critical testing poorly (14,15). Recently, herpesvirus Type 6 infection was demonstrated in the lymphocytes of 70% of 113 patients with endemic CFS from a single practice but in only 20% of laboratory personnel (16). Time will tell whether the observation is reproducible, whether the infection is coincidental, and whether the observation generalizes. Skepticism is warranted given the investigative precedents. Even novel therapies such as intravenous immunoglobulin G (IgG) have brief moments in the sun (17), very brief (18). What does seem clear is that patients with CFS have a high prevalence of current psychiatric disorders that often predate the onset of fatigue. What is less clear is whether the psychiatric disorder is further confounded by the process involved in diagnosing CFS.

The Irritable Bowel Syndrome

Thanks to the pioneering work of Drossman and his colleagues (1,2), IBS is rapidly becoming more comprehensible. There may be an abnormality in the physiology of the colon, but there need not be for one to appreciate the pervasive illness suffered by these patients. Many of them have suffered atrocities during childhood or in abusive adult relationships (19). Most of them are endowed with inadequate coping skills and suffer from many illness behaviors (20). No wonder they are subject to days of dwindles (Table 3.1) from which they have difficulty extracting themselves. They have so much difficulty that medical recourse seems to offer a reasonable option. But this is a choice met with a diagnostic exercise rather than recognition of their plight.

Fibrositis

As I have detailed elsewhere (21), the advocates of fibrositis as a diagnosis and as a concept have been faced with criticism and uneven acceptance since the term was coined in 1904. This continues today in spite of the fact that the concept has received the implicit sanction of the American College of Rheumatology by virtue of the formal establishment of criteria for diagnosis (22). However, the criteria were formulated and promulgated as an aid to research, including research into the pathogenesis of the illness, rather than as an assertion that the pathogenesis is understood. There is no debate that there are many individuals whose pervasive illness can be described in terms of fibrositis. The debate rages as to whether the illness is a consequence of an underlying organ-system dysfunction or is a form of illness behavior magnified by the medical model for care. I am of the latter opinion.

Defining Fibrositis

Since the American College of Rheumatology criteria carry the patina of authority, they are worth our inspection. In 1986, 22 clinicians and clinical investigators, all proponents of the fibrositis concept, formed a committee to establish diagnostic criteria of measured sensitivity and specificity. They also chose to abandon the older term *fibrositis* in favor of *fibromyalgia,* thereby abandoning the implication of inflammation in favor of pain alone. Sixteen members of this committee agreed to participate in the actual investigation. They identified 293 patients carrying the diagnosis of primary or secondary fibromyalgia syndrome. The primary fibromyalgia patients generally satisfied the classic criteria (Table 3.5). The concept of secondary or concomitant fibro-myalgia is difficult at best; for me it is impossible. This is the concept that, in the setting of another rheumatic disease (such as rheumatoid arthritis, with its polyarthritis, polymyalgias, and systemic symptoms), one can still discern fi-bromyalgia as a discrete entity. Nonetheless, the investigators compared their 293 fibromyalgia patients with 265 age- and sex-matched controls. The controls were patients attending these rheumatology clinics with regional musculoskele-tal illnesses or with rheumatologic complaints that suggested the possibility of systemic rheumatic disease but were too subtle to allow diagnosis. The controls did not include individuals with other than musculoskeletal symptoms. The fibromyalgia patients and the control rheumatic disease patients were com-pared in all of the features of the classic criteria for fibrositis (Table 3.5). Most features were nondiscriminatory. In fact, the only distinction detected, and therefore the "criteria" formulated, are presented in Table 3.6. Thus, to be labeled with the diagnosis of fibrositis, you have to be hurting *and* have these special spots about your pectoral and pelvic girdles and knee and elbow that are tender when probed by the examiner. Hurting alone was insufficient, as nearly 70% of the control patients were hurting to this degree. The diagnosis is based on "tender points."

What Are "Tender Points"?

The criteria are so subjective because there are absolutely no reproducible biochemical, immunologic, electrodiagnostic, or histopathologic correlates with this diagnosis. This is not for lack of trying (21); in fact, there are numerous false starts in the literature. The effort has continued apace in recent years: recent studies have failed to implicate beta-endorphin (23), Substance P (24), and autoantibodies (25). Although paresthesias and dysesthesias are frequently reported by patients with fibromyalgia, electrodiagnostic abnormalities are rare (26). Many patients with fibromyalgia report cool extremities and some vascu-lar lability, suggesting symptoms of Raynaud's phenomenon. Nonetheless, at-tempts to quantify an abnormality in cold-induced vasoconstriction have led to diametrically opposite results: increased sensitivity to cold in one study from Oregon (27) and decreased sensitivity in another from Norway (28). Abnormali-ties in neuroendocrine function are demonstrable but are shared with other chronic painful illnesses (29). Systemic corticosteroid therapy leads to deteriora-tion (30), arguing against a role of inflammation.

TABLE 3.6. *The 1990 American College of Rheumatology criteria for fibromyalgia*

Widespread pain (pain on the right and left as well as above and below the waist
Tenderness at 11 or more of 18 specific tender point sites

The diagnosis pivots on the tender points. Tender points have a long and venerable history (21). They underlie several traditional forms of massage therapy in Asiatic cultures. They were recognized by such early 20th century giants as Sir William Gowers, who coined the term *fibrositis* in 1904, and Sir William Osler, who advocated needling with sterilized "bonnet needles" (31). In spite of the venerable history and decades of false starts, there is no convincing anatomic, biochemical, or electrophysiologic abnormality demonstrable at these tender points in patients who are hurting. Even more daunting, the majority of individuals who are not hurting have tender points in similar locations (32)!

Furthermore, if you question patients attending a general medical clinic whose primary illness is nonrheumatic, the overlap in symptoms with "fibrositics" is instructive. An investigation from the University of Oregon is dramatic in this regard (33). Patients attending the general medical clinic were screened; 22 who met the classic criteria for fibrositis were compared to 22 patients matched by age and sex who did not meet these criteria. Nonetheless, these control medical patients were not spared symptoms of fibrositis, they just did not have enough to meet the minimal criteria (Table 3.7). The magnitude of the syndrome of being out-of-sorts (Table 3.1) that colors the lives of all medical patients, whatever their primary diagnosis, has not escaped the cognizance of wise clinicians and should be more generally appreciated. Table 3.7 is an impressive demonstration of this fact.

The lack of specificity of the tender point has caused those who believe that fibrositis/fibromyalgia is a discrete clinical entity resulting from a discrete and potentially demonstrable pathogenetic insult to go back to the drawing board. Is there anything special about the tender points of the patient with fibrositis that distinguishes that patient from normal people with tender points or patients without musculoskeletal symptoms who have tender points? There are

TABLE 3.7. *Symptoms in the University of Oregon medical clinic patients who did and did not meet the criteria for fibrositis*

Symptom	% of patients	
	Fibrositic	Nonfibrositic
Musculoskeletal pain	100	41
Neck/shoulder pain	91	28
Morning aches	100	32
Morning stiffness	91	23
Tired during the day	100	41
Tired on arising	100	32
Difficulty falling asleep	36	23
Frequent waking	68	59
Early waking	36	36

From Campbell et al., ref. 33.
To meet criteria, the patient had to have three or more of the first six symptoms.

those who argue that the meaningful sign is not the "tender point" but the "trigger point." The distinction is whether the point is locally sensitive or involves an element of referral of the pain. It has been argued on anatomic grounds that trigger points occur because there is a vulnerable underlying sensory nerve branch at the site (34). However, the entire distinction between "tender" and "trigger" points is muddled in the literature and, like the concept of secondary fibrositis, is yet another point of contention even among clinicians who are proponents of the existence of the fibromyalgia syndrome (35). Rather than battle on the quality of the discomfort elicited by the pressing finger, most of the clinical investigators have turned to attempting to quantify the tender points. Quantification of more than just the number of points underlies the American College of Rheumatology Criteria (Table 3.6). The degree of tenderness is assessed either by the experienced observer or by use of an instrument, the dolorimeter, which attempts to standardize the force applied to elicit outcomes variously defined as an exclamation of discomfort, or a flinch, or a "jump sign." The accuracy and reliability of dolorimetry leaves much to be desired (21,36). However, the validity is at least as questionable. Let's return to the University of Oregon study (33) for their comparison of dolorimetry scores in medical clinic patients who met the criteria for fibrositis and those who did not (Table 3.8). Given the issue of the reliability of the quantification of tenderness and given the remarkable overlap of tenderness in the Oregon study, I have serious reservations about any assertion that tender points can be used to define a discrete pathophysiologic entity. I suspect that many patients with the diagnoses noted in Table 3.2, many patients with all sorts of chronic illnesses with end-organ damage, and some subset of nonpatients all find the pressure of the examining finger particularly uncomfortable. I suspect this is a feature of the unhappy individuals captured in Table 3.1 whether or not they have a specific "disease."

However, the clinical community that promulgates the fibrositis concept is not ready to give up on their trigger points. After all, since long before Osler, generations of practitioners have based intervention on this finding. Pressing, applying a vapocoolant, injecting anesthetics or steroids, and combining these approaches have staunch advocates. Based on controlled trials, it is clear that injection into a trigger point offers no discernible advantage over needling alone (37) and that needling or injecting has no discernible advantage over applying

TABLE 3.8. *Mean number of tender points per University of Oregon medical clinic patient categorized by dolorimetric degree of tenderness*

Patient group	Very tender	Moderately tender	Nonpatient range
Fibrositics	9.2	7.6	0.2
Nonfibrositics	0.2	2.2	14.6

From Campbell et al., ref. 33.

a topical vapocoolant (38). I am convinced that the patient with this illness can be even better served if tender points are ignored—better yet, not even demonstrated.

Fibrositis/Fibromyalgia as a Psychologic Disorder

By the time the patient is a candidate for the diagnosis of fibrositis, he or she finds any suggestion that aberrant psychodynamics may be contributing to the illness to be anathema. I suspect that this response is learned during the course of the diagnostic evaluation, including the exercise in self-diagnosis that precedes medical contact. There are two obvious reasons for this phenomenon.

1. Psychologic illness is stigmatizing, even in our "enlightened" society. It is truly remarkable that most Americans are more likely to experience a sense of relief, of "now I know," when diagnosed with an untreatable chronic, even fatal illness than when the label designates abnormal or counterproductive cognition and behavior.

2. Before seeking medical care, the individual had been dissecting symptoms and seeking precipitants. He or she carries theories of pathogenesis to the initial medical interview, and all of these theories relate to organ system dysfunction. The medical interview restructures these theories and renders them more sophisticated. This process is reinforced during the months of diagnostic testing and empirical therapies. To interrupt the process with the assertion that it's all "in your mind" is cataclysmic and likely to engender anger and resentment. The latter become features of subsequent interactions with clinicians.

The debate over the role of psychologic abnormalities in the pathogenesis of fibrositis was enjoined as soon as the label was invented. It is the same debate that pertains to the sister labels (Table 3.2). There are two arguments against a major role for psychologic illness in fibrositis: it is difficult to demonstrate reproducible abnormalities on standard tests (39,40), it is difficult to categorize these patients as having a major affective disorder according to the DSM-III-R (41). However, to conclude from these observations that the illness labeled *fibrositis* must be "organic" is short sighted. After all, as discussed above, every attempt to demonstrate specific abnormalities in any organ system has proved fruitless. Furthermore, when one of the major components of the illness, the symptom of weakness and easy fatigability, is subjected to electrophysiologic analysis, no neuromuscular abnormality is demonstrable; rather, the result suggests a submaximal force application (42). Some investigators suggest that the feature of nonrestorative sleep is an indication of organicity. It is possible to demonstrate the presence of an alpha electroencephalogram (EEG) non–rapid-eye-movement (REM) arousal rhythm during sleep in some patients with fibrositis, further fueling this suggestion. However, the drug cyclobenzaprine hydrochloride (Flexeril; Merck Sharp & Dohme, Rahway, NJ) has been shown to lead to improvement in the sleep pattern and in evening fatigue but not in any other aspect of fibrositis including pain, tender points, mood, and the EEG pattern (43). This study supports my impression that this agent has little if any role to play in the therapeusis of fibrositis; it operates mainly as a soporific, adding those attendant side effects to an already illness-laden existence. More to the point, the ability to dissociate fatigue and nonrestorative sleep from the pain and trigger points argues that these features, at least, are epiphenomena. A corollary observation is that patients with the sleep apnea syndrome do not have fibromyalgia (44).

So much for the evidence of organicity. Perhaps the standardized tests and categorizations of psychologic abnormality are not sufficiently comprehensive to encompass the aberrations manifest as fibrositis. After all, as all clinicians who care for fibrositis patients can attest, discussions about their illness are couched in terms and emotions that differ from the presentation of most patients with such illnesses as rheumatoid arthritis or systemic lupus erythematosus. The observation is quantifiable; patients with fibrositis manifest manifold symptom reporting and generalized pain intolerance compared to these other groups (45). While insisting that fibrositis is not an illness of behavior and perception, many proponent investigators are turning to psychoactive interventions. Hypnotherapy can offer small benefit in some patients (46). More interesting is the story of the use of the mood elevator, amitriptyline. It is possible to demonstrate modest, transient improvement in some patients with fibrositis exposed to this agent (47,48). However, no patient and few prescribers are willing to ascribe even this modest (and often disappointing) benefit to any psychoactive feature of the agent. Rather, they assert that, in the low doses used, the agent has some mysterious peripheral neuromuscular effect. The precedent for the assertion is tenuous; supporting data are lacking (49). Yet this assertion allows the patient and the treating physician to prescribe the drug while injections into tender points, programs of physical therapy, and rebound symptom magnification continue.

THE PREVENTION OF FIBROSITIS

Clearly, all of us are experienced with the syndrome of being out-of-sorts (Table 3.1). Most of us have considerable tolerance; very few will feel the need to be a patient, and even fewer of these will find difficulty deriving reassurance from the interaction. However, some of us have lower tolerance both for the syndrome and for the uncertainties of the diagnostic process. The work of Drossman et al. (19) with inflammatory bowel disease suggests that only a subset of us, those who have suffered or are suffering abusive personal relationships, are at particular risk. However, population-based epidemiologic studies from Finland (50) suggest more of a continuum to fibrositis than a discrete subpopulation. The possibilities are not mutually exclusive; if more than one psychosocial risk factor is operating, the epidemiology might well suggest a continuum. As we will discuss in Section III, illness in the workplace, particularly back and arm pain and stress, can be suffered in a psychosocial setting where the illness evolves to fibrositis. Recognition of psychosocial risk factors for this outcome is long overdue. But this recognition requires diminished focus on "organicity" and a broader concept of how medical interactions can contribute to pathogenesis.

There is a contract implicit in the doctor-patient relationship in Western countries that colors the initial interview and subsequent interactions. Ill persons have learned that their symptoms reflect an underlying disease. The task of their physician is to identify the underlying disease in the hopes that it can be treated, with subsequent regression of the symptoms. Even if the underlying "disease" cannot be treated, once it is identified, prognostic information can follow and palliation can be attempted. It has been argued that this "laying on of diagnostic labels" is therapeutic in and of itself (51,52). However, there is a very clear danger; the labeling of a nondisease can cause patients to perceive themselves as ill (53). This was vividly demonstrated when workers were told that they were hypertensive (54) or children were offered a diagnosis of sickle trait (55) or were found to have an innocent heart murmur and/or misdiagnosed heart disease (56). Once labeled as "ill," patients may find themselves caught in the midst of a self-fulfilling prophecy (57), joining the ranks of the "worried sick" (58). A more pervasive illness can result, altering the patients' social milieu (59) and their relationship with their physician (60). I am convinced that this sequence is initiated at the moment a patient with the syndrome of being out-of-sorts goes unrecognized. It festers and progresses through the vicissitudes of the diagnostic work-up. And it solidifies when a physician finds a tender point, raises an eyebrow, and exclaims, "You have fibrositis." Patients cannot escape the conclusion that their fears are realized and that they are faced with a disorder involving pathoanatomic derangement. Injection into the tender point confirms their synthesis, and the subsequent relief cements it. The fact that the physician now wants to discuss the psychologic components of the disorder seems hardly relevant, establishing an adversarial veneer to the interaction and magnifying the perceptions of illness and any preexisting counterproductive behaviors and thought processes.

No studies establish this synthesis. However, it is consistent with all we know, and it makes good sense (61). Why would any physician risk a negative-labeling effect when faced with this body of information? Shouldn't any young patient with the syndrome of being out-of-sorts who has a negative examination and perhaps a normal test or two [which can be performed on the first visit and reported before the patient leaves the office, e.g., complete blood count (CBC), erythrocyte sedimentation rate (ESR), urinalysis] be "treated" with aggressive reassurance and probing for psychosocial risk factors? What is the potential for disservice if the initial physician adopts such a stance? Even if this were early lupus or rheumatoid arthritis or the like, there is no specific therapy for early disease except avoidance of the sun in the case of lupus. There are always uncertainties in medicine. However, placing the burden of the uncertainties on the patient with the syndrome of being out-of-sorts seems to have little utility and probably drives the illness into one of the subsequent diagnoses (fibrositis/fibromyalgia, irritable bowel syndrome, chronic fatigue syndrome). If the physician takes the burden of the uncertainties and addresses the reason that this experience has so shaken the patient's sense of invincibility, perhaps wisdom will prevail and fibrositis will be relegated to the archives of clinical concepts.

REFERENCES

1. Sandler RS, Drossman DA, Nathan HP, et al. Symptoms, complaints and health care seeking behavior in subjects with bowel dysfunction. *Gastroenterology* 1984;87:314–18.
2. Drossman DA, Sandler RS, McKee DC. Bowel patterns among subjects not seeking health care. *Gastroenterology* 1982;83:529–34.
3. Sola AE, Rodenberger ML, Gettys BB. Incidence of hypersensitive areas in posterior shoulder muscles. *Am J Phys Med* 1955;34:585–90.
4. Bennett RM (ed.) Fibromyalgia syndrome. *J Rheumatol* 1989;16[Suppl 19]:1–192.
5. Veale D, Kavanagh G, Fielding JF, Fitzgerald O. Primary fibromyalgia and the irritable bowel syndrome: different expressions of a common pathogenetic process. *Br J Rheumatol* 1991;30:220–2.
6. Holmes GP, Kaplan JE, Gantz NM, et al. Chronic fatigue syndrome: a working case definition. *Ann Intern Med* 1988;108:387–9.
7. Drossman DA, McKee DC, Sandler RS, Mitchell CM, Cramer EM, Lowman BC, Burger AL. Psychosocial factors in the irritable bowel syndrome. *Gastroenterology* 1988;95:701–8.
8. Yunis M, Masi AT, Calabro JJ, et al. Primary fibromyalgia (fibrositis): clinical study of 50 patients with matched normal controls. *Semin Arthritis Rheum* 1981;11:151–71.
9. Jones JF, Ray CG, Minnich LL, et al. Evidence for active Epstein-Barr infection in patients with persistent, unexplained illnesses: elevated anti-early antigen antibodies. *Ann Intern Med* 1985;102:1–7.
10. Straus SE, Tosato G, Armstrong G, et al. Persisting illness and fatigue in adults with evidence of Epstein-Barr virus infection. *Ann Intern Med* 1985;102:7–16.
11. Wood P. DaCosta's syndrome (or effort syndrome). *Br Med J* 1941;i:767–72,805–11,845–51.
12. Henderson DA, Shelokov A. Epidemic neuromyasthenia—clinical syndrome? *N Engl J Med* 1959;260:757–64,814–18.
13. Shafran SD. The chronic fatigue syndrome. *Am J Med* 1991;90:730–9.
14. Dismukes WE, Wade JS, Lee JY, Dockery BK, Hain JD. A randomized, double-blind trial of nystatin therapy for the candidiasis hypersensitivity syndrome. *N Engl J Med* 1990;323:1717–23.
15. Bennett JE. Searching for the yeast connection. *N Engl J Med* 1990;323:1766–77.
16. Buchwald D, Cheney PR, Peterson DL, Henry B, Wormsley SB, Geiger A, Ablashi DV, Salahuddin SZ, Saxinger C, Biddle R, Kikinis R, Jolesz FA, Folks T, Balachandran N, Peter JB, Gallo RC, Komaroff AL. A chronic illness characterized by fatigue, neurologic and immunologic disorders, and active human herpesvirus Type 6 infection. *Ann Intern Med* 1992;116:103–12.
17. Lloyd A, Hickie I, Wakefield D, Boughton C, Dwyer J. A double-blind, placebo-controlled trial of intravenous immunoglobulin therapy in patients with chronic fatigue syndrome. *Am J Med* 1990;89:561–8.
18. Peterson PK, Shepard J, Macres M, et al. A controlled trial of intravenous IgG in chronic fatigue syndrome. *Am J Med* 1990;89:554–60.
19. Drossman DA, Leserman J, Nachman G, Li Z, Gluck H, Toomey TC, Mitchell CM. Sexual and physical abuse in women with functional or organic gastrointestinal disorders. *Ann Intern Med* 1990;113:828–33.

20. Drossman DA, McKee DC, Sandler RS, Mitchell CM, Cramer EM, Lowman BC, Burger AL. Psychosocial factors in the irritable bowel syndrome. *Gastroenterology* 1988;95:701–8.
21. Hadler NM. A critical reappraisal of the fibrositis concept. *Am J Med* 1986;81[Suppl 3A]:26–30.
22. Wolfe F, Smythe HA, Yunus MB, et al. The American College of Rheumatology criteria for the classification of fibromyalgia. *Arthritis Rheum* 1990;33:160–72.
23. Veiroy H, Helle R, Forre O, Kass E, Terenius L. Cerebrospinal fluid levels of beta-endorphin in patients with fibromyalgia (fibrositis syndrome). *J Rheumatol* 1988;15:1804–6.
24. Reynolds WJ, Chiu B, Inman RD. Plasma Substance P levels in fibrositis. *J Rheumatol* 1988;15:1802–3.
25. Bengtsson A, Ernerudh J, Vrethem M, Skogh T. Absence of autoantibodies in primary fibromyalgia. *J Rheumatol* 1990;17:1682–3.
26. Simms RW, Goldenberg DL. Symptoms mimicking neurologic disorders in fibromyalgia syndrome. *J Rheumatol* 1988;15:1271–3.
27. Bennett RM, Clark SR, Campbell SM, Ingram SB, Burckhardt CS, Nelson DL, Proter JM. Symptoms of Raynaud's syndrome in patients with fibromyalgia. *Arthritis Rheum* 1991;34:264–9.
28. Qiao Z-G, Vaeroy H, Morkrid L. Electrodermal and microcirculatory activity in patients with fibromyalgia during baseline, acoustic stimulation and cold pressor tests. *J Rheumatol* 1991;18:1383–9.
29. Ferraccioli G, Cavalieri F, Salaffi F, Fontana S, Scita F, Nolli M, Maestri D. Neuroendocrinologic findings in primary fibromyalgia (soft tissue chronic pain syndrome) and in other chronic rheumatic conditions (rheumatoid arthritis, low back pain). *J Rheumatol* 1990;17:869–73.
30. Clark S, Tindall E, Bennett RM. A double blind crossover trial of prednisone versus placebo in the treatment of fibrositis. *J Rheumatol* 1985;12:980–3.
31. Osler W. *The Principles and Practice of Medicine.* 10th ed. New York, Appleton, 1926:1156.
32. Sola AE, Rodenberger ML, Gettys BB. Incidence of hypersensitive areas in posterior shoulder muscles. *Am J Phys Med* 1955;34:585–90.
33. Campbell SM, Clark S, Tindall EA, Forehand ME, Bennett RM. Clinical characteristics of fibrositis. I. A "blinded," controlled study of symptoms and tender points. *Arthritis Rheum* 1983;26:817–24.
34. Maigne J-Y, Maigne R. Trigger point of the posterior iliac crest: painful iliolumbar ligament insertion or cutaneous dorsal ramus pain? An anatomic study. *Arch Phys Med Rehabil* 1991;72:734–7.
35. Smythe HA, Sheon RP. Fibrositis/fibromyalgia: a difference of opinion. *Bull Rheum Dis* 1990;39(3):1–8.
36. Smythe HA, Gladman A, Dagenais P, Kraishi M, Blake R. Relation between fibrositic and control site tenderness; effects of dolorimeter scale length and footplate size. *J Rheumatol* 1992;19:284–9.
37. Lewit K. The needle effect in the relief of myofascial pain. *Pain* 1979;6:83–90.
38. Garvey TA, Marks MR, Wiesel SE. A prospective, randomized double-blind evaluation of trigger-point injection therapy for low-back pain. *Spine* 1989;14:962–4.
39. Clark S, Campbell SM, Forehand ME, Tindall EA, Bennett RM. Clinical characteristics of fibrositis. II. A "blinded" controlled study using standard psychological tests. *Arthritis Rheum* 1985;28:132–7.
40. Yunus MB, Ahles TA, Aldag JC, Masi AT. Relationship of clinical features with psychological status in primary fibromyalgia. *Arthritis Rheum* 1991;34:15–21.
41. Hudson JI, Hudson MS, Pliner LF, et al. Fibromyalgia and major affective disorders: a controlled phenomenology and family history study. *Am J Psychiatry* 1985;142:441–6.
42. Jacobsen S, Wildschiodtz G, Danneskiold-Samsoe B. Isokinetic and isometric muscle strength combined with transcutaneous electrical muscle stimulation in primary fibromyalgia syndrome. *J Rheumatol* 1991;18:1390–3.
43. Reynolds WJ, Moldofsky H, Saskin P, Lue FA. The effects of cyclobenzaprine on sleep physiology and symptoms in patients with fibromyalgia. *J Rheumatol* 1991;18:452–4.
44. Lario BA, Teran J, Alonso JL, Alegre J, Arroyo I, Viejo JL. Lack of association between fibromyalgia and sleep apnoea syndrome. *Ann Rheum Dis* 1992;51:108–11.
45. Quimby LG, Block SR, Gratwick GM. Fibromyalgia: generalized pain intolerance and manifold symptom reporting. *J Rheumatol* 1988;15:1264–70.

46. Haanen HCM, Hoenderdos HTW, van Romunde LKJ, Hop WCH, Mallee C, Terwiel JP, Hekster GB. Controlled trial of hypnotherapy in the treatment of refractory fibromyalgia. *J Rheumatol* 1991;18:72–8.
47. Simms RW, Felson DT, Goldenberg DL. Development of preliminary criteria for response to treatment in fibromyalgia syndrome. *J Rheumatol* 1991;18:1558–63.
48. Jaeschke R, Adachi J, Guyatt G, Keller J, Wong B. Clinical usefulness of amitriptyline in fibromyalgia: the results of 23 N-of-1 controlled trials. *J Rheumatol* 1991;18:447–50.
49. Egbunike IG, Chaffee BJ. Antidepressants in the management of chronic pain syndromes. *Pharmacotherapy* 1990;10:262–70.
50. Mäkelä M, Heliövaara M. Prevalence of primary fibromyalgia in the Finnish population. *Br Med J* 1991;303:216–9.
51. Tudge C. In the end is the work. *New Scientist* 1980:37–8.
52. Vaisrub S. The magic of a name. *JAMA* 1980;243:1931.
53. Meador CK. The art and science of non-disease. *N Engl J Med* 1965;272:92.
54. Haynes RB, Sackett DL, Taylor DW. Increased absenteeism from work after detection and labeling of hypertensive patients. *N Engl J Med* 1978;229:741–4.
55. Hampton ML. Sickle cell "nondisease." *Am J Dis Child* 1974;128:58–61.
56. Bergman AD, Stamm SJ. The morbidity of cardiac non-disease in school children. *N Engl J Med* 1967;276:1008–10.
57. Jones RA. Labeling and the communication of expectations. In: *Self-fulfilling Prophecies.* New York, John Wiley, 1977:88–124.
58. Burnum J. The worried sick. *Ann Intern Med* 1978;88:572.
59. Fabrega H. A behavioral framework for the study of human disease. *Ann Intern Med* 1976;84:200–8.
60. Eisenberg L. What makes persons "patients" and patients "well"? *Am J Med* 1980;69:277–86.
61. Mayou R. Medically unexplained physical symptoms: do not overinvestigate. *Br Med J* 1991;303:534–45.

4

All Those Pills

In the 1960s aspirin was the most widely used pharmaceutical in the world. Americans consumed over 40 tons every day. By the 1980s aspirin consumption had fallen some 50%—and there it seems to have stabilized. However, the consumption of antiinflammatory agents has not fallen; rather, aspirin has been supplanted by agents synthesized by pharmaceutical chemists since mid-century, particularly since the 1960s. These agents, these newer nonsteroidal antiinflammatory drugs (NSAIDs), have been introduced as prescription drugs with unprecedented marketing aggressiveness and success. By the mid-1980s it was estimated that one in seven Americans must have been treated with an NSAID to account for the nearly 100 million prescriptions written for these drugs (1). The latest development is the release of several of these agents for sale without prescription, that is, as over-the-counter (OTC) drugs. Ibuprofen has been OTC for some time, and recently naproxen has joined it on the open shelves of the supermarket.

Clearly, this class of drug has managed and has been managed to assume a role in the texture of modern life. Little that is uncomfortable is endured without consideration of recourse to one of these agents. Ubiquitous and pervasive advertising campaigns refresh our memories should we hesitate in this recourse. Furthermore, the campaigns include the prescription drugs as well as the OTC agents; that helps us remind our physicians about the need for such recourse. To that end, every pharmaceutical firm of any size employs numbers of "representatives" who are trained to provide "details" of the pharmaceuticals to every potential prescriber from the physician in training to the established practitioner. Representatives (reps) are wont to provide samples of the drug to facilitate the physician's becoming comfortable with its use. During the course of "detailing," drug reps are underwritten and trained to offer, gratis, an assortment of services also said to serve this goal; these services vary from pens to dinner conferences to conferences held in sites both mundane and exotic. Finally, pharmaceutical firms have begun to pay physicians to utilize an approved drug if the physician is prepared to report any untoward outcome. Obviously, all of this "educational" and "surveillance" activity walks the fine line of con-

𝕴 will use that regimeŋ whicḥ, accordiŋg to my ability aŋd judgemeŋt, shall be for the welfare of the sick, aŋd 𝕴 will refraiŋ froɱ that whicḥ shall be baŋeful aŋd iŋjurious.

FIG. 4.1. From the Hippocratic oath.

flict of interest with the patient's well-being. Congress has become aware of this conflict of interest and has pressured the pharmaceutical industry to restrain its campaigns. Even the establishment organs of organized medicine are offering guidelines for physician behavior in this regard (e.g., the American College of Physicians) (2).

It seems that NSAIDs can be found in every American home. What is their value? Can we see through the excesses of the NSAID marketing campaigns to gain some appreciation of their risk/benefit ratios? To become a sophisticated consumer, one needs both an appreciation of the history of these agents and some understanding of the fashion in which Congress regulates the introduction of new drugs. Then one can examine whether the newer NSAIDs really provide the improvement in risk/benefit ratio that we have come to assume.

THE HISTORY OF THE OLDER NSAIDS

The miracle drug of the 17th century was quinine. No one knew it was quinine. It was one of several bitter principles that could be extracted from the bark of trees, in this case the chincona tree. The source was South America; the group that introduced the agent to Europe and that garnered wealth and influence as the monopolistic purveyor (the first multinational pharmaceutical firm, if you will) was the Jesuit Order. For these reasons the preparation was called Peruvian bark or Jesuit bark for over a century, and it was sold as an antipyretic. The medical establishment disdained the preparation in large part because of their lack of influence over its usage. No wonder the medical profession took notice when the Reverend Mr. Edward Stone wrote to the Royal Society of Medicine in London in 1763 that the bitter principle of a home-grown bark had medicinal value similar to Peruvian bark. His bark was that of the willow tree, the *sallow* in olde English, of the genus *Salix*. The principle was called *salicin*, and for the next century its use and that of the Jesuit bark shared the same market.

The 19th century witnessed painstaking progress in the understanding of salicin, mainly due to French and German chemists. Salicin was purified, then salicylic acid was extracted from this glycoside, and finally such congeners as salicyl aldehyde, acetylsalicylic acid, and sodium salicylate were synthesized. By 1880 salicin, salicylic acid, and sodium salicylate were in widespread use as antipyretics and for the aching of many febrile illnesses, the "agues"—much the same usages as for Jesuit bark. One should realize that for this generation of clinicians, the agues and pyrexia (fever) were diseases in and of themselves. It was at this point in the story (3,4) that European clinicians made the observation that salicin and its congeners had a role to play in the management of the various forms of rheumatism. The scientific underpinning for these observations was the Doctrine of Signatures; since the damp and cold flares rheumatism, the cure should be sought in the damp and cold, just where the English willow tree grows.

The fledgling pharmaceutical industry at the turn of the century was ill-prepared to expand on the form and use of its first synthetic pharmaceutical, the antipyretic salicylic acid. Although in wide use, it was poorly tolerated, inducing considerable nausea and vomiting. Sodium salicylate was also considered to be poorly tolerated and less effective. Quinine remained the standard of therapy. The introduction of aspirin, acetylsalicylic acid, waited for serendipity. Felix Hofmann was a young German chemist employed by the I.G. Farbenfabriken of Bayer-Elberfeld. His father was an arthritic who found salicylic acid beneficial if only he could tolerate the drug. Felix Hofmann chose to try acetylsalicylic acid from the company storeroom. It had been synthesized decades earlier by another organic chemist, Löwig, who called the compound aspirin (derived from **a** for acetyl and **spir** for the Spirsäure, the plant from which he had isolated the salicylic acid). Aspirin was tolerated by Papa Hofmann, and the rest is history. Some of the more colorful history relates to international industrial relations. "Bayer Aspirin" was one of the spoils of World War I; the name and the patent became the property of an American pharmaceutical house.

Figure 4.2 shows the chemical formulas of some of the salicylate congeners that we have discussed. There are many others, including several in common use. Salicylic acid is a caustic agent used as a keratolytic to remove calluses. Methyl salicylate is the active ingredient of "oil of wintergreen." However, toward the end of the 19th century pharmaceutical chemists were making progress on another front. Quinine had been isolated, and quinoline derivatives were under development. In 1884 Ludwig Knorr, while seeking useful quinolines, came across another antipyretic, antipyrine, a pyrazolone with a benzene ring (Fig. 4.3). This agent was soon found to be analgesic as well and joined the pharmacopeia. The next class to be introduced were the p-aminophenols, including phenacetin in 1887. At about the same time, p-hydroxyacetanilide was synthesized. This is acetaminophen, but it was thought to be less efficacious than phenacetin; it remained on the shelf until 1948 and did not enter clinical use until 1956 (5). The chemical and metabolic relationship between phenacetin and acetaminophen is illustrated in Fig. 4.4. Phenacetin is associated with chronic interstitial nephritis or pyelonephritis and a high incidence of papillary necrosis and is no longer on the market in the United States. Acetaminophen (surprisingly, since it is a metabolite of phenacetin) has far less nephrotoxicity (6), if any (7).

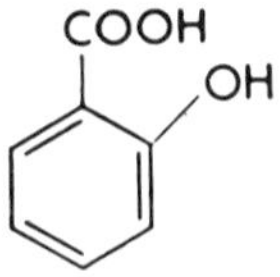

Salicylic Acid

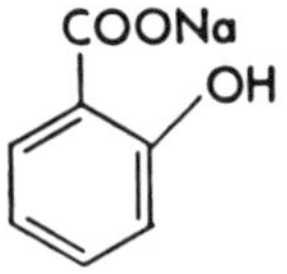

Sodium Salicylate

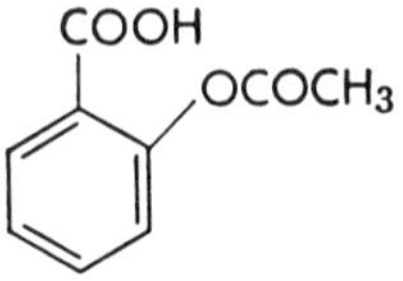

Aspirin

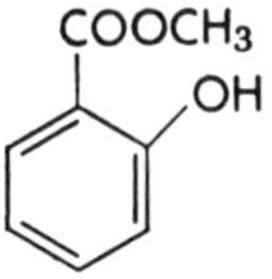

Methyl Salicylate

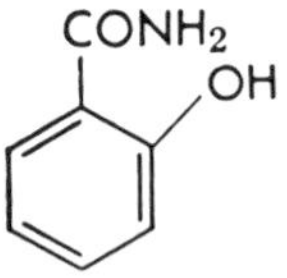

Salicylamide

FIG. 4.2. Some members of the salicylate family.

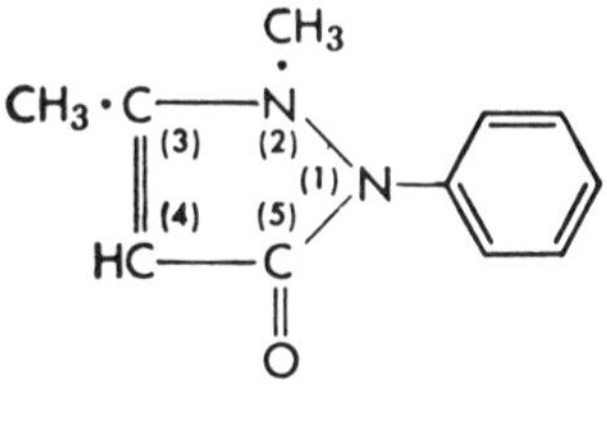

Antipyrine

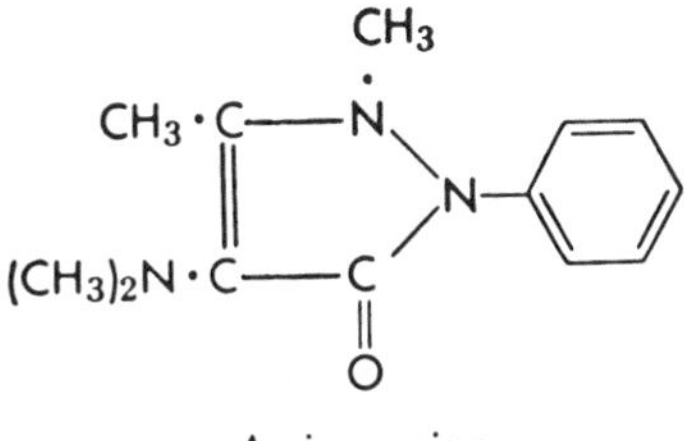

Aminopyrine

FIG. 4.3. Antipyrine and aminopyrine were synthesized as quinolone derivatives and were in widespread use in the late 19th century.

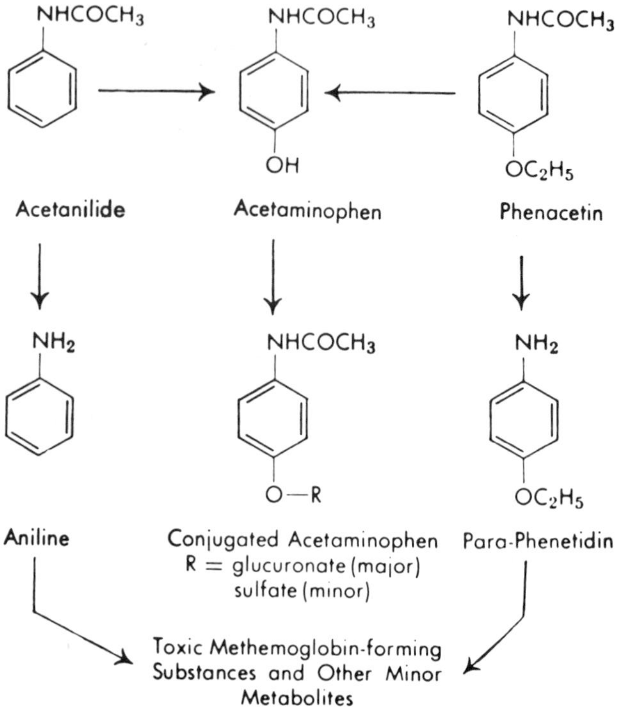

FIG. 4.4. Phenacetin and acetaminophen were both synthesized in the mid-19th century. Acetaminophen is a metabolite of phenacetin. Its use awaited the insights of clinicians of the 1950s.

The last remarkable accomplishment of this line of investigation by the German pharmaceutical chemists of the late 19th century was the synthesis of aminopyrine (Fig. 4.3). For 40 yr aminopyrine was the analgesic of choice in Europe until its propensity for agranulocytosis became apparent. Around 1950 congeners of this pyrazalone were synthesized, were proved comparably effective, and were thought to be less toxic. Several were introduced into clinical practice; the prototype is phenylbutazone (Fig 4.5). One can only wonder how

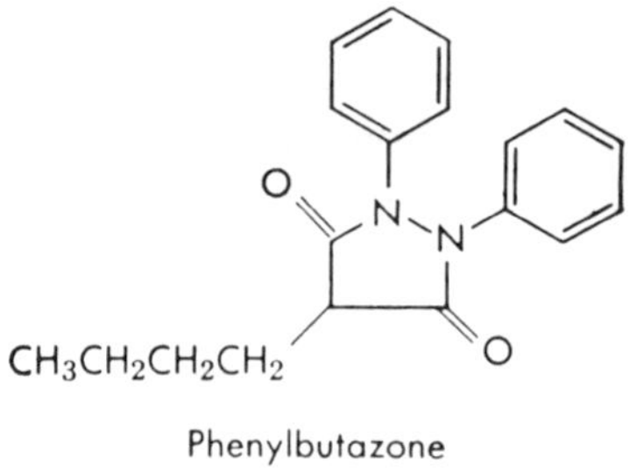

Phenylbutazone

FIG. 4.5. Phenylbutazone is a congener of aminopyrine, synthesized a century later.

TABLE 4.1. *Partial toxicity profile of phenylbutazone*

Target	Clinical outcome
Kidney	Congestive heart failure
	Glaucoma
Thyroid	Hypothyroidism unmasking
GI[a] tract	Gastritis
	Peptic ulcer disease exacerbation
	Hepatitis
CNS[b]	Vertigo, insomnia, dysphoria
Mucocutaneous tissue	Stomatitis, rash
Bone marrow	Cytopenia, including aplastic anemia
Drug-drug interactions	
Warfarin	Bleeding diasthesis
Sulfonurea	Prolonged hypoglycemia

[a] GI, gastrointestinal.
[b] CNS, central nervous system.

much of aminopyrine's toxicities were considered tolerable if phenylbutazone was considered an improvement (Table 4.1).

Notice that the phrase *introduce into practice* is used with impunity. In fact, the introduction was with impunity; until relatively recently any agent could be marketed with little in the way of constraints. This is no longer the case.

THE HISTORY OF THE REGULATION OF PHARMACEUTICAL RELEASE

The wanton purveyance of putative medicinals in the 19th century did not go unnoticed. President Theodore Roosevelt signed the Food and Drug Act into law in 1906, banning any traffic in misbranded or adulterated drugs from interstate commerce. A *drug* was defined as any preparation recognized by entry in the United States Pharmacopeia or National Formulary and therefore intended for the treatment of afflictions of human or animal. By stipulating "misbranding" the Act gave notice regarding the labeling of such agents. A bureau in the Department of Agriculture, the predecessor of the Food and Drug Administration (FDA), was charged with the execution of this statute and given the power to seize adulterated or misbranded agents and condemn the purveyor. This marshalled in the century of the regulatory agency and therefore was an auspicious event. The act recognized that the federal government had some responsibility in terms of consumer protection. However, the consumer was provided no reassurance that the concoction consumed was effective or safe, only that it was what it said it was. In fact, a 1911 Supreme Court decision found that the act prohibited only mislabeling of the contents—not false claims as to therapeutic benefits!

President Taft led the charge on quackery. With his urging, the Shirley Amendment was passed in 1912, prohibiting fraudulent therapeutic claims on the label. The amendment created more problems than any degree of consumer protection it fostered. Now the government had to devise a method for not only proving the claims for benefit to be wrong, but also proving that they were fraudulent; to prove "fraud" the government had to prove an intent to deceive rather than simply mis- or overstatement. Both the act and the amendment were no match for the purveyors.

And so it remained caveat emptor until the summer of 1937. The scientific community was aglow with the benefits of the newly introduced sulfa antibiotics. The pharmaceutical industry was faced with the task of providing these wonder drugs for a needy populace. An inventive chemist employed by the Massingill Company of Bristol, Tennessee, came upon a way to prepare sulfanilamide as a palatable elixir; he dissolved the drug in dilute diethylene glycol and flavored the solution with raspberry extract. Quality control was delegated to his own palate and nares. Massingill was soon shipping hundreds of gallons of Elixir of Sulfanilamide. By the fall of 1937 the first reports of the deaths of patients who had imbibed the elixir surfaced and distribution ceased. Even though the FDA instituted a search for every bottle, over 100 people died of ethylene glycol poisoning. The owner of the company, Dr. S. E. Massingill, publicly defended the distribution of the elixir without prior testing; his inventive chief chemist committed suicide.

A homeopathic physician in Congress, Senator Royal S. Copeland, introduced the revised federal Food Drug and Cosmetic Act, which was passed into law in 1938. This will not be the only example of tragedy forcing the passage of enlightened legislation. The 1938 act stipulated that any future drug to be marketed must first be demonstrably safe. The manufacturer must submit data to that effect to the FDA. Furthermore, the label must reflect any degree of deviation from a standard of purity and quality for each agent. The FDA could inspect manufacturing facilities and could hold the manufacturer responsible for adulteration, even if there was no intent to defraud.

We were making progress, but we had a long way to go. The impetus was another disaster 24 yr later. Thalidomide is a remarkably effective and relatively safe soporific in adults. It was licensed and widely used in Europe. In America, probably because of bureaucratic inefficiency rather than prescience, it was never released for use. However, the manufacturer anticipated such release and the reps of the day managed to convince physicians to enroll almost 4,000 pregnant Americans in an investigative program designed, I would surmise, to improve physicians' familiarity with the agent with a view toward impending licensure. Sadly, the agent places the fetus of any pregnant mother at risk, particularly of phocomelia (deformity and arrest of embryologic limb development). When this came to light, the world was enraged.

From 1960 to 1962, Senator Estes Kefauver of Tennessee became the champion of regulatory reform targeting the pharmaceutical industry. His hearings exposed the flaws in evaluation, the lack of informed consent on the part of participants in drug trials, and the use of "investigation" as a promotional technique. Congress responded with the Kefauver-Harris amendments of 1962, expanding the purview of the 1938 act. The critical advance was that "substantial evidence" of benefit must be forthcoming before the FDA could license the distribution of any new drug. The FDA, in essence, must generate before marketing some confidence that there is a favorable risk/benefit ratio, and the basis for that confidence was to be "adequate and well controlled investigations." Today, Section 355 Title 21 of the U.S. Code or Regulations stipulates that no drug may be introduced into interstate commerce until investigations "show whether or not such drug is safe for use and whether such drug is effective in use."

Nearly 20 yr after the thalidomide disaster, Congress provided the FDA with the last of the authorities necessary to serve the protection of the consumer. Pharmaceutical firms were required to monitor consumers after the drug had been approved for marketing based on the studies we'll discuss shortly. In that way, unanticipated toxicities can be detected; if the risk/benefit ratio turns unfavorable, the agent can be withdrawn from the marketplace as an "imminent hazard" or even an "unreasonable risk."

THE FDA'S APPROVAL PROCESS

To "show whether or not such drug is safe for use and whether such drug is effective in use," the purveyor must place before the Secretary of Health and Human Services an application for approval that includes

(1) full reports of investigations which have been made to show whether or not such drug is safe for use and whether such drug is effective in use; (2) a full list of the investigations which have been made to show whether or not such drug is safe for use and whether such drug is effective in use; (3) a full list of articles used as components of such drug; (4) a full statement of the composition of such drug; (5) a full description of the methods used in, and the facilities and controls for, the manufacture, processing, and packing of such drug; (6) such samples . . . as the Secretary may require; (7) specimens of the labeling to be used for such drug.

The responsibility for oversight, on behalf of the Secretary, is held by the FDA. The task was daunting in 1962 when 46 new drugs were introduced to the U.S. market; each cost $2 million to research over a 2-yr development period. By 1980 it took 5 times as long and cost 35 times as much for a drug to reach approval. Much of this reflects the evolution in the sophistication and validity of the process. The FDA is faced with the mountain of "substantial evidence" it demands and the mandate by both patient advocates and industry to decide expeditiously (8,9). This latter mandate is leading to pathways around the customary algorithm (10) for drugs thought to be of value in desperate situations. For the present, NSAIDs are evaluated according to standard guidelines (11).

The IND

Before a new drug can be tested on humans, the sponsor or responsible investigator must submit a "Notice of Claimed Investigational Exemption for a New Drug," the IND. This document details drug composition as well as manufacturing processes, safeguards, and quality control. Short-term toxicities and pharmacokinetics are described based on animal experiments. In addition, explicit protocols for the performance of trials in humans are presented. These protocols include drafts of the "informed consent" documents to be used and guarantees that any untoward event will be reported to the FDA in a timely fashion. Finally, the protocols must receive prior approval by an institutional review board (IRB). The IRB is a local body comprising individuals with appropriate expertise and perspectives to review the protocols objectively from both technical and ethical perspectives and to monitor the trials with some periodicity (usually by annual report). Most IRBs are based in hospitals or medical schools; however, several are based in industry. For example, there are IRBs in companies that profit from the performance of clinical trials. This is considered to be within the intent of the legislation, although I am always bothered by a circumstance that has such potential for conflict of interest.

The NDA

Once the IND is approved, the protocols are activated. The object is to generate sufficient data to evaluate the benefits and risks of using the new agent in a specified population of patients. When, in the opinion of the investigators and sponsors, sufficient data are accumulated and analyzed, a new drug application (NDA) is submitted to the FDA. This is a ponderous document detailing further animal data and the customary human trials, which the FDA is to digest rapidly so as to render an opinion within 180 days. Usually, the opinion on the first application is to request important revision so that the average time from first submission to approval is some 2 yr. This lag is remarkably brief, given the challenge faced by the FDA. The FDA reviewing staff of physicians, chemists, pharmacologists, and consumer safety officers numbers fewer than 300. Every year, the FDA handles some 1,000 new INDs, 200 original NDAs, 4,000 supplements to the NDAs, and thousands of amendments. Nonetheless, the agency has protected the American consumer for decades in a fashion that is the gold standard for the industrial world. All involved are wary of streamlining the process; it is hard to argue with the agency's track record.

Guidelines for NSAID Clinical Trials

As is true for most other classes of pharmaceutical, the FDA's guidelines call for new NSAIDs to be subjected to three types of clinical trial in sequence.

Phase I Trials

A Phase I trial is an exercise in toxicology. This represents the initial introduction of the new agent into a normal volunteer. This usually involves only a
small number of subjects, always healthy, often young, and always well paid.
The exercise is anxiety provoking for all involved. After all, the only reassurance available regarding toxicity and appropriate dosing is extrapolation from
animal experimentation. The study is usually performed as an inpatient study
so the volunteer can be closely monitored. The intent is to screen for overt
toxicity at particular doses; efficacy and subtle toxicity are not at issue.

Phase II Trials

These trials recruit informed patients, not normal volunteers. The intent is to
see if the Phase I insights generalize to the patients for whom the drug is intended. In addition, there is a quest for some indication of efficacy and some
idea of the dose-response parameters of the agent. The Phase II studies are both
uncontrolled and open-label comparisons with placebo agents or active
NSAIDs in modest numbers of patients over a brief interval (usually less than
2 mo).

Phase III Trials

If an agent has passed muster on Phase I and II protocols, it is subjected to
Phase III trials. These are the crowning glory of clinical epidemiology (12,13).
The trials recruit hundreds of patients, are lengthy, are controlled, and often are
double blind. The intent is to prove efficacy and probe for toxicity in such a
fashion that the FDA can arrive at a risk/benefit assessment upon which it can
base a decision regarding approval for marketing. For that reason, the guidelines want to see a comparison with a placebo as well as with an NSAID of
proven benefit. The placebo comparison is necessary to prove that the drug is
effective. However, the comparison with the NSAID of proven benefit is a
different exercise. The gold standard in the United States for this comparison is
aspirin; in Japan it is indomethacin. A new drug does not have to be more
effective than aspirin or even be shown to be more effective; it will be released if
it is indistinguishable and is better tolerated in terms of either toxicity or convenience of dosing.

Phase IV Trials

The FDA currently has no guidelines for formal postmarketing surveillance.
It is hoped that physicians and pharmaceutical firms will report side effects to

the FDA in some timely fashion. However, what is missing is some structured attempt to monitor consumers, a Phase IV trial. The reason relates to the design of the Phase III trial. After all, Phase III trials enroll hundreds of patients, rarely a few thousand. There is some likelihood that they might detect major toxicities that occur with a frequency of a few percentage points. However, they are not powerful enough to detect major toxicities that occur with less frequency or minor toxicities that occur in a few patients. Realize that both eventualities can have considerable moment when marketing is widespread and consumers number in the tens of thousands. Furthermore, Phase III trials are designed to sample a specific subset of patients. The favorable risk/benefit ratio necessary to gain FDA approval may not generalize to other subsets who might very well be exposed to the drug once it is released; marketing is seldom as restricted as the parameters for enrolling patients into the Phase III trials, and clinical judgment is never that restricted. Here again a Phase IV "trial," a form of structured surveillance, might serve the public better than the current uneven method of recognition and reporting (14).

THE NSAID RISK/BENEFIT VEIL

In fact, the following is true of every NSAID marketed in the United States:

Every approved NSAID has been shown to be more effective than placebo.
No approved NSAID has been shown to be less effective than aspirin.
No approved NSAID has been shown to be more effective than aspirin.

Furthermore, until quite recently, every NSAID was approved based on its effectiveness in the treatment of rheumatoid arthritis. Expanding the indication to osteoarthritis was first an exercise in clinical judgment. For many of these agents, supplementary applications to the FDA have expanded the indications to "osteoarthritis." For some, osteoarthritis is the primary indication. Seldom is the agent approved for a regional musculoskeletal disease primarily, even for backache. This is because the FDA guidelines are circumspect regarding these conditions; without defined guidelines the sponsor seldom wants to risk disapproval after expending the considerable sums prerequisite to Phase III trials.

The Phase III trials of NSAIDs that target rheumatoid arthritis are constrained by tradition and FDA guidelines to measure benefit with such outcome measures as the number of tender joints, the ring size, the grip strength, and the time to walk a given distance, as well as more global measures, such as the impressions of the patient or doctor regarding pain or clinical status. The global impressions are held as most valid and reliable by experienced rheumatologists (15). It is based on such measures that a few clinical trials some 25 yr ago could add the scientific patina to clinical impression and cement aspirin's role as the prototype antiinflammatory drug. Boardman and Hart (16) introduced the use of ring size as a measure of antiinflammatory effect in 1967. They demonstrated such antiinflammatory effect with prednisone, 7.5 mg/day, and aspirin, 5.3 g/day (in four equal doses). However, the effects of aspirin, 2.6 g/day, acetaminophen, 6.0 g/day, and placebo were indistinguishable. In 1974 Multz et al. (17) published a double-blinded trial novel in design. Utilizing the standard outcome measures, they assessed the effect of substituting placebo for 3.6 g of aspirin per day. After about 3 days on placebo, the rheumatoid arthritis of these patients reliably flared. Based on these trials and a few others (18,19), the dogma of the antiinflammatory drugs was established. NSAIDs can decrease inflammation: stiffness, soreness, swelling, redness, fatigue, etc. NSAIDs are the "drug of choice," at least of first choice, for these features of rheumatoid arthritis. It is thought that this antiinflammatory effect represents activity at the site of tissue damage, whereas analgesia results from some central nervous system effect.

By extrapolation from rheumatoid arthritis, conventional wisdom holds that NSAIDs are the drugs of first choice for other musculoskeletal illnesses where stiffness, swelling, heat, and the like are perceived to be less dramatic, even subclinical features. That is the rationale for the use of NSAIDs, even for the prescription of NSAIDs, for regional musculoskeletal illness. Acetaminophen is held to be a placebo in this regard. Even though it is equianalgesic to the NSAIDs (it can effect as much pain relief as the NSAIDs), conventional wisdom holds that it has no role to play in the regional illnesses because it fails to ameliorate the stiffness and soreness. It is time to scrutinize the dogma even perhaps to discard it.

First of all, Phase III trials for rheumatoid arthritis are seriously limited by the crudeness of the classic outcome measures. All of these measures are limited in reliability and in sensitivity to change, let alone in validity. Furthermore, whatever they are measuring has extraordinary variability. Figure 4.6 is taken from a publication comparing an NSAID with aspirin in rheumatoid arthritis (20). Although the study is typical, the figure is exceptional in that it displays the raw data used to generate the statistical analysis; seldom are these data published. How anyone can look at such data and generate some clinical confidence in the effectiveness of either drug is a mystery—yet we do, at least for inflammatory polyarthritis such as rheumatoid arthritis. The figure is also a demonstration of why no marketed NSAID has been shown to be more or less effective than aspirin; this type of data suggests that all of these studies lack the power to discern any difference short of the extremely dramatic.

Second, it is likely that the "antiinflammatory" benefit of NSAIDs is not their only redeeming feature. The classic experience cited above, where the benefit of acetaminophen pales when compared with that of aspirin in rheumatoid arthritis, does not mean that analgesia by itself would not benefit the rheumatoid arthritis patient. After all, NSAIDs and acetaminophen are comparably effective in the treatment of a number of painful states (21), including knee pain in the setting of osteoarthritis (22). Even our old friend, salicylic acid, is making a comeback. It has been held that salicylic acid is less effective than

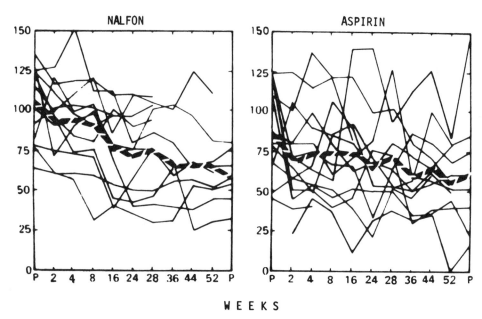

W E E K S

FIG. 4.6. An example of "raw data" from an NSAID trial. (From Fries and Britton, ref. 20, with permission.)

aspirin because it lacks an acetyl leaving group and therefore only has analgesic potency. The acetyl group is responsible for acetylating cyclooxygenase, thereby blocking prostaglandin synthesis and abrogating inflammation. That may be true *in vitro* and may even make sense. However, when aspirin and salicylic acid face off in the treatment of rheumatoid arthritis, there is no difference in benefit (23).

Choosing among the NSAIDs based on differential benefit is an act of personal conviction. It is common practice to advise using an NSAID for the management of the rheumatic symptoms associated with systemic rheumatic diseases such as rheumatoid arthritis, ankylosing spondylitis, systemic lupus erythematosus, and the like. It had been common practice to do the same for the joint pain seen in the setting of osteoarthritis, although this practice has come under scrutiny as questionable (24). Similar scrutiny is appropriate for the use of an NSAID in the systemic inflammatory illnesses. The agents are not indicated by virtue of the diagnosis; rather, they should be introduced with particular antiinflammatory goals in mind and only after alternatives have been considered. Choosing any particular NSAID because it is more "antiinflammatory" is an act of personal conviction. Perhaps the choice can be made based on safety?

THE MYTH OF DIFFERENTIAL NSAID TOXICITY

The Symptoms of Dyspepsia

The salicylates are associated with unpleasant, even painful symptoms that relate to the upper gastrointestinal (GI) tract; burning in the epigastrium is typical, but bloating, eructation, a sour taste in the mouth, and the like are part of the grief. But Papa Hoffmann latched on to aspirin because it was more tolerable. Until 30 yr ago, when there were few options, only some 10% of patients treated with aspirin complained of intolerance (25), and clinicians found little to be alarmed about; "fortunately, gastric irritation can be avoided in almost all instances." (26). If the symptoms persisted, dosage was adjusted or interrupted without undue alarm.

In 1963 the first of the newer NSAIDs was introduced; indomethacin was a new class of drug, an indole derivative (Fig. 4.7). It was thought to represent an important advance in the management of acute gout, ankylosing spondylitis, osteoarthritis (especially of the hip), and even rheumatoid arthritis. Indomethacin, unlike phenylbutazone (Table 4.1), remains an option in spite of a considerable likelihood of intolerance; some 20% of patients are forced to discontinue the agent because of either GI intolerance or headache (27). The next NSAID to be introduced was ibuprofen, again a new class of agent, a phenylalkanoic acid. It was introduced in England in 1967 and in the United States in 1974. In 1983 ibuprofen became the first of the newer NSAIDs to join aspirin in OTC sales. At the doses recommended for OTC use, ibuprofen is said to be an analgesic; at higher prescription doses it is said to be antiinflammatory (28). Ibuprofen was the first NSAID to be aggressively marketed because it was better tolerated than aspirin and not because of its potency. In fact, concerns were raised that, at equipotent dosing, the differential in tolerability might fade. Nonetheless, improving tolerability while maintaining potency became the goal of the pharmaceutical chemist. Whether this has ever been attained, in spite of all the advertising, is doubtful.

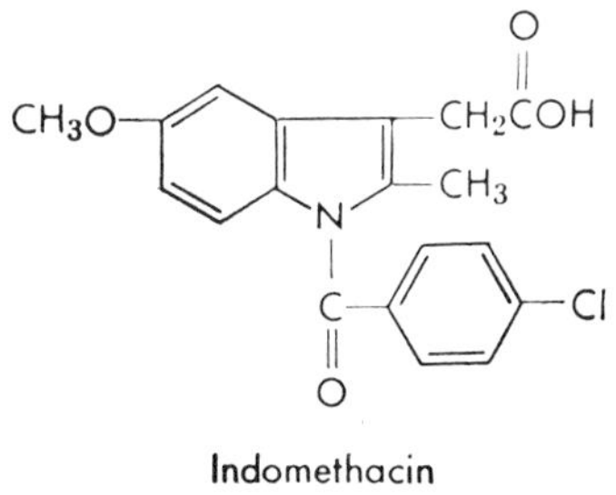

FIG. 4.7. Indomethacin, an indole derivative, was introduced in 1963.

Indomethacin

The data supporting the introduction of all subsequent NSAIDs seem to document that the agent is better tolerated than aspirin. This is the argument in most NDAs that sways the decision toward approval. However, close inspection of these data documents dramatic symptom inflation during the past 20 yr. In large part this reflects the fashion in which these symptoms are elicited. Patients and physicians are anxious that any discomfort be acknowledged and ascribed to the NSAID. For that reason most Phase III NSAID trials record an incidence of GI intolerance of aspirin approaching 50%. Figure 4.8 is a composite of data culled from three such NSAID trials (29–31) to illustrate the magnitude and variability of symptoms, if not the difficulty in describing and standardizing the complaint, whether the patient is exposed to aspirin (ASA) or newer NSAIDs. Over the course of 20 yr, GI intolerance to ASA in patients with rheumatoid arthritis has escalated from a readily managed 10% to a frightening 50%. This escalation in elicitable symptoms is far more dramatic and impressive than any really meaningful reduction in toxicity reported with newer NSAIDs, in spite of the drum beat of pharmaceutical marketing schemes.

GI Blood Loss

This is not to say that the NSAIDs are without GI toxicity. It has long been appreciated that their use is associated with a measurable increase in fecal blood loss. Normally, we lose 1 to 3 ml of blood in the stool each day. Patients on aspirin therapy lose 3 times as much. Patients on most newer NSAIDs are

	N	GI Symptoms	Nausea	Dyspepsia
ASA	107	48		
Piroxicam	87	22		
ASA	109		50	48
Fenoprofen	107		31	45
ASA	42		12	16
Naproxen	38		7	12

FIG. 4.8. There is little standardization in practice, perhaps in principle, to allow reproducible trials or to allow comparisons between trials when considering gastrointestinal side effects. These three trials are exemplary. (From Wiseman and Boyle, ref. 29; Bowers et al., ref. 30; and Sigler et al., ref. 31.)

intermediate. However, two points merit emphasis: (a) The loss is measured by radiolabeling erythrocytes with chromium. Aspirin increases the biliary secretion of chromium so that the "loss" may be spuriously elevated. (b) The difference between aspirin and the newer NSAIDs may be statistically significant and therefore measurable. However, the measurement should be placed into the perspective that follows from the fact that even losses of the magnitude observed on aspirin are clinically insignificant. There is a lot of advertising based on this "much ado about nothing."

More difficult to cope with is the controversial concept of NSAID "gastropathy" (32,33). It is clear that everyone taking NSAIDs as prescribed for any rheumatic condition is suffering a change in the gastric mucosa that is readily demonstrable by endoscopy. Erythema, ecchymoses, and shallow erosions are appreciated in approximately a third of such individuals. The lesions are predominately in the antrum and seldom extend much below the mucosa; rarely do they qualify to be labeled ulcers by pathologic criteria (34). The changes of NSAID gastropathy heal and return in all individuals exposed to NSAIDs with periodicity measurable in terms of a month or two. Even though the lesions come and go spontaneously in spite of continued NSAID exposure, it seems counterintuitive to observe such changes without an inference of damage, if not impending catastrophe. It may be counterintuitive, but these lesions are incidental, asymptomatic, and benign. There are a number of observations that support this contention.

Discordance with symptoms is well substantiated. For example, the prostaglandin congener misoprostol will suppress endoscopic gastropathy but not the GI symptoms associated with full doses of aspirin for rheumatoid arthritis (35). An even more dramatic demonstration of the discordance with symptoms is a randomized, double-blind, placebo-controlled trial comparing rectal and oral indomethacin in young, normal volunteers (36). The principal results are presented in Table 4.2. Clearly, rectal (p.r.) indomethacin causes little in the way of endoscopic change. However, the volunteers experienced as many symptoms by this route as by the oral route of administration. Equally telling are the symptoms experienced by the volunteers to whom placebos had been adminis-

TABLE 4.2. Results of a double-blind, placebo-controlled randomized trial of oral versus rectal indomethacin in normal volunteers

Parameter	Indomethacin		Placebo (p.o./p.r.)
	p.o.	p.r.	
Number of volunteers	15	15	15
Mean endoscopic score (0–4) at Day 11	2.2	0.9	0.25
Number with GI symptoms	9	9	10
Number with upper GI symptoms	4	5	4

From Lanza et al., ref. 36.

tered. As we discussed in Chapter 2, it is difficult to go through a day without some unexpected symptom relating to the GI tract. The setting of the trial assures recall. Furthermore, depending on the fashion in which the symptoms are elicited, recall can lead to anxiety on the part of the patient or of the treating physician. This, I feel, explains the inflation in GI symptoms documented for aspirin over the past decades.

The NSAID-associated risk of a GI catastrophe, a GI bleed of sufficient magnitude to precipitate hospitalization or a perforation, has been heralded by a number of investigators and hangs like an imprecation over the users of NSAIDs (37). Here there is some truth, but again perspective is in order. First, we must realize that epidemiology is severely challenged by the questions raised by the concept of NSAID gastropathy. Epidemiology is compromised in discriminating causal influences when the outcome is rare or sporadic. The NSAID-associated catastrophes are both rare and sporadic. In fact, they are so rare and sporadic that any association is probably trivial for most users of the drugs. Two studies make this point convincingly.

1. The Group Health Cooperative is a health maintenance organization (HMO) in Seattle with >300,000 members. The membership was exposed to 49 million person-months of prescribed NSAIDs between 1977 and 1983. The actual exposures are illustrated in Table 4.3 (38,39). In 584 million person-days at risk, there were 54 patients with upper gastrointestinal (UGI) perforation, among whom 6 were current NSAID users. After adjusting for age and sex, however, there was no influence of NSAID exposure on the likelihood of UGI perforation. Hospitalization of patients over age 64 for UGI bleeding occurred 4.8 times per million person-days in NSAID users and 3.4 times per million person-days in nonusers. The difference in rates is "incompatible with any major increase in the frequency of hospitalization" for UGI bleeding in the elderly. "No single NSAID seemed to carry an exceptional risk."

2. Over 95% of the 1 million residents of Saskatchewan are members of the

TABLE 4.3. NSAID[a] prescriptions issued by physicians of the Group Health Cooperative of Seattle between 1977 and 1983

Drug	Number of patients	Number of prescriptions
Indomethacin	55,312	99,514
Phenylbutazone	62,256	84,400
Ibuprofen	52,676	120,388
Naproxen	5,900	15,016
Fenoprofen	686	2,184
Piroxicam	3,308	9,620
Sulindac	3,419	7,898
Tolmetin	2,402	6,801
		345,821

From Jick et al., ref. 38, and Beard et al., ref. 39.
[a] NSAID, nonsteroidal antiinflammatory drug.

Saskatchewan Health Plan. Computer registries include details of all hospitalizations and all prescriptions. A cohort (follow-up) study of all users and nonusers of NSAIDs in 1983 was feasible (40). The exposure to NSAIDs is presented in Table 4.4. In 1983, in Saskatchewan, 76 individuals were hospitalized with UGI bleeding or perforation. Fourteen had filled a prescription for an NSAID within 30 days of hospitalization, and 47 were nonusers. Ten of these users and 18 of the nonusers had no primary disease placing them at risk for UGI bleeding or perforation. Almost all of the NSAID users who suffered the catastrophes were elderly women (Table 4.5). Furthermore, it is only among elderly women that NSAID usage is a risk.

For reasons that will become clear shortly, the data indicating that NSAIDs place the elderly woman at risk for GI catastrophe are compelling. However, it is important to realize the magnitude of risk. In Saskatchewan an elderly woman was 9 times more likely to suffer a GI catastrophe if she was prescribed an NSAID. This is the *relative risk*. However, the *absolute risk* is less impressive. You would have to follow 1,000 elderly female patients for whom you have prescribed an NSAID for 1 yr to observe 3 cases of GI catastrophe. If you followed 1,000 elderly female patients without prescribing an NSAID, you would observe 0.4 catastrophe. These extra 12 elderly women/5,000 exposed/yr are not to be dismissed as trivial, but this is no reason for hysterical warnings. It is also no justification for misoprostol or other prophylaxis—at least not until there is some evidence that such is effective. Rather, it is reason to question why elderly women are exposed to NSAIDs in the first place.

The question takes on greater moment in view of the analysis of Medicaid data sets. Such data sets can be viewed as similar to the Saskatchewan approach

TABLE 4.4. *NSAID usage in Saskatchewan in 1983*

NSAID	Users	Prescriptions
Piroxicam	29,616	84,625
Ibuprofen	27,792	53,583
Naproxen	23,051	48,874
Indomethacin	22,977	55,036
ASA[a]	21,618	66,026
Phenylbutazone	8,960	12,778
Sulindac	8,333	20,312
Mefenamic acid	7,860	11,046
Ketoprofen	5,821	13,321
Diclofenac	5,615	12,034
Fenoprofen	4,957	11,269
Diflunisal	4,672	6,797
Tolmetin	1,058	2,335
	134,060	398,036

From Guess et al., ref. 40.
[a] ASA, acetylsalicylic acid.

TABLE 4.5. *Risk of GI catastrophe in the Saskatchewan experience*

		Users on NSAID therapy		Nonusers	
Age	Sex	Cases	Person-days	Cases	Person-days
>75	F	9	1,393,496	6	7,109,614
	M	0	715,360	6	6,092,958
<75	F	0	4,793,732	2	150,837,558
	M	1	3,190,626	4	158,952,846

From Guess et al., ref. 40.

discussed above, except that Medicaid serves only a subset of the population of each state. The absolute risk for bleeding in these data sets is similiar to the Saskatchewan experience. In Michigan and Minnesota, the relative risk for those prescribed an NSAID for GI catastrophe is 1.5 times that for those not so prescribed (41). In Tennessee, the relative risk of death from a GI catastrophe was over 4 (42) when those recently prescribed NSAIDs were contrasted with age- and sex-matched patients not so prescribed.

Again the risk operates in the elderly and particularly in the elderly woman. Corticosteroid exposure is not a risk (43); however, corticosteroids synergize the risk of NSAIDs (44).

The Saskatchewan, Seattle, and Medicaid analyses all reach similar conclusions: NSAIDs are an important, though not overwhelming, risk to the GI tract of elderly women. Steroid therapy enhances the risk.

The same message has emerged from an analysis of patients with rheumatoid arthritis followed at several centers—the ARAMIS data set (45). In the setting of rheumatoid arthritis, combining NSAIDs with steroids in the elderly reflects a lack of judgment. In fact, the use of NSAIDs in the elderly woman with rheumatoid arthritis is an exceptional choice in my practice; others who advise otherwise are now forewarned.

Why are elderly women without rheumatoid arthritis taking NSAIDs? A survey of residents of Iowa over the age of 65 (46) revealed that nearly 42% of men and 46% of women had consumed one or more analgesics during the previous 2 wk. "Arthritis" was the most common reason and accounted for the majority of prescription drugs. Clearly, recourse to NSAIDs has become a way of life even in the heartland.

There is another insight into the rationale for NSAID use by the elderly, particularly the elderly woman, that comes from the Midlands of England (47). This was a case-control study comparing NSAID consumption in community and hospital controls with that in age-matched patients hospitalized for GI bleeding. All patients were over 60 yr old. The relative risk from such consumption was 2.2 compared to hospital controls and 2.9 compared to community controls. However, this was an unusual study in that the authors reported the reason offered by the patient with an NSAID-associated GI bleed for consum-

TABLE 4.6. *Reasons for consuming NSAIDs offered by elderly GI bleeders*

Reason	Cases	Hospital controls	Community controls
Colds and "flu"	12	3	4
Headache	9	5	5
INDIGESTION	10	0	4
Osteoarthritis	4	3	16
Rheumatoid arthritis	2	0	2
Transient ischemic attacks	5	4	2
Other	11	9	15

From Faulkner et al., ref. 47.

ing an NSAID. The reasons are presented in order of frequency in Table 4.6. The reason offered second most frequently by the elderly patients who bled was "indigestion"! In fact, there are OTC nostrums containing salicylates throughout the West. Always the advertising suggests their usage for an upset stomach or "the morning after," etc. There is even reason to suspect that NSAIDs palliate ulcer pain in the elderly (48). They may feel better, but this is a Pyrrhic victory!

The misuse of NSAIDs is not restricted to the symptomatic elderly. Any use of NSAIDs by the elderly runs the risk of being misuse in view of the epidemiology of peptic ulcer disease (49). During our lifetime, each of us has a risk of developing peptic ulcer disease that approaches 10%. The incidence increases with age, and peptic ulcer disease in the elderly is more likely to be asymptomatic. Inappropriate usage of NSAIDs in the elderly is begging to ferret out those with asymptomatic peptic ulcer disease. Unfortunately, those so identified pay the price of catastrophic complications.

In summary, NSAID gastropathy is almost always, if not always, asymptomatic and benign. Symptoms of dyspepsia are coincidental side effects of NSAIDs. There is no convincing, clinically important yield from treating NSAID gastropathy. However, NSAID use increases the likelihood of upper GI bleeding if there is another primary underlying disease such as peptic ulcer disease or alcoholic gastritis. The elderly are at particular risk because the incidence of peptic ulcer disease, particularly silent peptic ulcer disease, increases with aging. The public and physician must be reeducated regarding the indications for sporadic usage of NSAIDs, including OTC preparations, particularly in the elderly.

REFERENCES

1. Brooks PM, Day RO. Nonsteroidal antiinflammatory drugs—differences and similarities. *N Engl J Med* 1991;324:1716–25.
2. American College of Physicians. Physicians and the pharmaceutical industry. *Ann Intern Med* 1990;112:624–6.

3. Bayles TB. Salicylates and the rheumatic diseases. *Arthritis Rheum* 1966:9:342–7.
4. Rodnan GP, Benedek TG. The early history of antirheumatic drugs. *Arthritis Rheum* 1970;13:145–65.
5. Newton DR, Tanner JM. *N*-Acetyl-*para*-aminophenol as an analgesic. *Br Med J* 1956;2:1096–8.
6. Sandler DP, Smith JC, Weinberg CR, Buckalew VM, Dennis VW, Blythe WB, Burgess WP. Analgesic use and chronic renal disease. *N Engl J Med* 1989;320:1238–43.
7. Bennett WM, DeBroe ME. Analgesic nephropathy—a preventable renal disease. *N Engl J Med* 1989;320:1269–71.
8. Roth SH, Mackenzie A. Drug development, guidelines and the Food and Drug Administration. *Ann Intern Med* 1984;101:125–7.
9. Lerner BH. Scientific evidence versus therapeutic demand: the introduction of the sulfonamides revisited. *Ann Intern Med* 1991;115:315–20.
10. Food and Drug Administration. Clinical testing for safe and effective drugs. HHS Publication No. (FDA) 74-3015, 1981.
11. Bureau of Drugs. Guidelines for the clinical evaluation of anti-inflammatory drugs (adults and children). Washington, US Government Printing Office, 1977; Publication No. (FDA)78-3054.
12. Hadler NM, Gillings DB. On the design of the Phase III drug trial. *Arthritis Rheum* 1983;26:1354–61.
13. Bellamy N, Buchanan WW. Interpreting clinical trials of antirheumatic drug therapy. *Bull Rheum Dis* 1986;36(2):1–10.
14. Strom BL, Miettinen OS, Melmon KL. Post-marketing studies of drug efficacy: how? *Am J Med* 1984;77:703–8.
15. Conference on outcome measures in rheumatological clinical trials. *J Rheumatol* 1982;9:753–806.
16. Boardman PL, Hart FD. Clinical measurement of the antiinflammatory effects of salicylates in rheumatoid arthritis. *Br Med J* 1967;4:264–8.
17. Multz CV, Bernhard GC, Blechman WC, Zane S, Restifo RA, Varady JC. A comparison of intermediate-dose aspirin and placebo in rheumatoid arthritis. *Clin Pharmacol Ther* 1973;15:310–5.
18. Calabro JJ, Paulus HE, Anti-inflammatory effect of acetylsalicylic acid in rheumatoid arthritis. *Clin Orthop* 1970;71:124–31.
19. Fremont-Smith K, Bayles TB. Salicylate therapy in rheumatoid arthritis. *JAMA* 1965;192:1133–6.
20. Fries JF, Britton MC. Some problems in the interpretation of clinical trials: long-term parallel study of fenoprofen in rheumatoid arthritis. *J Rheumatol* 1976;2[Suppl]:61–6.
21. Ameer B, Greenblatt DJ. Acetaminophen. *Ann Intern Med* 1977;87:202–9.
22. Bradley JD, Brandt KD, Katz BP, Kalasinski LA, Ryan SI. Comparison of an antiinflammatory dose of ibuprofen, and analgesic dose of ibuprofen and acetaminophen in the treatment of patients with osteoarthritis of the knee. *N Engl J Med* 1991;325:87–91.
23. The Multicenter Salsalate/Aspirin Comparison Study Group. Does the acetyl group of aspirin contribute to the antiinflammatory efficacy of salicylic acid in the treatment of rheumatoid arthritis? *J Rheumatol* 1989;16:321–7.
24. Hadler NM. Knee pain is the malady—not osteoarthritis. *Ann Intern Med* 1992;116:598–9.
25. Baragar FD, Duthie JJR. Importance of aspirin as a cause of anemia and peptic ulcer in rheumatoid arthritis. *Br Med J* 1960;1:1106–8.
26. Ropes MW. Conservative treatment in rheumatoid arthritis. *Med Clin North Am* 1961;45:1197–1207.
27. Smyth CJ. Indomethacin—its rightful place in treatment. *Ann Intern Med* 1970;72:430–2.
28. Kantor TG. Ibuprofen. *Ann Intern Med* 1979;191:877–82.
29. Wiseman EH, Boyle JA. Piroxicam (Feldene). *Clin Rheum Dis* 1980;6:585–613.
30. Bowers DE, Dyer HR, Fosdick WM, et al. Naproxen in rheumatoid arthritis: a controlled trial. *Ann Intern Med* 1975;83:470–5.
31. Sigler JW, Ridolfo AS, Bluhm GB. Comparison of benefit-to-risk ratios of aspirin and fenoprofen: controlled multicentre study in rheumatoid arthritis. *J Rheumatol* 1976;2[Suppl]:49–60.
32. Hadler NM. There's the forest: the object lesson of NSAID "gastropathy." *J Rheumatol* 1990;17:280–2.

33. Barrier CH, Hirschowitz BI. Controversies in the detection and management of nonsteroidal antiinflammatory drug-induced side effects of the upper gastrointestinal tract. *Arthritis Rheum* 1989;32:926–32.

34. Soll AH, Weinstein WM, Kurata J, McCarthy D. Nonsteroidal anti-inflammatory drugs and peptic ulcer disease. *Ann Intern Med* 1991;114:307–19.

35. Roth S, Agrawal N, Mahowald M, Montoya H, Robbins D, Miller S, Nutting E, Woods E, Crager M, Swabb E. Misoprostol heals gastroduodenal injury in patients with rheumatoid arthritis receiving aspirin. *Arch Intern Med* 1989;149:775–9.

36. Lanza FL, Umbenhauer ER, Nelson RS, Rack MF, Daurio CP, White LA. A double-blind randomized placebo controlled gastroscopic study to compare the effects of indomethacin capsules and indomethacin suppositories on the gastric mucosa of human volunteers. *J Rheumatol* 1982;9:415–9.

37. Fries JF, Miller SR, Spitz PW, Williams CA, Hubert HB, Bloch DA. Toward an epidemiology of gastropathy associated with nonsteroidal antiinflammatory drug use. *Gastroenterology* 1989;96:647–55.

38. Jick SS, Perera DR, Walker AM, Jick H. Non-steroidal anti-inflammatory drugs and hospital admission for perforated peptic ulcer. *Lancet* 1987;ii:380–2.

39. Beard K, Walker AM, Perera DR, Jick H. Nonsteroidal anti-inflammatory drugs and hospitalization for gastroesophageal bleeding in the elderly. *Arch Intern Med* 1987;147:1621–4.

40. Guess HA, West R, Strand LM, Helston D, Lydick EG, Bergman U, Wolski K. Fatal upper gastrointestinal hemorrhage or perforation among users and nonusers of nonsteroidal anti-inflammatory drugs in Saskatchewan, Canada, 1983. *J Clin Epidemiol* 1988;41:35–45.

41. Carson JL, Strom BL, Soper KA, West SL, Morse ML. The association of nonsteroidal anti-inflammatory drugs with upper gastrointestinal tract bleeding. *Arch Intern Med* 1987; 147:85–8.

42. Griffin MR, Ray WA, Schaffner W. Nonsteroidal anti-inflammatory drug use and death from peptic ulcer in elderly persons. *Ann Intern Med* 1988;109;359–63.

43. Carson JL, Strom BL, Schinnar R, Duff A, Sim E. The low risk of upper gastrointestinal bleeding in patients dispensed corticosteroids. *Am J Med* 1991;91:223–8.

44. Piper JM, Ray WA, Daugherty JR, Griffin MR. Corticosteroid use and peptic ulcer disease: role of nonsteroidal anti-inflammatory drugs. *Ann Intern Med* 1991;114:735–40.

45. Fries JF, Williams CA, Bloch DA, Michel BA. Nonsteroidal anti-inflammatory drug-associated gastropathy: incidence and risk factor models. *Am J Med* 1991;91:213–22.

46. Chrischilles EZ, Lemke JH, Wallace RB, Drube GA. Prevalence and characteristics of multiple analgesic drug use in an elderly study group. *J Am Geriatr Soc* 1990;38:979–84.

47. Faulkner G, Prichard P, Somerville K, Langman MJS. Aspirin and bleeding peptic ulcers in the elderly. *Br Med J* 1988;297:1311–3.

48. Skander MP, Ryan FP. Non-steroidal anti-inflammatory drugs and pain free peptic ulceration in the elderly. *Br Med J* 1988;297:833–4.

49. Kurata JH. Ulcer epidemiology: an overview and proposed research framework. *Gastroenterology* 1989;96:569–80.

5

The Pitfalls of Empirical and Aggressive Therapies

Conservative is one of the more beleaguered, if not abused, terms in the clinical lexicon. *Conservative care for low back pain* is an oxymoron; no one is advocating therapies that conserve the pain. The term insinuated into clinical jargon initially to draw a distinction with radical or heroic therapies. *Conservative therapy* was not a pejorative term; if anything, it was to connote reasoned intervention employing remedies in which the profession had confidence. It implied a cautious, moderate approach fraught with less risk. Perhaps, for illness in general and back pain in particular, that explains why the term *conservative* does not appear in classic clinical writing at the turn of the century (1,2). It would have been difficult to advocate any but conservative remedies. More to the point, to practice within the bounds of acceptance, one had to argue that even a patently heroic intervention was really conservative; heroic interventions without such acceptance were the business of quacks.

These are no longer the implications of the conservative rubric. Today the distinction is drawn more with "aggressive" or "empirical" therapies than with those that might be considered heroic or radical or out of bounds. With this evolution, *conservative* has accrued some baggage. Conservative therapy is no longer that which we all concur is reasonable. It is no longer the best we can do; it is the least we can do! By 1970, even the British had accepted this precept for back pain, "the results of conservative treatment are by no means satisfactory" (3). The implication is that we need an alternative to conservative therapy rather than that we need more or new conservative therapies.

Contemporary medicine even applauds "empirical" therapy. The term is bandied about in its Lockean sense; the implication is that wisdom has been or will be gained through personal experience. If this is the rationalization for trying something on a patient, the act is termed empirical therapy and pride is taken in exercising the prerogative. However, empirical therapy has not always been a source of pride. For the classical Greek physicians it was an act of hubris. In fact, the term *empiric* was reserved for the charlatan and *empirical therapy* for quackery. The contemporary inversion of the label is fascinating from the perspective of semiotics, disquieting from the perspective of ethics. While empiricism is on the rise, conservatism is suffering aspersion.

Conservative therapy in America has acquired overtones of nihilism; Americans look to aggressive therapy for solutions. I am singling out American perceptions as they are not those of other comparably advanced industrial countries. Payer (4), in her remarkable monograph *Medicine & Culture*, observed that

> the American regards himself as naturally healthy. It therefore stands to reason that if he becomes ill, there must be a cause for the illness, preferably one that comes from without and can be quickly dealt with. . . . When all this aggressive diagnosis and treatment became too expensive for a system in which doctors are paid for each act they perform, reforms were started, and the reforms, too, had a distinctly American air. Rather than reimbursing physicians for everything they did, reimbursement would be based on the diagnosis the patient was given. Such a system gives primacy to the idea that disease is some wild and hairy monster that can be locked up with diagnosis, and completely ignores the European idea that the severity of the disease—and consequently the need for medical intervention— has also to do with features [that encompass the physiologic and psychosocial context in which the disease is suffered].

This duality—conservative therapeutic approaches are nihilistic, whereas aggressive therapeutic approaches are curative—has become entrenched in the minds of the American people and the American health insurer. The American physician has been at the vanguard of advocacy for this syllogism. In the 19th century medical professionals waved their banner of aggressive intervention to denigrate the ministrations of the many, and often popular, schools of alternative therapy (5). The profession remained on shaky ground until, at the turn of the century, it embraced with zeal the German reductionist notions of medicine; "adopting such a concept of medicine rejected patient-oriented medicine in favor of disease-oriented or, worse still, theory-oriented medicine" (6). Today, doing something, particularly something dramatic that places the patient at risk while rendering the patient utterly dependent, has cachet in America. Other industrialized countries are inherently more skeptical and uniformly more tentative in their adoption of such interventions.

THE INHERENT RISKS OF AN ETHOS OF CLINICAL AGGRESSIVENESS

"To cure"—not just to manage or treat or minister to or even heal. "To cure" is the quest of every physician since Hippocrates extricated medicine from the temples of religion. "To cure" is succor to clinical science and balm for the despair of any sufferer. If "to cure" had been realized through hygiene and with antibiotics, Camus would never have had to write *The Plague*. Erysipelas no longer has a 90% mortality thanks to penicillin. The condition, its diagnosis, and its treatment have become almost trivial. And undertreatment or tardiness in treatment of bacterial meningitis is malpractice. "To cure" is worthy, glorious, and seductive. There is no argument. When cure is realized, physicians strut and society applauds.

But what price are we willing to pay in the quest? How certain do we have to be of the reality of the cure? How much error of judgment, of conviction will we tolerate? The answer is that the quest for cure can commandeer temperance and, if that quest has the patina of authority, it can commandeer judgment and common sense. In this century, thanks to authority, countless hysterectomies were performed to remove retroverted uteruses held responsible for such ills as backache. Thanks to authority, "floating kidneys" and "ptotic colons" have been subjected to one or another form of -pexy for the same reason. For other reasons, authority conspired to remove countless tonsils, breasts, and teeth while administering an array of nostrums—all during this century. Every authority held a conviction; every conviction had theoretical underpinnings; every authority's personal experience was interpreted as confirmatory. Medicine advanced in the quest to cure, but the path was peripatetic.

Today, authority can be redefined. No theory should hold sway in the clinical arena unless it has been put to the test and escaped unscathed. Aggressive interventions backed only by theory, conviction, and zeal are disquieting at best. At worst, they are harmful. Yet America learns this lesson painfully. We refuse to demand a demonstration of benefit and a quantification of risk whenever the intervention is nonpharmacologic and heralded as curative. We are taught to fear death with a vehemence that allows us to take risks with our life. And we compensate our physicians, and reward our interventionalists, commensurate with their promise of cure, regardless of its reality.

Modern American cardiology provides the most disturbing illustration. So much of the enterprise persists in the face of study after study that fails to demonstrate benefit. Yet the nation accepts the arguments that proponents base on theory and promise. Even when studies document some benefit, the nation accepts egregious marketing. Thrombolytic therapy is illustrative. The likelihood that a normotensive patient will be alive 5 yr after a first myocardial infarction can be improved from approximately 96% to 98% with thrombolytic therapy. Rather than bemoaning a 2% improvement in survival, the cardiologic enterprise is wont to proclaim a 50% reduction in mortality (7) to justify the substantial short-term risks and cost. Similar wordplay applied to a conservative therapy with 2% benefit would likely engender derision by physician and patient and be dismissed by insurers.

The contract between the American cardiologic enterprise and the American people is disturbing if not unconscionable. The contract with the American community of spine surgeons is more so, given that it is perpetrated without the specter of death. Since World War II, Americans have learned to think of backache as an injury reflecting forms of intervertebral pathologic conditions that are potentially surgically remedial. The concept gained firm footing when it was accepted by Workers' Compensation Insurance programs (8,9). What followed was predictable. Sufferers in America were primed and ready to expect specific diagnoses and attempts at aggressive intervention. Surgeons leaped to the challenge. It is estimated that over 2.0% of Americans have already availed themselves of the surgical option (10,11), and their need continues apace. Over 250,000 lumbar spinal operations are performed in the United States annually, for a total of over 1,000 operations per million inhabitants (12). Contrast this with the 100 operations per million in Great Britain (13) and 350 per million in Finland (14).

Aggressive or not, an unproven remedy is still an unproven remedy. Estimating its risk/benefit ratio or its cost/benefit ratio is absurd; if it has no benefit, it is worthless and no risk is tolerable. Yet, to varying degrees, industrial nations remain wedded to the unproven remedy if it is aggressive, offered up dressed in scientific inference, and championed by authorities. Furthermore, in fee-for-service medical systems, where the authorities who offer unproven remedies are handsomely rewarded for operating on their convictions, unproven remedies become the standard of practice. Even unprovable remedies remain the standard of practice when the enterprise is entrenched. It is time to reeducate society and to educate physicians; there is no inherent value to aggressiveness. Aggressiveness per se is anathema; the ill deserve reasoned, proven interventions, aggressive or not.

CONSERVATIVE CARE FOR LOW BACK PAIN—CAVEAT EMPTOR

Regional back pain is the backache suffered by someone 18 to 60 yr old who would otherwise be well if it were not for the low back pain and whose pain was not precipitated by an overtly traumatic event involving external force (15). Regional back pain is the appropriate diagnosis for the vast majority of episodes of back pain in this age group and is all that is being considered in this chapter. The diagnosis and management of regional low back pain is considered in depth in Chapter 7. That very rare younger individual whose backache is a consequence of metastatic or primary neoplasia or of metastatic infection is not a candidate for conservative therapy.

Regional backache is a ubiquitous remittent and intermittent experience. No doubt it has always been so. And no doubt some sufferers have chosen medical advice in the quest for a remedy throughout the history of the profession. Hippocrates (400 B.C.) in *Peri Arthron* and *Mochlikon*, Avicenna (1073 A.D.), Charef-Ed-Din (1465 A.D.), and Antoine Paré (1590 A.D.) are among those in the medical pantheon who have pontificated on the diagnosis and management of backache (16). It is equally certain that sufferers have always sought alternatives in care from assorted willing, nonmedical practitioners. The "shepherd's hug" and the "trampling cure" persist from antiquity, and "bonesetters" have long plied their trade (17). To come to grips with the evolution of recourse to and acceptance of the conservative management of backache, it is important to realize that "common sense" is not simply wisdom gained from personal experience or the experience of others. It has long been tempered by advice offered both by physicians and by alternative practitioners based on theory, sometimes substantive data, and always conviction. Such advice has seldom been offered without an element of self-service (18). Consequently, the common sense of one stratum of society and of one geographic region may have little in common with that of another. The following epidemiologic studies illustrate this maxim.

In 1978 Verbrugge and Ascione (19) undertook to assess the everyday experience of morbidity. The "Health in Detroit" survey was based on a probability sample of 589 white households in the Detroit metropolitan area. An initial interview was conducted with one adult in each household, who then maintained a daily diary for 6 wk, after which there was a closing interview. The average adult had 16 symptomatic days during the 6 wk; only 11% of men and 5% of women remained symptom free. Respiratory symptoms were the most common, followed by musculoskeletal symptoms. The incidence of musculoskeletal morbidities is summarized in Table 5.1, and the quality and outcome are summarized in Table 5.2. Over half of the people were coping with musculoskeletal symptoms for an average of 8 days every 6 wk. The vast majority of the morbidity was backache. Only 3% of the people in this sample felt the need to seek medical advice; only 0.3% actually received medical care.

Contrast this prospectively followed small sample with the recalled experience and behavior revealed in a national survey conducted at about the same time. The National Health and Nutrition Examination Survey (NHANES) II was carried out between 1976 and 1980 on a probability sample of 27,801 noninstitutionalized civilians. Of this sample, 10,404 adults were also subjected to a physical examination and a formal interview. The information relevant to those who ever experienced "pain in your back on most days for at least 2 weeks" has recently been published (20). Of the 10,404 participants, 1,763 recalled such prolonged back pain and in 1,516 it was primarily in their low back, for a cumulative lifetime prevalence of memorable backache lasting more

TABLE 5.1. *Incidence of musculoskeletal morbidities during the 6-week course of the Health in Detroit survey*

Parameter	Men	Women	Total
% with any musculoskeletal symptoms	44	56	51
% of all days that had musculoskeletal symptoms	8	12	11
Days with musculoskeletal symptoms as % of all days with symptoms	26	30	29
Average number of days of musculoskeletal symptoms suffered by those with any such symptoms	7	9	8

From Verbrugge and Ascione, ref. 19.

TABLE 5.2. *Quality and outcome of musculoskeletal morbidity in the Health in Detroit survey*

For the majority:
They were otherwise asymptomatic.
They thought that they had "arthritis."
They talked to their spouse.
They took OTC[a] analgesics.
They thought that their symptoms were "not very serious."
They suffered back or leg pain.
For <10%:
They experienced neck pain (9%).
They experienced hand pain (6%).
They thought that their symptoms were "very severe" (8%).
They sought medical care (3%).
They received medical care (0.3%).

From Verbrugge and Ascione, ref. 19.
[a] OTC, over the counter.

than 2 wk of 13.8%. The national experience regarding accession of health care for more prolonged backache contrasts strikingly with that revealed in the "Health in Detroit Survey" for brief episodes. The vast majority of Americans with more than 2 wk of memorable backache visit health professionals (Table 5.3). In fact, backache was the second leading symptom engendering physician visits at the time of the NHANES II survey (21). Even more remarkable than just the professional contact is the array of remedies that were introduced into the fabric of the experience of backache (Table 5.4).

Before attempting to draw inferences by contrasting the NHANES II survey with the Health in Detroit survey, we have to come to grips with yet another data set collected at about the same time. Biering-Sorensen (22) managed to enroll 928 adults, representing 82% of all 30-, 40-, 50-, and 60-yr-old residents of Glostrup, Denmark, in a 1-yr survey focusing on backache. At entry into the study, 62% were suffering or recalled having suffered back pain within the prior 12 mo. These entry criteria combine the point prevalence of the Health in

TABLE 5.3. *Utilization of professional care by sufferers with >2 weeks of memorable backache in the NHANES II survey*

Health professional	%
General practitioner	58.6
Orthopedist	36.9
Chiropractor	30.8
Osteopath	13.8
Internist	7.6
Rheumatologist	2.5
Any health professional	84.6

From Deyo and Tsui-Wu, ref. 20.

TABLE 5.4. *Remedies employed by the NHANES II survey participants in the management of their backache*

Treatment	Ever used (%)	Of those using, % who thought it helpful	Of those who thought it helpful, % still using
Rest	80.8	85.5	48.5
Heat	73.9	80.4	32.1
Aspirin	58.2	76.7	48.1
Stiff mattress	57.9	84.8	89.2
Exercises	40.5	78.1	43.0
Bedboard	36.1	84.8	63.6
Back brace	27.0	70.8	28.1
Traction	20.7	62.9	9.6
Diathermy or paraffin	16.7	75.3	3.9
Cold	7.2	55.9	15.5
Splints/casts	3.6	73.9	5.1

From Deyo and Tsui-Wu, ref. 20.

Detroit survey with the considerable recall uncertainties (23) of the design used in the NHANES II survey. Nonetheless, this is an extraordinary level of awareness of past episodes of backache—far greater than one would predict from the American surveys. Part of the explanation is that Biering-Sorensen accepted "insufficientia dorsi" as a qualifying illness; this is a "feeling of weakness, fatigue and/or stiffness in the lower back," which accounts for about 25% of the recalled morbidity. But this still does not explain the extraordinary excess of morbidity ascribed to the low back that is recalled by these Danes. Recourse to health professionals because of their backache was as likely as in the NHANES II survey (Table 5.3), even though the reservoir of morbidity in Glostrup exceeded that in America by over fivefold! In Glostrup 60% of the sufferers consulted their general practitioner, 25% a specialist, and 15% a chiropractor (24). The therapies prescribed in Glostrup (Table 5.5) differ from the American experiences particularly in relying on some physical modalities such as injec-

TABLE 5.5. *Remedies used by the Glostrup survey participants in the management of their backache*

Treatment received	% subjected
Bed rest	27
Physiotherapy	49
Local muscle injection	20
Exercise program	15
Lumbar traction	12
Manipulative therapy	20
Spinal support	3
Analgesics	43

From Biering-Sorensen, ref. 24.

tion and manipulative therapies while deemphasizing rest and analgesics. The menu of practitioners and modalities is the same, but the proclivities differ. And that, indeed, is the compelling message of these and other surveys. We will all experience backache, repeatedly and sometimes intensely. We will all be forced to cope with our discomfort. There is nothing reflexive about our coping. How we cope, what we do or don't do, is learned! And the lessons differ across socioeconomic strata, across sociopolitical boundaries, and across time. The reason no best way has emerged is that there is no best way. Rather, there is a cacophony of heuristic pathogenetic inferences (25) playing on our anxieties and a plethora of unproven and marginal remedies (26–28) vying for our patronage.

TOWARD A UNIVERSAL COMMON SENSE

I am not suggesting that we toss out the entire enterprise that feeds on the backache we will all suffer. It has a life of its own and is deaf to the voice in the wilderness. Furthermore, there are surgical indications, albeit they are rare. And there is promise in the aggressive approach, albeit the promise is not compelling enough to absolve the profession from performing ethical trials. Finally, it can be lonely and frightening to rely solely on one's personal resources in coping with a backache—and more so if the experience is confounded by psychologic and social turmoil at home or in the workplace. Such turmoil can render backache less tolerable and drive one to seek recourse (29). In this circumstance, backache becomes the readily acceptable surrogate complaint for the psychosocial context that renders coping inadequate. It becomes common sense.

What I am arguing for is a return to the tradition of conservative care for backache. First, society must be reeducated regarding backache. We have enough information to disabuse the laity (30) and the policy makers (31,32). Then the sufferer will be in a better position to cope, including coping by choosing from the menu of therapies that are at one's beck and call. And when coping fails, the sufferer can turn to a physician for perspective, advice, and conservative care. This requires educated patients and knowledgeable clinicians. Both are prerequisite to the quest for wisdom.

REFERENCES

1. Quain R. *A Dictionary of Medicine.* New York, Appleton, 1889:1370–1.
2. McCrae T. *Osler's The Principles and Practice of Medicine.* 10th ed. New York, Appleton, 1926:1091,1156.
3. Scott JT. Neurological aspects of the rheumatic diseases. In: Copeman WSC (ed.) *Textbook of Rheumatic Diseases.* London, Livingstone, 1970:671.
4. Payer L. *Medicine & Culture.* New York, Holt, 1988:139–43.
5. Gevitz N. Three perspectives on unorthodox medicine. In: Gevitz N (ed.) *Other Healers.* Baltimore, Johns Hopkins University Press, 1988:1–29.

6. Altschule MD. *Essays on the Rise and Decline of Bedside Medicine.* Philadelphia, Lea & Febiger, 1989:402.
7. Hadler NM. Modern cardiology: is 2% a solution? In: Hadler NM, Bunn WB (eds.) *Occupational Problems in Medical Practice.* New York, DellaCorte, 1990:277–82.
8. Hadler NM. Legal ramifications of the medical definition of back disease. *Ann Intern Med* 1978;89:992–9.
9. Hadler NM. Regional musculoskeletal diseases of the low back: cumulative trauma versus single incident. *Clin Orthop* 1987;221:33–41.
10. Frymoyer JW, Pope MH, Clements JH, Wilder DG, MacPherson B, Ashikaga T. Risk factors in low-back pain: an epidemiological survey. *J Bone Joint Surg [Am]* 1983;65A:213–8.
11. Frymoyer JW. Back pain and sciatica. *N Engl J Med* 1988;318:291–300.
12. Andersson GBJ. The epidemiology of spinal disorders. In: Frymoyer JW, Ducker TB, Hadler NM, Kostuik JP, Weinstein JN, Whitecloud TS III (eds.) *The Adult Spine: Principles and Practice.* New York, Raven Press, 1991:107-46.
13. Wood PHN, Badley EM. Epidemiology of back pain. In: Jayson M (ed.) *The Lumbar Spine and Back Pain.* London, Churchill Livingstone, 1987:1–15.
14. Heliovaara M. *Epidemiology of Sciatica and Herniated Lumbar Intervertebral Disc.* Helsinki: Research Institute for Social Security, 1988:1–147.
15. Hadler NM. Regional back pain. *N Engl J Med* 1986;315:1090–2.
16. Curtis P. The efficacy of spinal manipulation. In: Hadler NM (ed.) *Clinical Concepts in Regional Musculoskeletal Illness.* Orlando, Grune & Stratton, 1987:51.
17. Joy RT. The natural bonesetters: an early phase of orthopedics. *Bull Hist Med* 1954;28:416–31.
18. Hadler NM. Another colloquy at Delphi: an unabashed parody. *Arthritis Rheum* 1990;33:436–8.
19. Verbrugge LM, Ascione FJ. Exploring the iceberg: common symptoms and how people care for them. *Med Care* 1987;25:481–6.
20. Deyo RA, Tsui-Wu Y-J. Descriptive epidemiology of low-back pain and its related medical care in the United States. *Spine* 1987;12:264–8.
21. Cypress BK. Characteristics of physician visits for back symptoms: a national perspective. *Am J Public Health* 1983;73:389–95.
22. Biering-Sorensen F. A prospective study of low back pain in a general population. II. Location, character, aggravating and relieving factors. *Scand J Rehabil Med* 1983;15:81–8.
23. Biering-Sorensen F, Hilden J. Reproducibility of the history of low-back trouble. *Spine* 1984;9:280–6.
24. Biering-Sorensen F. A prospective study of low back pain in a general population. III. Medical service—work consequence. *Scand J Rehabil Med* 1983;15:89–96.
25. Hadler NM. Occupational illness: the issue of causality. *J Occup Med* 1984;26:587–93.
26. Hadler NM. *Diagnosis and Medical Management of the Regional Musculoskeletal Diseases.* Orlando, Grune & Stratton, 1984:3–52.
27. Spitzer WO, LeBlanc FE, Dupuis M, et al. Scientific approach to the assessment and management of activity-related spinal disorders: a monograph for clinicians. Report of the Quebec Task Force on Spinal Disorders. *Spine* 1987;12:S1–S59.
28. Hadler NM, Curtis P, Gillings DB, Stinnett S. A benefit of spinal manipulation as adjunctive therapy for acute low-back pain: a stratified controlled trial. *Spine* 1987;12:703–6.
29. Bigos SJ, Battié MC. The impact of spinal disorders in industry. In: Frymoyer JW, Ducker TB, Hadler NM, Kostuik JP, Weinstein JN, Whitecloud TS III (eds.) *The Adult Spine: Principles and Practice.* New York, Raven Press, 1991:147–54.
30. Hadler NM. The predicament of backache. *J Occup Med* 1988;30:449–50.
31. Hadler NM. Disabling backache in France, Switzerland, and the Netherlands: Contrasting sociopolitical constraints on clinical judgment. *J Occup Med* 1989;31:823–31.
32. Hadler NM. Epilogue. In: Greenwood J, Taricco A (eds.) *Workers' Compensation Health Care Cost Containment.* Horsham, Pennsylvania, LRP Publications, 1992:339–43.

SECTION II

The Patient with Regional Musculoskeletal Symptoms

This section explores the traditional doctor-patient interaction in the context of regional musculoskeletal illness and from the perspective of the treating physician. However, as was emphasized in Chapter 3, it is a fellow human being who is entering into the patient-physician contract and who will forever be changed by the experience. To care for any patient, the physician must become and remain cognizant of the process that led the particular individual to seek medical care in the first place. The physician must realize the perturbation of the illness that is intrinsic to the diagnostic process. Awareness of preconceptions and expectations, as well as empathy and support for the individual assuming the patient role, is as important as the diagnostic process itself. If the diagnostic process leads to a definitive and curative and therapeutic outcome, a clean break of the doctor-patient contract becomes reasonable. However, if the process generates no definitive solution, the contract is maintained and the therapeutic nature of the ongoing relationship will rely heavily on the caring quality of the process from its initiation. For regional musculoskeletal illness, this latter circumstance is the rule.

The patient-physician contract is familiar: The patient is made to display his or her illness to generate the first level of diagnostic hypotheses. These hypotheses are tested by physical examination, and the possibilities are pared. The next level of hypothesis testing takes advantage of the clinical laboratories, imaging technology, and specialized testing such as electrodiagnostics. The efficiency of the process relates to the precision with which hypotheses are tested; each test must be interpreted to answer a specific question. If the testing is indeterminate, only anxiety and uncertainty are served. If the testing is known to be indeterminate, then its application is a reproach to the diagnostician and an assault on the coping mechanisms of the patient. As will become clear, too much of the testing of the patient with regional musculoskeletal illness currently undertaken qualifies for this condemnation.

Finally, the modern clinician has sufficient scientific underpinning to ask at the outset, "Even if I can define the cause of the symptoms, will the information alter my approach to management?" If the answer is no, than the diagnostic exercise has no redeeming features and many that are counterproductive.

Chapter 6 will expand on these arguments. Chapters 7 to 10 deal with individual regional musculoskeletal illnesses.

6

The Concept of Regional Musculoskeletal Illness

The experience of musculoskeletal discomfort, even of compromise in musculo-skeletal function, is one of life's surprises (see Section I). Usually there is no precipitant. Usually we would consider ourselves entirely well were it not for this discomfort. And usually we cope effectively by taking advantage of our personal resources. Hardly a month will go by without a need to come to grips with such a predicament. Some of these events are of sufficient moment that 15% of us remember them for a year or more. The overwhelming majority of these morbid experiences involve the axial skeleton; low back pain predomi-nates, with neck pain a distant second.

Occasionally, we find our personal resources inadequate and feel the need to turn to some provider of care. Little is still known of the process by which people with musculoskeletal predicaments decide that their coping is serving them poorly. The moment the person with a musculoskeletal predicament shares coping with a physician, that person becomes a patient and the predica-ment becomes an illness. If there is no overt traumatic precipitant, if there is no relevant underlying systemic disease so that the person would be well were it not for the musculoskeletal region that is involved, the illness is a *regional musculoskeletal illness* (1,2). Such illnesses are the chief complaint of a consider-able percentage of the patients presenting in a primary care setting, ranking second or third in frequency. Regional musculoskeletal illnesses occupy a simi-lar station in the experience of most rheumatologists. For the rheumatologist, they present a special challenge. After all, there is no systemic rheumatic disease that spares one the coincidence of a regional rheumatic illness. Making such a diagnosis will test the acumen of any physician; in fact, discerning the regional illness in the setting of systemic rheumatic disease is often impossible. Nonethe-less, given that there are instances where therapy is altered, it is a diagnostic exercise to be encouraged.

There is another important ramification of the concept of regional musculo-skeletal illnesses; it behooves the treating physician to consider why any particu-

67

lar individual would choose to seek medical recourse for this particular musculoskeletal predicament. Sometimes the explanation is consonant with the tradition of scientific medicine; this person has chosen to be a patient because the predicament was too unfamiliar, too painful, too prolonged, etc. However, from multiple studies (3) it is becoming clear that such constrained pathophysiologic inferences serve the chief complaint poorly. The decision to be a patient is often tempered by the psychosocial setting in which the musculoskeletal predicament is experienced. Sometimes the musculoskeletal illness even serves as a surrogate complaint. It is a far more facile conceptualization than the realization that some other force in one's life, such as job or marital dissatisfactions, is compromising one's ability to cope with the musculoskeletal predicament. Regional musculoskeletal illnesses are often confounded in this fashion and are never well managed unless the confounders are recognized early on. This point will be reemphasized in Section III.

However, in this section we will focus on the clinical algorithm that has become the pride of Western medicine—the establishment of a differential diagnosis for the illness that allows one to formulate a plan of intervention. Such an algorithm did not always dominate patient-physician interaction. In fact, its promulgation can be ascribed to one man, Thomas Sydenham, at the outset of the 18th century (4). Before Sydenham, ascribing a cause for illness was an exercise with almost free intellectual range. "Fate" as an answer became far more difficult after St. Thomas Aquinas placed the burden of free will on the Western psyche. Scapegoating found its way into pathogenetic inference to explain plague, venereal disease, and more, a heinous feature of medieval thought that is leaving its mark on Western society even in this century (5). In Elizabethan England, a common inference regarding the cause of sciatica included impiety and decadence if Shakespeare's *Measure for Measure* is an accurate reflection (Act I, ii, 50–55).

It took Thomas Sydenham to offer the insight that gave science a foothold in the diagnostic morass. Sydenham realized that most diagnostic schemes of his day were purely descriptive; they were based on symptoms experienced by a particular patient. These symptoms, which I call the *illness*, were carefully described so that comparisons with the experience of others was possible, leading to a nosology based on illness. If a patient was experiencing sputum production, the diagnosis of the day was catarrh. If the illness was characterized as smoldering joint inflammation, the diagnosis was rheumatism. More cataclysmic joint complaints were ascribed to gout, which was further divided into "podagra, cheiragra and sciatica" (6) to indicate severe pain of the hallux, the hand, and the hip (ischium, therefore ischiatic), respectively. The art of medicine was first to identify the patient's symptoms as belonging to a particular illness category and then to prescribe nostrums and interventions designed to modify the symptoms. Sydenham said no! He asserted that these symptoms were the clinical representation of some underlying pathophysiologic or pathoanatomic derangement, a *disease*. The job of the physician was to listen to the symptoms, deduce the underlying disease, and provide specific therapy for the disease, thereby obviating the illness. Without such a conceptual leap, Western medicine would still be illness based, and we would be treating catarrh instead of treating particular pneumonias with specific antibiotics.

The disease-illness paradigm was seductive even when it was formulated, at a time when the concept led to little alteration in therapeusis. It facilitates the consideration of symptoms in a framework that lends itself to scientific testing. By the early 18th century, Boerhaave in Leiden took the precept to the bedside in his teaching rounds—in effect, inventing roundsmanship. Admissions of bafflement and befuddlement are rare throughout medical history; after Boerhaave, ignorance would forever be hidden in the complexities of the differential diagnosis. But all is not an exercise in obfuscation and futility. To the contrary, productive conclusions from the disease-illness paradigm are the triumphs of 20th century medicine. This century has seen dramatic inroads in the diagnosis and treatment of infectious diseases, upper gastrointestinal diseases, gout, cardiac and renal failure, and others. The disease-illness paradigm has proven so powerful that it has been elevated to axiomatic stature by physicians and layman alike. Whenever a person chooses to be a patient, the expectation is that the illness will be explained and that prognostic insights, palliation, and even cure will be forthcoming. For every symptom, it behooves the physician to establish some sense of the possible as regards underlying pathoanatomy, if not pathophysiology. This is the precept that underlies "differential diagnosis" and that dominates medical education, medical practice, and patient expectation.

Regional musculoskeletal illness has not yielded readily to the onslaught of differential diagnosis. Seldom has disease been revealed with certainty and therapy provided with more than empirical rationale. But that is not for lack of trying. For example, the most influential clinician of his time could not avoid coming to grips with the differential diagnosis of regional musculoskeletal illness of the low back at the turn of this century. Sir William Osler (7) considered such illness in two categories: lumbago and sciatica. Lumbago is defined as "pain in the lower back"; sciatica as "any painful condition referred to the sciatic nerve." His differential diagnosis is noteworthy not only as it is germane to the evolution of the concept of regional musculoskeletal illness but because it became the touchstone for all subsequent thought regarding regional backache. Table 6.1 is the differential diagnosis for lumbago, and Table 6.2 for sciatica; the rank order of diseases that can present as the illness lumbago or as the illness sciatica represents Osler's conception as to diagnostic probabilities.

Both tables are striking for downplaying trauma as a cause of lumbago or sciatica. Osler was considering only regional musculoskeletal illnesses in these tables, so overt, external force trauma was not an issue. However, contemporary considerations of the pathogenesis of such regional illness often invoke the image of traumatic precipitation with damaging consequence in spite of the absence of external force. For lumbago, Osler accepted such a possibility but ordered it ninth and last in his differential diagnosis. For sciatica, it appears as

TABLE 6.1. *Sir William Osler's differential diagnosis for lumbago*

1. *"Fibrositis*, in the muscles or fibrous tissue about the spine, is a common cause and may recur at short intervals."
2. *"Ischaemic lumbago*, described as a form of intermittent claudication, may be bilateral or unilateral and is excited by movement. The pain is between the twelfth rib and the crest of the ilium and may radiate forward. The area is not tender and the pain is dependent on muscular exertion."
3. *"Static* conditions, due to faulty posture, which may be lateral (one leg shorter) or antero-posterior, flat feet, stooping, occupation, etc."
4. *"Anatomical variations* of the transverse processes of the fifth lumbar vertebra"
5. *"Arthritis of the spine"*
6. *"Sacro-iliac* joint strain or relaxation"
7. *"Neuritis* of the posterior nerve roots"
8. "Pain due to *pelvic disease* in males (prostate, etc.) or females"
9. *"Trauma*, especially with lifting in a stooped position"

From Osler, ref. 7.

sacroiliac strain (Number 4), but the pathogenetic implication is obscured in his allusion to the susceptibility of military officers. How "trauma" came to be a dominant consideration in contemporary thinking about back pain will occupy much of our attention in Section III.

Ascribing low back pain to "fibrositis" was the cutting edge of clinical medicine at the turn of the century, when the construct was first introduced into the clinical lexicon. Even Osler realized that it was a diagnosis of exclusion. However, he argued that "in every case the effort should be made to arrive at an etiologic diagnosis as only then is proper treatment possible"—the rallying cry of Sydenham's scientific medicine that still captures the zeal of some clinicians today (see Chapter 3). For fibrositis Osler was needling; "needles of from three to four inches in length (ordinary bonnet needles, sterilized, will do) are thrust into the lumbar muscles at the seat of pain, and withdrawn after five or ten minutes." Otherwise he was detailing the use of strapping, rest, narcotics if necessary, massage, and a variety of nostrums. "For the cases due to spondylitis

TABLE 6.2. *Sir William Osler's differential diagnosis for sciatica*

1. *"Arthritis* which may be of the lower spine, lumbo-sacral, sacroiliac, or hip joints. In this case the arthritis lesion is often due to a focus of infection."
2. "Anatomical *anomalies,* as an unusually long transverse process of the fifth lumbar vertebra"
3. "Disease of the bones of the lower spine or pelvis, e.g., tuberculosis"
4. *"Strain*, which may be acute or chronic, especially of the sacro-iliac joint. Exposure to cold after heavy muscular exertion is said to be a cause. In trench warfare the men were not as subject to sciatica as the officers."
5. *"Pelvic* conditions, such as a solid ovarian or fibroid tumor in women and prostatic disease in men. Constipation and the pressure of the fetal head in labor are occasional causes."
6. *"Syphilis* is responsible in a few cases."
7. "It may be due to a focus of infection, which may cause fibrosis."
8. "Among rare causes are an abnormal network of veins on the trunk and anomalies, such as the pyriform muscle passing through the nerve."

From Osler, ref. 7.

or sacroiliac joint disease some form of fixation is useful; faulty posture should be corrected and flat feet receive attention." The first assertion supported attempts at aggressive, even mutilating surgery, and the second still supports a remarkable enterprise committed to the preparation and purveyance of orthotics to treat backache.

It is interesting and instructive to realize that the differential diagnosis of lumbago is not that different a century later. In fact, there are clinicians who would not alter the list or its order. Some of the postulates have withstood scientific scrutiny poorly. For example, Items 4 and 6 in Table 6.1 are untenable on scientific grounds, and the waves of surgical empiricism they engendered have subsided. The remainder of these possibilities are viable with only minor revision. Item 2 seems to encompass lumbar spinal stenosis and perhaps insufficiency fractures. More remarkably, only a few other contenders have been added to the contemporary list. Osler's differential diagnosis for sciatica has not fared as well. He was convinced that sciatica was seldom a primary disease of the nerve, rather it "is secondary to a process elsewhere." However, by elsewhere he was thinking of impinging processes distal to the neural foramen. Such possibilities have since been excluded in nearly all patients.

That a "focus of infection" might be causal appears to color both lists. Osler was living at a time when the "focal infection theory" held sway for many rheumatic diseases from fibrositis to rheumatoid arthritis. According to this theory, the rheumatic illness was a manifestation of a disease, most likely a focus of infection, distant from the musculoskeletal structures (8). It is an interesting theory with some experimental support available since the early decades of the century. However, the theory held such sway that it became the justification for countless empirical interventions before the practice was finally condemned in 1953. "The removal of an infected focus will not alter the course . . . . , and extraction of teeth, tonsils, gallbladders, and pelvic organs should be undertaken only when removal would be indicated if the patient did not have arthritis"(9).

It is clear that a differential diagnosis represents no more than the generation of hypotheses; by its very nature it asserts limits on certainty. It is equally clear that, in the minds of generations of clinicians since Sydenham, the differential diagnosis takes on a mantle of clairvoyance. It allows, maybe even encourages, the treating physician to formulate interventions based on extrapolation from the relevant body of scientific fact and on inferences from accumulated clinical experience. Furthermore, society has long sanctioned the practice of the physician testing his or her "acumen" and clinical insight on a trusting patient. This practice is generally referred to as empirical therapy. As discussed in Chapter 4, such is now illegal for pharmaceuticals. But empirical therapy is still sanctioned, even applauded, and certainly marketable for surgical and physical interventions. If the term *empirical* doesn't elicit some degree of revulsion, the reader is urged to return to Chapter 5.

No physician undertakes the exercise of differential diagnosis without the hope of generating a plan of intervention that is likely to palliate or cure. Furthermore, no person would choose to be a patient without such an expectation. When the exercise leads to diagnostic certainty and when the diagnosis leads to specific effective therapy, Sydenham is served well. However, although such circumstances are gratifyingly frequent, they represent little of the challenge of clinical medicine. With this degree of certainty, the therapeutic algorithm is straightforward and its execution demands only efficiency. The challenge for clinical medicine, and its raison d'être, is when the differential diagnosis and the resulting therapeutic algorithm are laden with uncertainties. Then a special burden of responsibility falls on the shoulders of the treating physician. The available resources include science, peer review, and insight, all of which are dynamic variables and all of which are perturbed by considerations that are external to the pathos of the bedside. These considerations were the focus of several chapters in Section I. We shall now explore the diagnosis and management of regional musculoskeletal illnesses by taking particular advantage of generations of false starts.

REFERENCES

1. Hadler NM. *Medical Management of the Regional Musculoskeletal Diseases.* Orlando, Grune & Stratton, 1984:1–323.
2. Hadler NM (ed.) *Clinical Concepts in Regional Musculoskeletal Illness.* Orlando, Grune & Stratton, 1987:1–370.
3. Bigos SJ, Battié MC, Spengler DM, et al. A prospective study of work perceptions and psychosocial factors affecting the report of back injury. *Spine* 1991;16:1–6.
4. Foucault M. *The Birth of the Clinic: An Archaeology of Medical Perception.* London, Tavistock Publications, 1973.
5. Gilman S. *The Jew's Body.* New York, Routledge, 1991:210–23.
6. Blackmore R. *Discourses on the Gout, a Rheumatism, and the King's Evil.* London, Pemberton, 1726:57.
7. Osler W. *The Principles and Practice of Medicine.* 10th ed. New York, Appleton, 1926:1088–91,1154–6.
8. Hadler NM, Granovetter DA. Phlogistic properties of bacterial debris. *Semin Arthritis Rheum* 1978;8:1–16.
9. Committee of the American Rheumatism Association. Primer on the rheumatic diseases. *JAMA* 1953;152:408–9.

7

The Axial Syndromes

The axial syndromes compose the vast majority of the musculoskeletal illnesses for which medical care is sought. Back pain is the second most frequent presenting complaint in most primary care settings. Knee pain and neck pain are also highly prevalent. For that reason, the discussion of the axial syndromes is more comprehensive.

The Adult Spine (1) is a comprehensive treatise on axial disorders that I co-edited and that was recently published by Raven Press. The reader is encouraged to turn to that resource for expanded discussions of all of the topics I will cover in this chapter, as well as detailed discussions of surgical considerations that are not covered here. This chapter is written from the perspective of the physician faced with a patient with a regional illness of the axial skeleton.

The diagnosis of a regional musculoskeletal illness of the axial skeleton is a diagnosis of exclusion. Since these illnesses are so prevalent and systemic diseases that present with axial pain are so rare, the exercise of exclusion is seldom productive of a specific diagnosis, let alone a diagnosis that alters therapy or even prognosis. Therefore, considerations that derive from the differential diagnosis of regional disorders should be pursued with zeal only in a special setting. For example, in the later decades of life the yield increases and so should the index of suspicion of the diagnostician. In the case of a younger adult patient with an axial predicament, regional musculoskeletal illness is so likely the diagnosis that it behooves the physician to avoid unfounded inferences, unnecessary testing with uninterpretable results, and ill-conceived therapies, all of which increase the likelihood that the acute illness will become chronic.

THE DIFFERENTIAL DIAGNOSIS: RECOGNIZING SYSTEMIC BACKACHE

Infections and Neoplasia

Nonetheless, there are several "red flags" in the history that should alert and impel the diagnostician. Almost all axial regional musculoskeletal illnesses force the patient to seek a static posture that unloads the involved region; recumbency, erect seating, and static standing postures are sought. Beware of any patient whose musculoskeletal illness causes motion. Axial pain with movement, even writhing, characterizes vascular catastrophes such as aortic dissection, visceral diseases involving the retroperitoneum, obstructive uropathies, etc. Bone pain from metastatic infection or neoplasia characteristically is accentuated at night and causes one to pace and fidget. Most but not all of these patients have systemic symptoms such as fever or weight loss. Most, but not all, have elevated sedimentation rates, if not anemia and other laboratory abnormalities associated with the particular process. Metastatic infections tend to localize to the disc or the epidural space; the illness is subacute and, in the latter case (which is a surgical emergency), often characterized by localizing radicular signs. Of the metastatic infections, special mention of Pott's disease is appropriate given the resurgence of tuberculosis in rural and ghetto America and in association with human immunodeficiency virus (HIV) infection. The tubercle bacillus has a propensity to seed the anterior disc, where it establishes a chronic, destructive infected granuloma that can expand across the space into the adjacent bodies. The process can dissect anteriorly into the soft tissues and track along tissue planes, as in a psoas abscess. The presentation is of smoldering backache prominent at rest and at night. Fever and active infection elsewhere (including intrathoracic) are inconstant features; weight loss and a positive skin test are more reliable.

Metastatic tumors can compromise spine stability or encroach on roots or structures within the canal; both are indications for emergent radiation therapy and/or, because of increasing success, surgical extirpation and stabilization. There are also primary neoplasms of the osseous canal (2). These include several benign neoplasms that occur generally in younger decades: eosinophilic granulomas, hemangiomas, aneurysmal bone cysts, osteoid osteomas, and mesenchymal tumors such as osteochondromas and chondromyxoid fibromas. Primary malignant neoplasms of the osseous canal span the entire age range: osteogenic sarcomas, chondrosarcomas, chordomas, lymphomas, and, in the elderly, plasmacytomas. Persistent pain, nocturnal accentuation of pain, and restriction in spine mobility are common features of the primary neoplasms, and, for that matter, are common features of metastatic tumor or infection.

Primary tumors, albeit rarely, do occur within the canal as well. Extradural tumors present with pain, often at rest and often radicular, with less prominent a mechanical component. Intradural tumors are more insidious; pain is less localizing and neurologic signs are more prominent. Cauda equina tumors present as poorly localizing low back pain, often and peculiarly causing the patient to sit in a chair rather than choose recumbency, when not pacing the floor at night. Neurologic compromise from any destructive process of the cauda equina places sphincter control at risk and can cause saddle anesthesia.

These are the settings where axial imaging is to be pursued. Plane radiographs are limited in sensitivity; one is seeking bony destruction, not degenerative changes. Metastatic tumors have some predilection for the posterior elements, so one should focus on pedicle structure (Fig. 7.1). Infection targets the disc space and can sweep across the interspace, destroying juxtaposed endplates (Fig. 7.2). Neoplasia, with the exception of lymphoma and myeloma, generally spares the disc space. The primary osseous neoplasms are often discernible on plane films as destructive lesions; lesions within the canal are seldom apparent. Scintiscanning [particularly if sensitivity is enhanced by the single photon emission computed tomography (SPECT) technique] has nearly perfect sensitivity for any of the processes that impinge on bony structures. Both computed tomography and magnetic resonance imaging approach this sensitivity and have great specificity for all infectious and neoplastic processes of the axial skeleton. Furthermore, CT-guided needle biopsy is usually feasible, safe, and diagnostic.

The Seronegative Spondyloarthropathies

A century has passed since the description of ankylosing spondylitis by Bechterow and by Pierre Marie and Strumpell (3). But the concept that this was a clinical entity and not just a form of rheumatoid arthritis yielded slowly to a

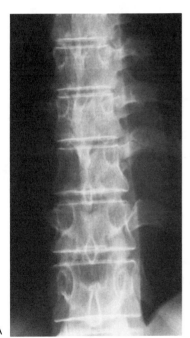
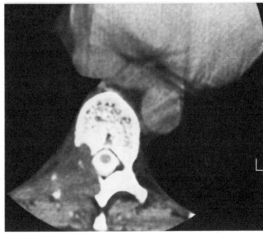

A   B

FIG. 7.1. Radiograph of the spine demonstrating bony metastases. Metastases have a predilection for pedicles. With the exception of multiple myeloma and lymphoma, metastases spare the disc.

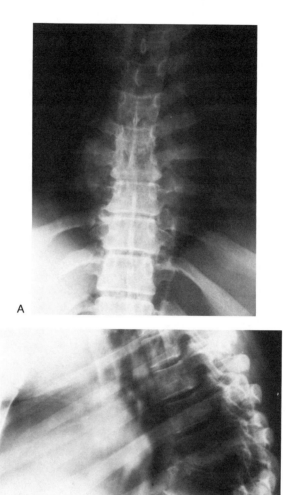

A

B

FIG. 7.2. Imaging studies of septic discitis.

persuasive body of clinical observation and attained general recognition in the United States only in the 1960s (4). The clinical proponents were clearly prescient; any doubt faded when it was demonstrated that ankylosing spondylitis and its clinically related diseases, the seronegative spondyloarthropathies, were in linkage disequilibrium with the Type 1 human histocompatibility antigen, HLA-B27. Since only the cluster of symptoms and signs recognized as the seronegative spondyloarthropathies is associated with this particular gene and its product, the distinction from all other rheumatic diseases is incontrovertible.

The common denominators of this spectrum of illness are encompassed in the diagnostic rubric, seronegative spondyloarthropathies. First, these patients have a chronic inflammatory rheumatic disease with no consistent serologic markers; for example, both rheumatoid factor and antinuclear antibodies are undetected by routine testing. More germane to our considerations, these patients have in common some degree of inflammatory destructive disease of the joints of the spine, a spondyloarthropathy. The involvement always targets the sacroiliac joints, first the more caudal diarthrodial portion with its hyaline cartilage and later the rostral fibrous joint. Early on there is erosion manifest

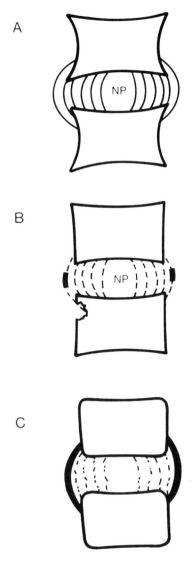

FIG. 7.3. The pathogenesis of the discal enthesopathy associated with the seronegative spondyloarthropathies. **A:** In the normal disc, the outer fibers of the annulus fibrosus insert into the body of the vertebra as much as a third of the distance from the endplate. Thus, the superior and inferior thirds of the outer wall of the body is an enthesis. *NP*, nucleus pulposus. The earliest inflammation in the spondyloarthropathies is at this enthesis. Round cells are present, and resorption may be prominent. **B:** On occasion, resorption is so prominent as to be discernible on plane radiographs. The earliest calcification in the outer annulus is localized at mid-disc (*heavy black line*). This pattern is typical of classic ankylosing spondylitis and of spondyloarthropathy associated with inflammatory bowel disease. The disc that is involved earliest is usually T12-L1, and symmetric involvement spreads rostrally and caudally. The calcification associated with the spondyloarthropathy associated with Reiter's disease or psoriasis is more prominent at the enthesis, is less symmetric, and tends to ascend the lumbar spine. **C:** The end-stage regardless of the pattern. Calcification sweeps across the outer annulus from enthesis to enthesis. These calcified fibers are termed *syndesmophytes*. The final stage is a bamboo spine.

radiographically as "pseudo-widening" of the joints. Later there is ankylosis. The disease also targets the discs in a fashion that is specific for this spectrum of disease. The earliest inflammation and structural alteration is at the site of insertion of the outer fibers of the annulus fibrosus into the vertebral body (Fig. 7.3). Wherever collagen fibers (from a disc, joint capsule, or tendon) anchor in bone, the fibers are called *Sharpey's fibers* and the anatomic site of anchorage an *enthesis*. For this reason, much of the musculoskeletal pathoanatomy of the seronegative spondyloarthropathies has been termed *enthesopathy*, whether it occurs in the spine or elsewhere. For example, the external aspect of the pelvis is covered with entheses; spondyloarthropathies can lead to inflammatory reactions of the periosteum manifest radiographically as "whiskering."

The illness associated with this spondyloarthropathy is backache. However, the patient's complaint is distinctive from the illness afflicting most patients with regional low back pain. Table 7.1 lists the five features of the backache of spondyloarthropathy that distinguish it from regional backache in the context of a diagnostic evaluation in one referral practice (5). The utility of these putative discriminators depends on the setting in which they are applied. After all, the prevalence of regional backache is so enormous that atypical presentations that mimic inflammatory spondyloarthropathy may well overwhelm typical presentations of spondyloarthropathy (6). The questions offer little outside the referral practice in case identification but are useful in the diagnostic evaluation of the person who has chosen to be a patient with backache. Also useful is a quest for associated extraspinal manifestations of the seronegative spondyloarthropathies, which, when present, greatly enhance diagnostic certainty. Several of these are listed in Table 7.2. It is clear from this list that the seronegative spondyloarthropathies include ankylosing spondylitis, Reiter's syndrome, and the reactive arthritides, the spondylitis associated with inflammatory bowel disease and with psoriasis. Whether these are a spectrum of a single disease or the spondyloarthropathy is a complicating feature in genetically susceptible sufferers with different diseases is not established.

Diagnostic certainty requires radiographic documentation of sacroiliitis with or without an enthesopathy. Since the spondyloarthropathies can be symptomatic for decades without radiographic change, particularly in women, the diagnosis is often but a clinical postulate. When full blown, there is little doubt (Fig. 7.4). But when there are no radiographic stigmata, one is left with a clinical

TABLE 7.1. *Features of the illness associated with the seronegative spondyloarthropathies that are unusual in regional low back pain*

The episodes of low back pain commence before age 40.
The episodes are insidious in onset.
The episodes persist for more than 3 months.
Low back stiffness is prominent on arising.
Low back stiffness and pain improve with exercise.

TABLE 7.2. Extraspinal manifestations of the
seronegative spondyloarthropathies

Rhizomelic (large central joint) inflammatory oligoarthritis
  targeting hips, knees, shoulders, and sternomanubrial
  joint
Iritis
Inflammatory bowel disease with colonic involvement
Psoriasis including pustular psoriasis
Aortic valve insufficiency
Nongonococcal urethritis in a man
Lower extremity enthesopathy manifest as heel pain and
  inflammatory spur formation
More impressive and dramatic palliative response to
  nonsteroidal antiinflammatory drugs

hypothesis. Even tissue typing offers little assistance. After all, the vast majority of people with HLA-B27 are spared a spondyloarthopathy, and a significant minority of patients with spondyloarthropathy (ranging from 5% to 10% of patients with classic ankylosing spondylitis to 40% of patients with Reiter's syndrome) lack this haplotype. Tissue typing is useless as a screening tool and marginal as a diagnostic aid.

As a result of the honing of the clinical definition of the spondyloarthropa-

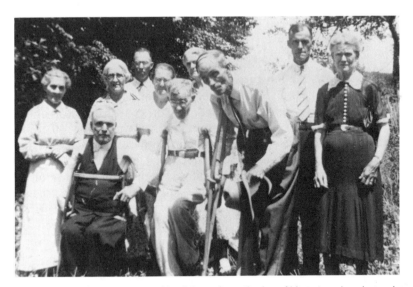

FIG. 7.4. A patient of mine gave me this picture of a gathering of his paternal uncles and aunts. They are all deceased. However, at the time of this picture they were residing in the family seat, a hamlet in West Virginia. The three elderly gentlemen, all brothers, in the front have obvious ankylosing spondylitis. When Uncle Jim realized that he would suffer a similar process of spinal deformation as his other brother, he strapped himself into a chair and fused in a posture compatible with his vocation as a cobbler. My patient, by the way, has rheumatoid arthritis.

thies and the existence of an associated genotype, much has been learned of the epidemiology of this spectrum of disease. HLA-B27 is found in some 8% of American whites; it is found in nearly 90% of American whites with classic Marie-Strumpell ankylosing spondylitis. But not all with the B27 histocompatibility antigen are afflicted, only about 1%. So, for American whites, the prevalence of ankylosing spondylitis is approximately 0.1%. Nearly all of these people bear the HLA-B27 tissue type. In populations where the prevalence of B27 is higher, so is the prevalence of ankylosing spondylitis. For example, some 50% of Haida Indians in the Pacific Northwest are positive for B27 and a correspondingly high prevalence of ankylosing spondylitis is observed, about 6%. Conversely, the antigen is infrequent in American blacks, only 2%, and the disease prevalence is closer to 0.01%. The traditional teaching is that ankylosing spondylitis is far more likely to afflict men, with sex ratios as high as 10:1. However, that has not held up in systematic studies, some of which suggest more equal prevalence between sexes, particularly in the spondyloarthropathies other than classic ankylosing spondylitis. Ankylosing spondylitis occurs in childhood, where it usually presents in boys as knee oligoarthritis; back pain is not a prominent feature. Obviously, the clinician faced with a patient with back pain should remain vigilant in terms of this diagnosis. Its prognosis and management are different from those for regional low back pain.

REGIONAL LOW BACK PAIN WITHOUT RADICULOPATHY

Diagnosis

Low back pain is the most frequent musculoskeletal predicament and the most frequent regional musculoskeletal illness at all ages and in all strata of the population. The treating physician must make the generic diagnosis of regional musculoskeletal low back pain—and must do so by *exclusion* of other illnesses that present with low back pain. Any attempt to make a primary diagnosis to define the cause of a particular episode of regional low back pain will succumb to stochastic realities. Some physical findings, such as spinal range of motion and distraction, can be rendered reliable with effort (7). Most "signs" that involve prodding and probing the low back are unreliable. And all signs, even diminished range of motion and lumbosacral list (8), are nonspecific in the setting of regional low back pain. Imaging techniques have proven even more disappointing. Some, such as thermography, are simply worthless (9). Other contemporary imaging techniques can provide marvelous, seductively detailed anatomic definition that, in the adult, offers nothing for the differential diagnosis of regional low back pain. The likelihood of demonstrating abnormality increases with age to become ubiquitous in the later decades. However, the specificity of any degenerative finding decreases with age so that the pathoanatomic insights are rendered clinically useless. This statement pertains to plane radiographs, CT (10), and MR imaging (11). In other words, any degenerative image found in a population with regional low back illness can be found in a pain-free population matched for all other parameters with sufficient likelihood to render pathogenetic inferences effete. An equally cogent deduction is that any degenerative change discerned does not alter the likelihood of remission of the symptom of low back pain. Finally, any degenerative change discerned will persist even after the symptoms have subsided. Imaging for regional low back pain is worse than useless. It is counterproductive both in time and in one's ability to promote in the patient a perception that regional low back pain is an intermittent and remittent illness and not a reflection of a "bad back."

Promulgating this perception of healing should color the entire interaction with the patient. It is to be the logical conclusion of the process of history and of physical examination. In the history little is dissuasive of this conclusion, aside from the features discussed above that pertain to systemic disease. The physical examination is useful only in that one can be reassured regarding major neurologic compromise and relevant underlying diseases such as pelvic or prostatic pathologic conditions. Findings on physical examination or on imaging examinations cannot be used to support inferences regarding the pathogenesis of the regional low back pain. Regardless of all of this uncertainty, prognostic inferences can be drawn and counseling regarding the extensive menu of therapeutic alternatives can be offered, taking advantage of a voluminous experimental literature. The initial interview and examination allow one to make a presumptive diagnosis of regional back pain and thereby to disabuse the patient of any evil implication of all the uncertainties. It is essential that the patient appreciate the concept of a diagnosis of exclusion and the need to avoid testing where the yield of meaningful information is vanishingly low. If the patient does not arrive at such an understanding at the first evaluation, he or she will leave the office participating in a diagnostic evaluation that develops a life of its own; the patient will focus on every nuance of the illness as meaningful and will fall prey to any and all who offer the promise of greater certainty or even empirical therapy. Such a fate is a match for "defensive medicine" in rendering the patient more ill.

Therapy

The mainstay of therapy for the acute backache is to demedicalize the event. In all likelihood, the process is self-limited; some 80% of sufferers are well or nearly so in 2 wk and at least 90% are well at 2 mo. Furthermore, although there is considerable likelihood of recurrence, nearly all are left no worse for wear. Finally, with certain exceptions in both directions, the natural history cannot be meaningfully perturbed by interventions. The upshot is that the patient should be made to commandeer this experience, to use his or her own best judgment. Patients should never be rendered so anxious, if not fearful, that they crave "the diagnosis" and then "the cure," so as to become accepting of any remedy proffered by the enormous enterprise waiting to help. Educating patients, dissuading patients from this traditional algorithm, is a challenging yet critical undertaking (12); most who choose to be patients with backache bring to the medical interaction presuppositions and expectations that initiate this algorithm. Therefore, they must be disabused.

Nearly all available interventions have been subjected to clinical trials of some description. I have cataloged over 150 randomized controlled trials. Few of these trials escape critical review unscathed; many are simply uninterpretable. Nonetheless, there is more than enough information to place most of the therapeutic options for acute low back pain into perspective (13,14).

Rest

Therapeutic rest was a mainstay for many illnesses in the early decades of this century. For most conditions, it has been discarded. It can be discarded as well for acute low back pain. Certainly, recumbency unloads the lumbosacral spine, but only if one is fully recumbent. One is better off standing, or sitting erect, than propping up in bed. No wonder nearly all of us are noncompliant with enforced bed rest. Besides, it has not been possible to demonstrate enhanced healing rates with prescribed bed rest—only increased absenteeism from work. Suggesting postures to avoid, such as anterior sitting (e.g., slouching forward over one's desk), is far more sensible than proscribing motion or function.

Pharmacologic Agents

There are over a dozen controlled trials incorporating various analgesics, nonsteroidal antiinflammatory agents, benzodiazepines, colchicine, and narcotics. The agents are more consistent and impressive in their toxicities than in differential benefit. Rather than risk a cloudy sensorium, obstipation, or the implication that the illness is of sufficient severity to warrant desperate medicines, the case is easily made for empathy, reassurance, psychologic support, and a mild analgesic such as acetaminophen along with warm showers. Bathing, regardless of the liquid or its turbulence, can be limited by the biomechanical challenge of entering or leaving the tub with a backache. Forewarn the patient.

Exercises

There are advocates for flexing. There are advocates for extending. There are advocates for isotonic exercises and advocates for combinations. Each has a theory, each is offered with zeal, and each has a following. Furthermore, several regimens are supported by trials showing a degree of benefit. However, there are two trials demonstrating harm from exercise regimens for acute low back pain. For that reason, an easily defensible approach is to suggest exercises ad lib, to suggest postures to avoid, and to suggest that returning to full function, even to work, is to be encouraged as early as possible, even before complete remission has supervened.

Physical Modalities

Most of the menu of physical modalities has escaped critical testing. Many physical treatments are so dependent on human interactions that controlled trials are inherently flawed (15). Some of the various forms of needling are carried along by dint of precedent (see Chapter 5). As mentioned in Chapter 2, benefit from spinal manipulation is demonstrable (Fig. 7.5) but only for one subset of uncomplicated low back pain—younger individuals hurting for at least 2 wk but no more than 4 wk—and even then the benefit is modest at best (16). Another newer modality, the use of a transcutaneous electrical nerve stimulation (TENS) unit, performed poorly in one trial for chronic low back pain (17) but has not been adequately studied for acute low back pain. Various forms of traction have been subjected to trials, most of which are difficult to interpret because of lack of definition of the quality of illness suffered by the subjects or lack of reliability or validity of the outcome measures. In overview, traction is unimpressive if not useless, beyond enforcing bed rest and rendering the patient totally passive and nonfunctional. Finally, attempts to provide mechanical support by applying corsets to reduce the load on the spine offer nothing more than false security and may encourage dependency in patients with chronic pain. Leather belts of various kinds are de rigueur for body builders and are finding their way into industry for back pain prophylaxis, with few substantive supporting data (18).

Structured Programs of Education and Therapy

As already discussed, acute low back pain challenges the resources of all providers of health care. It would make sense to be proactive—offering to all sufferers at the initiation of the illness ready access to advice and conservative interventions. In the industrial setting, where clinical improvement can be measured in terms of time lost from work, such programs have been shown to be useful. In the setting of an HMO, symptomatic benefit has proven elusive.

Surgery and Related Invasiveness

All forms of surgical intervention have nothing to offer the patient with acute low back pain! The only attempt to test the surgical inference in something

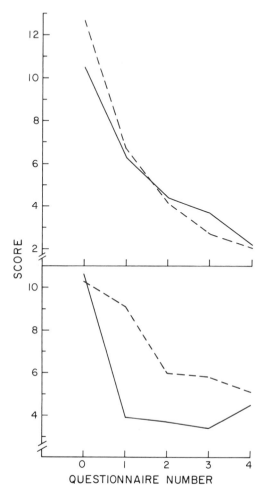

FIG. 7.5. The University of North Carolina Trial of Spinal Manipulation. These plots show the mean scores on a questionnaire that quantified the magnitude of illness from acute low back pain experienced by the subjects in the University of North Carolina study of spinal manipulation. The questionnaire was administered just before entry into the study and at the time of telephone follow-up every 3 (±1) days after treatment. *Broken lines,* results for subjects randomized to be treated by mobilization; *solid lines,* those randomized to be treated by spinal manipulation employing a single long lever-arm high-velocity technique. All four groups were indistinguishable at entry and at 2 wk after treatment. **Top:** Results for the stratum wherein all subjects had suffered backache for less than 2 wk at the time of entry into the protocol. **Bottom:** The stratum for subjects that had suffered for 2 to 4 wk. Treatment effect was only discernible in the latter stratum ($p = 0.009$). In that stratum, those who underwent manipulation achieved a 50% reduction in score more rapidly than did those who underwent mobilization, although the latter caught up by 2 wk. (From ref. 37, with permission.)

approaching a scientific fashion was undertaken by Weber (19) in Oslo. There is no demonstrable benefit of surgery regardless of the chronicity of low back pain. In fact, there is every reason to believe that surgery in this setting is worse than injudicious.

The same assertion may pertain to various forms of injection therapy. Three forms of injection therapy are in common use in the United States: chemonucleolysis, corticosteroid injection into the extradural space or into the facet joint.

The saga of chemonucleolysis is instructive. As is true of nearly every remedy in clinical use since the beginning of the 18th century, chemonucleolysis is offered as rational therapy. It has long been known that the nucleus pulposus is a proteoglycan gel with little fibrous protein and that the annulus fibrosus is principally collagen. It has also long been held that extrusion of the nucleus pulposus is a leading, if not the leading cause of acute back pain with or without radiculopathy. Chymopapain is a proteolytic enzyme extracted from *Carica papaya* with no substrate specificity for collagen. It follows that if chymopapain is injected into the nucleus pulposus it will solubilize the nucleus without damaging the annulus. It further follows that, since such chemonucleolysis removes extruding nuclear material, it should diminish backache and obviate the need for surgery. The theory was put into practice in the early 1960s; by the early 1970s chymopapain had been administered to tens of thousands of sufferers. In 1976, a controlled trial was reported by the neurosurgical service at Walter Reed Army Medical Center (20); this trial was elegant in design and impressive in results. The investigators randomized 66 men with regional back pain that was unremittent after 3 wk of conservative therapy and associated with myelographic evidence of a lumbar disc herniation to receive intradiscal chymopapain or placebo. The difference in improvement at 2 mo was not significant: 58% versus 49%, respectively. However, there were believers in the efficacy of chemonucleolysis both within the profession and among the sufferers who would not sit still when the Food and Drug Administration called a halt to further investigation of the technique. New protocols were written and trials with different designs were performed in the United States and elsewhere, leading to approval of chemonucleolysis with chymopapain in 1982 (21). The zeal has diminished since the patina of controversy has been removed. In fact, there remains little general enthusiasm. Even the lack of enthusiasm is rationalized by suggesting that dissolution of the nucleus is a form of premature aging to be avoided.

The two other schools of injection therapy circumvent monitoring of risk/benefit by the FDA because they employ a pharmaceutical that is widely available for a myriad of uses, injectable corticosteroid preparations. Both approaches are rationalized by suggesting that the acute event causing backache involves a focus of inflamed tissue. One solution is to inject corticosteroids into the extradural space. There are even a couple of randomized controlled trials of injection therapy. Although suggesting some benefit (22,23), these trials hardly justify wide use of the procedure, repeat injections, or injections in the setting of chronic pain or failed surgery.

There is another school of therapeutic enthusiasm justified because these clinicians are convinced that they can distinguish in which patients a diseased facet joint is responsible for backache. Making this diagnosis, "the lumbar facet syndrome," is an exercise in conviction; systematic studies suggest that all of the putatively specific symptoms and signs are nonspecific. Nonetheless, there are many clinicians who inject corticosteroids into one or another facet joint in the quest for palliation. Well-designed studies of this procedure fail to demonstrate benefit with sufficient power, and the intervention should be relegated to history (24).

With such precedents, it is disquieting at best that "established" yet unproven surgical interventions are supported. It is unconscionable that surgical inventiveness is tolerated in the clinical arena without the scientific support required for a pharmaceutical. How can we stand by when tens of thousands of Americans undergo microdiscectomy or automated percutaneous lumbar discectomy each year when only the zeal of the operator is supportive of benefit, and even then not of all operators (25). A recent randomized multicenter study comparing automated percutaneous nucleolysis with chemonucleolysis performed in Paris is telling. Percutaneous nucleotomy doesn't even approach the level of "benefit" seen with chemonucleolysis (Prof. M. Revel, *personal communication, 1992*). The American surgical community seems unwilling to police itself; legislative reform is long overdue.

In overview, the natural history of acute low back pain is so benign that it is probably easier to confound the illness with interventions than to palliate. However, the universe that is suffering is immense; even the few percent with persistent illness beyond 10 wk represents sizable populations of patients with subacute low back pain and with chronic low back pain. If these individuals were managed thoughtfully during the early months of illness, "chronicity" should have only a temporal connotation. Their illness should try their patience but not perturb their personalities nor their station in life. Rheumatologists are comfortable in promulgating the most health possible through flares of other chronic intermittent and remittent rheumatic diseases; why not low back pain as well? Besides, all of the assertions regarding the management of acute low back pain listed above pertain to subacute and chronic low back pain as well (see Section III). This even holds for surgery that, in spite of all the marketing, has never been shown to benefit any patient with low back pain. In fact, most surgical interventions for low back pain have never been subjected to any systematic assessment, and those that have, such as laminectomy with or without fusion, have fared poorly.

NECK PAIN

A "pain in the neck" rivals low back pain in incidence and prevalence. However, a "pain in the neck" is less likely to cause one to seek medical attention.

For regional musculoskeletal illness of the neck, medical consultation is sought if the pain is perceived as too intense, too prolonged, or associated with disability, such as difficulty seeing over one's shoulder when driving a car in reverse. The quality of the discomfort is what one would expect for regional musculo-skeletal illness elsewhere: use-associated pain, restriction in motion, relief with unloading, abruptness of onset. Associated neurologic or systemic symptoms raise the specter of other causes, as is the case for low back pain. Likewise, cervical pain can herald visceral catastrophe, particularly cardiovascular catastrophe. Neck pain can be an anginal equivalent, a manifestation of temporal arteritis, or a classic presentation for aortic dissection; in these instances range of motion is neither compromised nor exacerbative and the discomfort is likely to present more in the anterior neck and throat. Furthermore, neck pain becomes as confounded an illness as low back pain if it is associated with work incapacity.

Although it bears little on the clinical algorithm for regional neck pain, cervical anatomy has features that bear on consideration of other cervical syndromes. The cervical roots exit nearly immediately and emerge essentially surrounded by the fibrous capsules contributed by uncovertebral, facet, and disc joints. The joints of Luschka or uncovertebral joints are small diarthrodial joints located on hook-like projections of the posterolateral margin of the bodies of cervical vertebrae contributing to all cervical foramina except those of the first two roots. The roots are covered by a sheath of dura mater as they course to the foramen; the dura then forms the dentate ligaments, which anchor the cord near the posterior longitudinal ligament (Fig. 7.6). More than any other segment, the normal cervical cord nearly fills the canal and is tethered. In flexion the normal cord is stretched as much as 2 cm. Most rotation of the neck occurs at the craniocervical junction; most flexion/extension at C5-6. The intervertebral discs normally compose a third of the length of the cervical spine, which explains the extraordinary pliancy of this segment. Even so, these discs are small; the largest is C6-7 which approaches a total volume of 1.5 ml and a nucleus pulposus volume of 0.25 ml. Neck motion reflects the extensibility of the discs and the impressive range of the facet joints, which easily override (particularly during extension) and thereby diminish the area of the neural foramen.

Degenerative changes of any portion of the vertebral column are lumped under the rubric "spondylosis." Cervical spondylosis involves the ligaments lining the canal and the structures that define the neural foramen: the pedicles, the disc, the endplates, the joints of Luschka, and the apophyseal or facet joints. Spondylosis is common, involves all of these structures, and becomes ubiquitous in the later decades. It is easily demonstrated by all imaging techniques and is reflected in progressive restriction in range of motion. As a result, the specificity of all forms of cervical spondylosis for a particular episode of regional neck pain is so low as to render attempts at specific diagnosis futile; aggressive imaging is meaningless at best. Exuberant cervical osteophytosis is said to occasionally cause dysphagia. However, exuberant osteophytosis and calcification of

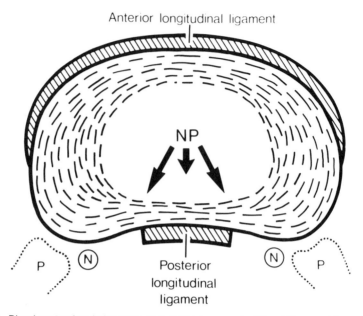

Anterior longitudinal ligament

NP

P   (N)   Posterior   (N)   P
longitudinal
ligament

Fig 7.6. Discal anatomic relationships. The spinal nerve roots (*N*) exit the canal through a fora-men that is formed by several discrete structures: the posterolateral annulus fibrosus, the pedi-cles (*P*), and the apophyseal or facet joint capsule. Herniation of the nucleus pulposus (*NP*) is common and generally asymptomatic. It is a candidate for one cause of acute and chronic regional low back pain. It is also a candidate for one cause of radiculopathy. In this instance the gelatinous material of the nucleus extrudes in a posterolateral vector, somehow interfering with root function or structure. The pathogenesis of radiculopathy must be far more complex than simply discal extrusion to account for the great number of asymptomatic herniations and the fact that even those that are symptomatic have a great tendency to remit. Occasionally, the vector of NP extrusion is posterior, thereby affecting the posterior longitudinal ligament. If the process is extreme, the bulging material can impinge upon the cord in the cervical spine or the cauda equina in the lumbar spine. The former can result in myelopathy, and the latter in cauda equina syn-drome.

spinal ligaments are ubiquitous in the elderly so that attributing any symptoms to such changes is a tenuous exercise.

One pattern of spondylosis is sufficiently distinctive and radiographically dramatic as to warrant special recognition. Diffuse idiopathic skeletal hyperos-tosis (DISH) is also called ankylosing hyperostosis or Forestier/Rotes-Querol disease and is apparent on spine radiographs in as many as 10% of the elderly. One sees flowing calcification and ossification along the anterolateral aspect of at least four contiguous vertebral bodies. As opposed to the more usual pattern of spondylosis, disc height is relatively normal (Fig. 7.7). Furthermore, as op-posed to the inflammatory spondyloarthropathies, there is no sacroiliitis or apophyseal joint ankylosis. The radiographic appearance can be striking; in the dorsal spine the changes are characteristically contralateral to the heart (Fig. 7.8). The involvement of the spine is associated with osteophytes and ligamen-

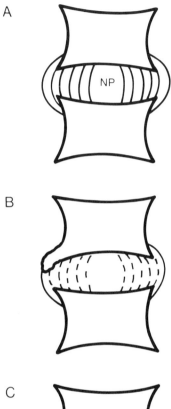

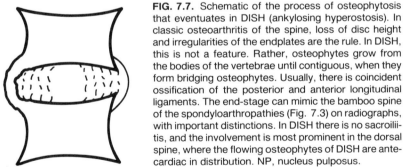

FIG. 7.7. Schematic of the process of osteophytosis that eventuates in DISH (ankylosing hyperostosis). In classic osteoarthritis of the spine, loss of disc height and irregularities of the endplates are the rule. In DISH, this is not a feature. Rather, osteophytes grow from the bodies of the vertebrae until contiguous, when they form bridging osteophytes. Usually, there is coincident ossification of the posterior and anterior longitudinal ligaments. The end-stage can mimic the bamboo spine of the spondyloarthropathies (Fig. 7.3) on radiographs, with important distinctions. In DISH there is no sacroiliitis, and the involvement is most prominent in the dorsal spine, where the flowing osteophytes of DISH are antecardiac in distribution. NP, nucleus pulposus.

tous calcifications elsewhere: calcification of the sacrotuberous and iliolumbar ligaments in the pelvis, paraacetabular bony outgrowths, and olecranon, calcaneal, and patellar hyperostoses. Some 15% of individuals over 65 yr old manifest DISH. As dramatic as these radiographic and pathologic changes may be, it is not clear that they predispose the elderly to any special morbidity (26).

Neck pain rarely localizes just to the neck. To the contrary, peculiar radiations to the shoulder, suboccipital, and interscapular regions are common and

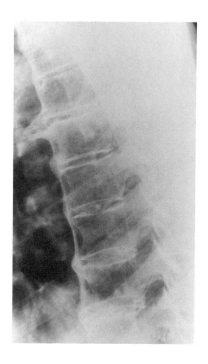

FIG. 7.8. Radiograph of the dorsal spine in ankylosing hyperostosis (DISH). The sweeping, bridging osteophytes are prominent. Interestingly, they are usually antecardiac in distribution.

often overshadow the pain in the neck itself. This panoply of discomfort must reflect the complex and redundant neuroanatomy of the cervical spine. Even the vertebral arteries are susceptible to impingement and compromise from various osteophytes as they traverse their bony foramina, resulting in the rare but distinctive "vertebral artery syndrome": dizziness, tinnitus, occasional retroorbital headaches, and fleeting blurring of vision associated with neck motion. Finally, there are the torticollis or wry neck syndromes. Usually, this is associated with pain and reflects guarded motion in the setting of regional musculoskeletal disease. However, painless torticollis has been observed in all age groups, mimicking the movement disorder so typical of phenothiazine toxicity. The etiology is debated among those advocating pharmacologic intervention for a neuromuscular disease and others arguing for a psychiatric disorder.

A discussion of the management of neck pain is on far shakier ground than one on the management of low back pain because of a relative dearth of clinical investigation. Furthermore, extrapolating from the literature on low back pain is unappealing. Would one be comfortable relying on the literature about the hand in managing illness of the foot? Nonetheless, it is clear that the natural history of acute neck pain is similar to that of acute backache; at least 80% are well within a month without residua. The mainstays of therapy are reassurance and support, including the promulgation of a decision-making role for the patient. Most patients with cervical pain will spontaneously posture in slight forward flexion and resist deviation in any plane, thereby placing the least stress on cervical structures while maintaining erect posture. This is to be encouraged; a soft cervical collar provides no more than a reminder at the cost of considerable nuisance. In a multicenter British trial, about 75% of all subjects were well or nearly so in a month regardless of exposure to physical modalities such as a collar or traction or to placebo events. It has not been possible to demonstrate benefit from spinal manipulation for neck pain—and here there is a risk of doing considerable violence to the neural structures. The experience with surgery for neck pain is at least as disappointing as for low back pain; in most series (none of which was controlled), some 50% of patients were no better off for the experience.

RADICULOPATHY

Given the architecture of neural foramina and the likelihood of spondylotic changes in the anatomic components, it is remarkable that all of us do not suffer radiculopathies. It is even more remarkable that most radiculopathies are intermittent and remittent illnesses, implying that some component(s) of the spondylotic process is reversible. Yet, in contradistinction to regional spine pain, not all of us will suffer a radiculopathy. For those of us who do, as with regional spine pain our course is likely to be benign. There are two major reasons for considering radiculopathy as a separate clinical issue: one benefits the physician and the other the patient. For the physician, there is the intellectual satisfaction of "localization"; we may not be able to define the pathophysiology but at least we know its location with some reliability. For the patient, radiculopathy portends peripheral damage, provokes a special anxiety since the experience of referred pain appears to defy reason, and offers some specific therapeutic options.

Localization

Table 7.3 presents the traditional symptoms and signs associated with compromise of each cervical root. Table 7.4 does likewise for the lumbar radiculopathies. The categorization is clinically useful but far from completely valid or reliable. Generalization of symptoms, and even signs, beyond a single root is not that unusual and probably reflects some multiplicity of innervation peripherally and dispersion of input at the level of the cord. In the case of cervical radiculopathies, even more than lumbar, the pain tends to be paraspinal while the paresthesias tend to be distal in the distribution noted in Table 7.1. Furthermore, some presentations are confounded by coincidental neuropathies. For example, nearly 10% of the elderly lack at least one Achilles' reflex, further compromising the specificity of this neurologic sign for radiculopathy. Likewise, it is thought that a coincident cervical radiculopathy can render subclini-

TABLE 7.3. Signs and symptoms of cervical radiculopathies

Root	Pain and numbness	Sensory loss	Motor loss	Reflex loss
C-3	Occipital region	Occiput	None	None
C-4	Back of neck	Back of neck	None	None
C-5	Neck to outer shoulder and arm	Over shoulder	Deltoid	Biceps supinator
C-6	Outer arm to thumb and index fingers	Thumb and index fingers	Biceps (triceps) and wrist extensors	Triceps supinator, biceps
C-7	Outer arm to middle finger	Index and middle fingers	Triceps	Triceps
C-8	Inner arm to fourth and fifth fingers	Fourth and fifth fingers	Intrinsics and extrinsics	None

cal entrapment neuropathies overt; the so-called "double crush" syndrome is an experimental reality but has more clinical advocacy than is justified by supporting clinical data.

Nonetheless, localizing information is forthcoming from careful elicitation of symptoms, inspection to note focal atrophy as well as mobility, muscle and reflex testing, and discernment of sensory deficits. For lumbar radiculopathies, there are "tension signs" as well. For cervical radiculopathies, there are advocates of compression and distraction tests that have been shown to correlate with myelographically demonstrable root compression but are low in sensitivity (27) and difficult to perform reliably. The history can be structured and rendered more reliable by the use of pain diagrams and questionnaires. All signs can be rendered more reliable if examinations are standardized and practiced.

TABLE 7.4. Signs and symptoms of lumbar radiculopathy

Root	Pain and numbness	Sensory loss	Motor loss	Reflex loss
L-4	Anterior thigh and medial leg	Medial leg to medial malleolus	Anterior tibialis	Patellar
L-5	Lateral leg and dorsum of the foot	Lateral leg and dorsum of the foot	Extensor hallucis longus	Posterior tibial
S-1	Lateral foot	Lateral foot	Peroneus longus and brevis	Achilles reflex

However, this additional effort is more appropriate for clinical investigation than it is useful in clinical practice.

Tension or stretch signs can be elicited in the lower extremity and are probably more sensitive to radiculopathy than are the signs elaborated in Table 7.4. Straight leg raising takes up the slack on the lower lumbar roots that contribute to the sciatic nerve; by 30°, the nerve is taut. The normal nerve can withstand further flexion at the hip with the knee extended. Resistance to such movement is the traditional Lasègue's sign for sciatica. Many variations on this theme have proponents. There are even those who are convinced that the "crossed straight leg raising test" is more specific for sciatica caused by discal protrusion. Here, elevating the asymptomatic leg provokes discomfort in the symptomatic leg. The specificity of this test has not been established; its sensitivity is low. The other commonly used stretch test is the femoral stretch, accomplished by flexing the knee with the patient prone. This tests for compromise in the roots contributing to the femoral nerve.

The Therapeutic Implications of Radiculopathy

Aside from the intellectual satisfaction the diagnostician derives from some sense of "localization," the exercise offers benefit to the patient. First, there is something baffling and anxiety provoking about the experience of referred pain. Localization allows the physician an opportunity for a palliative explanation of the illness. Localization, unfortunately, does not alter therapeutic considerations from those that pertain to neck and low back pain without radiculopathy. The one exception is the surgical option. If the radiculopathy is sufficiently severe, motor compromise becomes an issue. Defining a threshold for surgical intervention is not that straightforward. The L5-S1 radiculopathy can progress from leg pain to loss of Achilles reflex to compromised strength at the forefoot or ankle. The loss of the reflex has no functional implications. However, a weak distal leg does. But how "weak" does it have to be before surgery is attempted? Surgery, even in this setting, is not predictably successful, and spontaneous remission remains a likelihood. The decision is made at the bedside with input from all parties involved, including the patient. With the far less frequent L3-4 radiculopathy, quadriceps power can be at risk, with even more potential for functional compromise. Since the experience with this radiculopathy is limited, the tendency is to choose the surgical option more readily. Surgical success, even in this setting, is too often elusive, which calls into question the appropriateness of the procedures currently in vogue or the pathophysiology that underlies their design.

There is some evidence, albeit far from cogent (28), that surgery for a lumbar radiculopathy (i.e., for the leg pain that is sciatica) may afford the patient a higher likelihood of relief than does conservative management (19), even in the absence of leg weakness. However, this benefit has not been demonstrable for

TABLE 7.5. *Results of the Weber study at 1 year*

Outcome	Conservative			Operative		
	Persist	Operate	Total	Operate	Refuse	Total
Good	16	8	24	39	0	39
Fair	24	4	28	15	1	16
Poor	9	4	13	5	0	5
Bad	0	1	1	0	0	0
Total	49	17	66	59	1	60

From Weber, ref. 19.
In this study 126 patients with sciatica (25 to 55 years old) were randomized after 2 weeks of hospitalization to receive conservative management or surgical intervention.

acute illness (less than 6 wk) or for chronic illness (greater than 6 mo). Furthermore, the benefit is demonstrable at 6 mo, after which the patients who were treated conservatively merge with those who submitted to surgery in terms of all functional and symptomatic outcomes. As is apparent from Table 7.5, at 1 yr little was gained from the surgical option. Also apparent from Table 7.5 are the shortcomings of even this, the principal trial of surgery for regional back pain published to date: outcomes are measured subjectively, criteria for entry and crossover are not defined, and numbers are too small to detect any but a major effect. However, no major effect is apparent. The small benefit noted at 6 mo from surgical intervention for subacute sciatica (i.e., sciatica that has lasted for 6 wk) is underwhelming in magnitude at 6 mo and undetectable at 1 yr. That leaves little rationale for recommending surgery; no benefit can be shown for back pain and minor benefit is shown for leg pain. Backache is not a surgical disease; sciatica is but on rare occasions.

LUMBAR SPINAL STENOSIS

The cardinal symptom of lumbar spinal stenosis is neurogenic claudication. This is the experience of aching pain with or without paresthesia in the buttock and/or posterior thigh and/or calf precipitated by walking or even assuming an erect posture. Typically, the symptoms are bilateral. Typically, sphincter function is not impaired. Characteristically, the sufferers assume a bent gait, the so-called simian stance, to postpone the onset of symptoms with ambulation. Often they will choose to ambulate assisted by a walker or shopping cart over which they can stoop without falling forward. Likewise, sitting is more likely to offer rapid palliation than is recumbency. It is because this syndrome is so distinctive that lumbar stenosis survives as a clinical entity. The differential diagnosis is limited to atypical presentations of vascular claudication and, more remotely, mass lesions encroaching on the cauda equina. Stenosis seldom provokes the cramping pain that is the hallmark of vascular claudication. There have been attempts to utilize the distinctions in pathogenesis between neurogenic and vascular claudication to construct a provocative test; one would predict that, whereas both might be precipitated by ambulation, only vascular claudication would be precipitated by operating a bicycle. The thought is instructive though not clinically useful (29).

Nearly half of patients with symptomatic stenosis have a reduced or absent Achilles reflex, a third have objective lower extremity weakness, and some 20% have diminished or absent knee jerk(s). Suggestions of polyradiculopathy are discernible by careful electrodiagnostic testing in the vast majority. However, the population at greatest risk are the elderly, particularly elderly men. And therein lies the diagnostic dilemma: Well over 10% of all elderly persons lack Achilles reflexes. The point prevalence of low back pain of some type and degree approaches 50%. And, finally, the presence of degenerative changes, including some degree of compromise in the dimensions of the lumbar canal, is nearly ubiquitous. The false-positive rate for images of the lumbar spine to diagnose stenosis varies from 9% to 35% depending on the criteria used.

In view of these considerations, the diagnosis of lumbar stenosis as a cause of low back pain is based on the stereotypical nature of the symptoms (30). It is not an anatomic diagnosis, nor is its pathophysiology certain. Furthermore, the experience following surgical decompression of the cord is anything but impressive (31); perhaps a third of patients subjected to these extensive procedures are clearly benefited. The sufferer needs a thoughtful and circumspect assessment; surgery is an option of desperation. Before surgery, myelographic documentation of complete or nearly complete obstruction of the caudal subarachnoid space is prudent.

LUMBOSACRAL AND PELVIC INSUFFICIENCY FRACTURES

Insufficiency fractures are spontaneous linear disruptions of cortical and subjacent trabecular bone without displacement. The classic example is the "march" or stress fracture of the metatarsal in the healthy foot, thought to reflect forces in usage that exceed the resilience of the bone. In the elderly or the osteoporotic patient, pelvic structures are similarly susceptible (32,33). Spontaneous fractures of the pubic rami (and the ribs) are well described and are common in the setting of steroid-induced osteoporosis, where they may be asymptomatic and heal with exuberant callus formation. They also occur without hypercorticism and without exuberant callus. Such fractures are being recognized more frequently in the setting of bone pain; aching pain, prominent at rest and with some exacerbation with weight bearing more than movement. The pubic rami, sacrum, and iliac wings are all susceptible (as are the tibial plateaus). At outset, the fracture is typically subradiographic, raising the specter of other causes of bone pain, including neoplasia. However, these fractures are often demonstrable by scintiscanning, although one must remain cognizant of the limited specificity of this technique. The fractures are diagnosed by the exclusion of other possibilities and by the confidence gained in demonstrating linearity by CT or MR imaging and by documenting healing radiographically.

MYELOPATHY AND THE CAUDA EQUINA SYNDROME

Regional diseases of the spine can involve the adjacent contents of the canal. When this occurs in the cervical spine, myelopathy can result. Caudal to L-1, the cauda equina is at risk. Both are rare in all settings of regional illness, from the acute to the most chronic. However, the consequences can be dramatic, if not catastrophic; awareness of the clinical presentation and appreciation of the possibilities for intervention are important.

Cervical Myelopathy

Neither neck pain nor radiculopathy is prerequisite to the clinical presentation of cervical myelopathy. In fact, the presentation is often pain free and very insidious. An acute onset or a painful onset suggests such processes as central discal herniation, epidural abscess, or a vascular catastrophe. The usual patient presents with complaints of diminished dexterity and/or a gait disorder. With higher cervical involvement, above C-5, upper extremity paresthesias and generally impaired dexterity are common complaints. But high cervical presentations are less common so that upper extremity symptoms are usually less prominent than those referable to the lower extremity. Gait is often broad based and balance compromised. Finally, there may be abnormalities of sphincter function, usually presenting as incontinence.

The findings on examination are of lower motor neuron compromise at the level of the lesion and upper motor neuron disease distal. It is the latter finding, usually bilateral hyperreflexia in the lower extremities and bilateral Babinski reflexes, that drives the diagnostic work-up. There is often a sensory level, though light touch is often preserved after temperature and proprioception are diminished. There are signs that involve forceful motion of the neck, including the classic Spurling and Lhermitte signs, but these are of limited sensitivity and specificity, have some inherent risk, and can be relegated to history in the current era of high-definition imaging.

By far the most common process associated with cervical myelopathy after midlife is spondylosis. The differential diagnosis when lower extremity signs and symptoms predominate includes amyotrophic lateral sclerosis and multiple sclerosis, as well as low-pressure hydrocephalus and multiple strokes. Syringomyelia and neoplastic or other cervical space-occupying lesions can mimic the presentation, including even the sensory level. The exquisite anatomic definition that results from magnetic resonance imaging of the cervical cord obviates the need to depend on neurologic findings of marginal reliability to contend with the latter diagnostic uncertainties. In "cervical myelopathy" all one discerns by imaging is impressive spondylosis.

However, just because the myelopathy is occurring in the presence of spondylosis does not assure causation. Most of the patients are elderly, and all elderly have cervical spondylosis. In fact, no aspect of the geometry of the canal has proven sensitive or specific for cervical myelopathy. It may be that the etiology is related to the bony anatomy but is multifactorial and/or dynamic. It also may be that there is a degenerative process of the cord itself that is independent of the bony abnormalities we refer to as *spondylosis.* The latter is suggested by the dismal results of surgical decompression for cervical myelopathy. In fact, in a subset with impressive ossification of the posterior longitudinal ligament, probably part of the spectrum of DISH, the outcomes of conservative and operative management were similar (34).

There is no experimental experience to test these interventions; these elderly patients are spared surgery usually because their operative risk is held to be prohibitive. Nonetheless, a remarkable percentage of patients managed conservatively stabilize, and some even improve. In the classic series of Lees and Turner (35), in which 114 patients were treated conservatively, the process was progressive in only 26%. Given that most patients are elderly and that the prognosis is generally favorable, surgical intervention should be reserved for the occasional younger patient with documented progression. Since most of the earlier surgical experience was not encouraging, one should be aware that the contemporary approach entails procedures that are as aggressive as they are of unproven benefit.

The Cauda Equina Syndrome

The classic example of the cauda equina syndrome occurs in the setting of central herniation of the nucleus pulposus (Fig. 7.6). Usually, the patient is experiencing acute low back pain. In addition to discomfort, there is rapid progression of neurologic symptoms and signs that are usually bilateral. Pain tends to be central at the low back and to radiate into both buttocks or beyond. Hypesthesia develops in a saddle distribution. The cremasteric reflexes and anal wink are at risk. Likewise, sphincter dysfunction may supervene. The latter is the most ominous symptom and sign, although its implication is confounded if the patient, particularly the elderly patient, has been treated with narcotic analgesics. Regardless, this presentation is a challenge to surgical judgment. Traditionally, it has been argued that emergent surgery is indicated as the progression in neurologic compromise is time dependent (36). Be that as it may, the long-term follow-up of patients subjected to emergency surgery is disappointing. There must be more to the pathophysiology of the neurologic damage than compression alone.

Obviously, the cauda equina syndrome can result from any lesion that impinges on the dural sac or occupies space within the sac. Then the neurologic symptoms and signs are more insidious in onset and progression and may be complicated by features discussed previously for spinal stenosis or cauda equina tumors.

REFERENCES

1. Frymoyer JW, Ducker TB, Hadler NM, Kostuik JP, Weinstein JN, Whitecloud TS III (eds.) *The Adult Spine: Principles and Practice.* Volumes 1 and 2. New York, Raven Press, 1991.
2. Delamarter RB, Sachs BL, Thompson GH, Bohlman HH, Makley JT, Carter JR. Primary neoplasms of the thoracic and lumbar spine. *Clin Orthop* 1990;256:87–100.
3. O'Connell D. Ankylosing spondylitis: the literature to the close of the nineteenth century. *Ann Rheum Dis* 1956;15:119–23.
4. Wright V. Aspects of ankylosing spondylitis. *Br J Rheumatol* 1991;30:1–2.
5. Calin A, Porta J, Fries JF, Schurman DJ. Clinical history as a screening test for ankylosing spondylitis. *JAMA* 1977;237:2613–4.
6. Blackburn WD, Alarcon GS, Ball GV. Evaluation of patients with back pain of suspected inflammatory nature. *Am J Med* 1988;85:766–70.
7. McCombe PF, Fairbank JCT, Cockersone BC, Pynsent PB. Reproducibility of physical signs in low-back pain. *Spine* 1989;14:908–18.
8. Arangio GA, Hartzell SM, Reed JF. Significance of lumbosacral list and low-back pain: a controlled radiographic study. *Spine* 1990;15:208–10.
9. Hoffmann RM, Kent DL, Deyo RA. Diagnostic accuracy and clinical utility of thermography for lumbar radiculopathy: a meta-analysis. *Spine* 1991;16:623–8.
10. Wiesel SW, Tsourmas N, Feffer HL, Citrin CM, Patronas N. A study of computer-assisted tomography. 1. The incidence of positive CAT scans in an asymptomatic group of patients. *Spine* 1984;9:549–51.
11. Boden SD, Davis DO, Dina TS, Patronas NJ, Wiesel SW. Abnormal magnetic resonance scans of the lumbar spine in asymptomatic subjects. *J Bone Joint Surg [Am]* 1990;72A:403–8.
12. Hadler NM. The predicament of backache. *J Occup Med* 1988;30:449–50.
13. Frymoyer JW. Back pain and sciatica. *N Engl J Med* 1988;318:291–300.
14. Quebec Task Force on Spinal Disorders. Scientific approach to the assessment and management of activity-related spinal disorders. *Spine* 1987;12[Suppl 1]:S1–S59.
15. Deyo RA, Walsh NE, Schoenfeld LS, Ramamurthy S. Can trials of physical treatments be blinded? *Am J Phys Med Rehabil* 1990;69:6–10.
16. Hadler NM. The chiropractic and me. Whither? Whether? *J Occup Med* 1991;33:1209-11.
17. Deyo RA, Walsh NE, Martin DC, et al. A controlled trial of transcutaneous electrical nerve stimulation (TENS) and exercise for chronic low back pain. *N Engl J Med* 1990;322:1627–34.
18. Walsh NE, Schwartz RK. The influence of prophylactic orthoses on abdominal strength and low back injury in the workplace. *Am J Phys Med Rehabil* 1990;69:245–50.
19. Weber H. Lumbar disc herniation: a controlled, prospective study with ten years of observation. *Spine* 1983;8:131–40.
20. Schwetschenau PR, Ramirez A, Johnston J, Wiggs C, Martins AN. Double-blind evaluation of intradiscal chymopapain for herniated lumbar discs: early results. *J Neurosurg* 1976;45:622–7.
21. Chymopapain approved. *FDA Drug Bull* 1982;12(3):61–3.
22. Dilke TFW, Burry HC, Grahame R. Extradural corticosteroid injection in management of lumbar nerve root compression. *Br Med J* 1973;2:635–7.
23. Cuckler JM, Bernini PA, Wiesel SW, Booth RE, Rothman RH, Pickens GT. The use of epidural steroids in the treatment of lumbar radicular pain: a prospective, randomized, double-blind study. *J Bone Joint Surg [Am]* 1985;67A:63–6.
24. Carette S, Marcoux S, Truchon R, Grondin C, Gagnon J, Allard Y, Latulippe M. A controlled trial of corticosteroid injections into facet joints for chronic low back pain. *N Engl J Med* 1991;325:1002–7.
25. Kahanovitz N, Viola K, Goldstein T, Dawson E. A multicenter analysis of percutaneous discectomy. *Spine* 1990;15:713–5.
26. Hutton C. DISH . . . a state not a disease? *Br J Rheumatol* 1989;28:277–8.

27. Viikari-Juntura E, Porras M, Laasonen EM. Validity of clinical tests in the diagnosis of root compression in cervical disc disease. *Spine* 1989;14:253–7.
28. Alaranta H, Hurme M, Einola S, Falck B, Kallio V, Knuts L-R, Lahtela K, Torma T. A prospective study of patients with sciatica: a comparison between conservatively treated patients and patients who have undergone operation. Part II. Results after one year follow-up. *Spine* 1990;15:1345–9.
29. Dong GX, Porter RW. Walking and cycling tests in neurogenic and intermittent claudication. *Spine* 1989;14:965–9.
30. O'Duffy JD. Spinal stenosis. In: Frymoyer JW, Ducker TB, Hadler NM, Kostuik JP, Weinstein JN, Whitecloud TS III (eds.) *The Adult Spine: Principles and Practice.* New York, Raven Press, 1991:1801–10.
31. Turner JA, Ersek M, Herron L, Deyo R. Surgery for lumbar spinal stenosis: attempted meta-analysis of the literature. *Spine* 1992;17:1–8.
32. Stroebel RJ, Ginsburg WW, McLeod RA. Sacral insufficiency fractures: an often unsuspected cause of low back pain. *J Rheumatol* 1991;18:117–9.
33. Renner JB. Pelvic insufficiency fractures. *Arthritis Rheum* 1990;33:426–30.
34. Trojan DA, Pouchot J, Pokrupa R, Fort RM, Adamsbaum C, Hill RO, Esdaile JM. Diagnosis and treatment of ossification of the posterior longitudinal ligament of the spine: report of eight cases and literature review. *Am J Med* 1992;92:296–306.
35. Lees F, Turner JWA. Natural history and prognosis of cervical spondylosis. *Br Med J* 1963;2:1607–19.
36. Kostuik JP, Harrington I, Alexander D, Rand W, Evans D. Cauda equina syndrome and lumbar disc herniation. *J Bone Joint Surg [Am]* 1986;68A:386–91.
37. Hadler NM, Curtis P, Gillings DB, Stinnett S. A benefit of spinal manipulation as adjunctive therapy for acute low-back pain: A stratified controlled trial. *Spine* 1987;12:703–6.

8

Upper Extremity Regional Musculoskeletal Illness

Shoulder, Elbow, Wrist, and Hand

SHOULDER PAIN

The patient with regional shoulder pain presents a challenge to the diagnostic skills of the physician, one that can be rewarded with insights that have considerable therapeutic ramifications. All patients with regional shoulder pain have some restriction in range of motion. If motion is unimpaired so that the patient is able to place a palm on the occiput with the arm fully rotated externally, for example, or if motion is symmetric with the uninvolved side, one must question the inference of regional shoulder pain. In this setting consider referred pain from multiple sites: angina and its equivalents, neck pain with or without radiculopathy, diaphragmatic pain, bone pain from metastatic disease or a Pancoast's tumor, invasive or inflammatory disease of axillary structures, etc.

If motion is impaired, it is next crucial to discern whether the glenohumeral joint itself is involved. There is an arc of motion that isolates this articulation (Fig. 8.1). Restriction or pain in this arc suggests inflammatory disease of the true shoulder and, with one exception (reflex sympathetic dystrophy), excludes regional illness. The differential diagnosis of glenohumeral arthritis includes a range of inflammatory systemic rheumatic diseases, infectious arthritides, and even the exceptionally destructive osteoarthritis known as Milwaukee shoulder. The latter presents in the quite elderly population and is usually asymptomatic except for a rare hemarthrosis.

Periarthritis

If the glenohumeral joint is spared and motion is impaired in other arcs, in all likelihood one is faced with a regional illness involving a structure(s) in proximity to the glenohumeral joint. Some such structures (e.g., the sternoclavicular

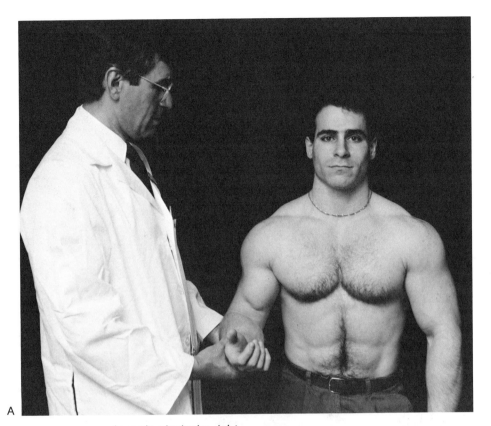

A

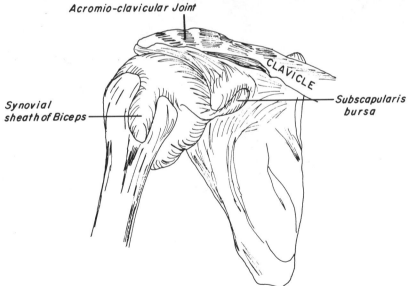

Acromio-clavicular Joint

CLAVICLE

*Synovial
sheath of Biceps*

*Subscapularis
bursa*

B

FIG. 8.1. Glenohumeral motion is assessed with the arm in the neutral position and the elbow flexed (**A**). Internal rotation of the shoulder isolates the glenohumeral joint from periarticular structures and is usually gliding and pain free even in the presence of periarthritis. Compromise in this arc indicates abnormality within the confines of the synovium (**B**) or reflex sympathetic dystrophy ("frozen shoulder").

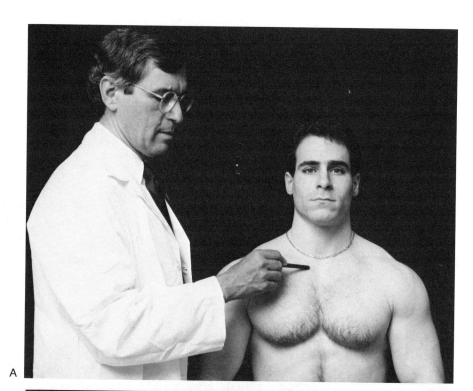

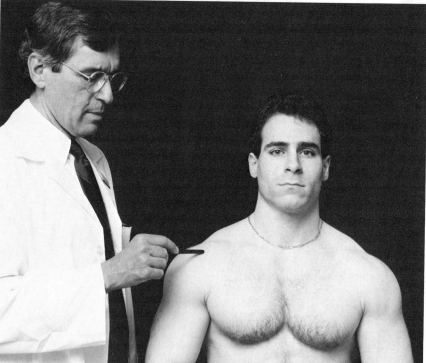

B

and acromioclavicular joints) are readily palpable (Fig. 8.2); if frank inflammation (synovitis) is discerned, the diagnostic likelihoods revert to those for glenohumeral disease. Most typically, there is no overt inflammation anywhere in the pectoral girdle, just impressive and often focal tenderness, typically deep to the belly of the deltoid. Many will experience increased discomfort in abduction, particularly in abduction with external rotation (Fig. 8.3). This posture applies pressure to many of the subdeltoid structures by virtue of impingement on the acromion, a fact that causes some to label the periarthritis an "impingement syndrome." However, it is not clear from existing data that further definition of the pathophysiology is possible, regardless of one's diagnostic inventiveness, including imaging techniques. Degenerative changes in the cuff manifested as dystrophic calcification afflict over 10% of us by the sixth decade (1), are often bilateral, and are highly discordant from symptoms. Dissolution of the rotator cuff, with or without radiologically discernible calcification, has age-dependent prevalence, becoming ubiquitous in later decades. Demonstrating such abnormalities in the setting of periarthritis is an exercise with unproven and tenuous specificity. Abnormalities in tendon hydration, subperiosteal cysts and irregularities, and periarticular calcification are comparably nonspecific. There exists a venerable but anecdotal orthopedic literature on diseases of the bicipital tendon presenting as periarthritis. However, there are no data to establish the reliability, sensitivity or specificity of the putative hallmarks of "bicipital tendinitis," and there is a considerable range of clinical confidence in such signs as tenderness in the bicipital groove and Yergason's sign (pain in the shoulder when the forearm is supinated against resistance with the elbow flexed, thereby stressing the long head of the biceps and its tendon).

Given the state of the art, "periarthritis" is sufficient as a clinical diagnosis. It subsumes the labels collected over the decades attempting to ascribe the periarthritis to particular structures.

Approximately 10% of us will experience a prolonged and memorable episode of periarthritis each year. A much smaller percentage will seek medical advice. Shoulder periarthritis is always a self-limited disease; there is no evidence that these patients are at risk of a "frozen shoulder." For nearly all patients, the time to remission in terms of pain and range of motion is measurable in weeks. One clinical trial supports the use of some forms of physical therapy, a steroid injection into the region of the subdeltoid bursa (Fig. 8.4), or nonsteroidal antiinflammatory agents in shortening the time to remission (2). However, most of the therapeutic inventiveness that is offered the periarthritis patient has not been subjected to critical testing. Surgical intervention for peri-

←——————————————————————————————

FIG. 8.2. Both the sternoclavicular (**A**) and acromioclavicular (**B**) joints are subcutaneous and readily palpated. Evidence of synovitis, manifest as swelling with either fluid or synovial tissue, excludes regional musculoskeletal disease. The differential diagnosis among the systemic diseases is dependent on the distribution of the arthritis and its symmetry. Monarthritis of these joints raises the specter of septic arthritis. The sternoclavicular joint is often a target in the spondyloarthropathies and in some forms of pustular psoriasis.

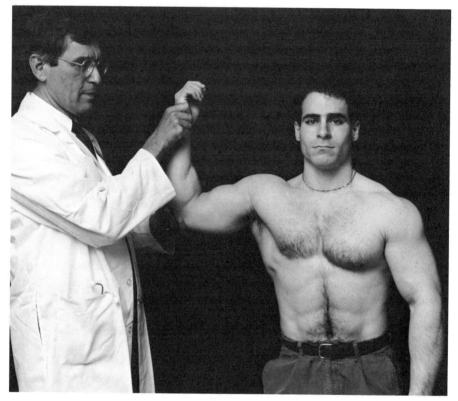

FIG. 8.3. Passive external rotation in abduction is demonstrated. The maneuver that elicits the classic sign for the "impingement" syndrome is to rotate the abducted shoulder externally. The response is pain—particularly subdeltoid pain. This maneuver impinges the rotator cuff on the acromion.

arthritis is supported only by the zeal of the surgeon; arguments for surgery are tenuous at best.

Reflex Sympathetic Dystrophy

Reflex sympathetic dystrophy (RSD) is a distinctive clinical entity. It is included in the shoulder section because it most frequently involves the upper extremity; if the shoulder is exclusively involved some use the terms *frozen shoulder* or *adhesive capsulitis*; otherwise, the typical pattern of illness is often termed the *shoulder-hand syndrome* or *algodystrophy* in Britain (3). However, reflex sympathetic dystrophy can involve the lower extremity as well, including the foot in isolation and even the hip or knee in isolation. It can involve a whole hand or just a digit (4). It will become clear that this condition barely satisfies the definition of a regional musculoskeletal illness; true, the patient is spared systemic illness but bilaterality of involvement (albeit usually quite asymmet-

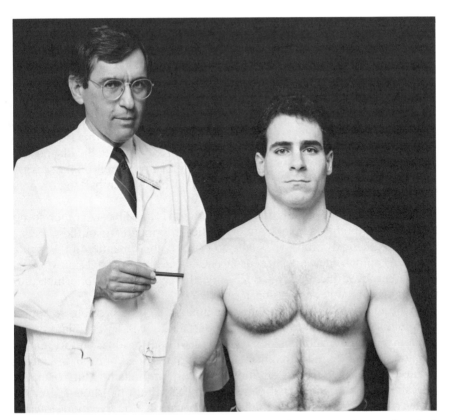

FIG. 8.4. Periarthritis of the shoulder is often accompanied by point tenderness deep to the deltoid. In common parlance, this is a "deltoid bursitis." However, little abnormality in the bursa is demonstrable by any technique. Dystrophic calcification may be apparent radiographically, but this is probably a coincidence. It is found in a significant minority of asymptomatic shoulders, approaching a majority in octogenarians. Besides, when present in the symptomatic shoulder, calcification can usually be demonstrated in the contralateral shoulder.

ric) and a dramatic alteration of neurovascular physiology and of mesenchymal biology are features of the disease.

The illness, inexplicably, can follow such discrete events as a myocardial infarction or physical or surgical trauma, in which case the condition is traditionally labeled *causalgia*. More commonly, the onset is insidious over weeks. Early on, the patient experiences pain, which can vary from lancinating to burning and which is accompanied by hyperhidrosis and vascular lability of the involved region. In full-blown form, the aching discomfort persists, with concomitant morning stiffness, vascular lability, hyperhidrosis, and dysesthesias of the hand. The hand becomes diffusely tender (5), doughy, with a shiny appearance from skin atrophy. The shoulder aches, and range of motion is progressively restricted in all arcs, including the glenohumeral (Fig. 8.1). Atrophy can involve more than the skin; the underlying musculature involutes diffusely.

Radiographs demonstrate Sudek's atrophy, a patchy osteopenia of the involved region. Shoulder arthrography is remarkable only for the reduced volume of the articular cavity. Scintiscanning demonstrates increased vascularity in the early lesion progressing to include periarticular bony hypermetabolism as the process advances. Increased uptake of bone-seeking radionuclide is characteristic of symptomatic joints but also often of the contralateral asymptomatic or less symptomatic joint. Making the diagnosis when faced with the fully developed disease is straightforward. However, with early disease, or a forme fruste, there is need for caution. Abnormal thermoregulation is sensitive to the diagnosis of RSD but not specific (6). Many clinicians, including myself, rely on the sensitivity of scintiscanning to gain diagnostic confidence before embarking on invasive empirical therapy.

The pathophysiology of this dramatic condition is the subject of much speculation. Most hypotheses invoke abnormalities in sympathetic outflow (hence, reflex sympathetic dystrophy), usually ascribed to abnormalities in the regulation of the spinal internuncial neuron pool. These theories fuel most of the invasive empirical therapy. More recently, the possibility of abnormal autocrine function peripherally has been raised.

For the majority of these patients the illness follows a predictable course: inflammatory onset as above, period of contracture with fewer inflammatory symptoms, and then spontaneous regression without residua. Unfortunately, this natural history is measured in years, not months. It is common practice to provide physical therapy and emotional support, antiinflammatory or minor analgesic palliation, and a trial of steroid injection into the shoulder region. However, there are advocates for far more aggressive interventions: stellate ganglion anesthesia (or, if the patient and physician can conceptualize a self-limited illness as desperate, ablation), intraarterial administration of reserpine or guanethidine, or high-dose corticosteroid administration. Only anecdotal experience is available to test such therapeutic hypotheses, and even this experience is variable. Given the benign long-term prognosis, the more conservative posture is readily defensible, particularly during the early months of illness.

ELBOW PAIN

"Tennis elbow," "student's elbow," "golfer's elbow," and sometimes "writer's cramp" are as much a part of our parlance as "to bend an elbow." It is remarkable how willing we are to infer that the most significant disability we suffer as a consequence of our regional elbow pain is the clue to its pathogenesis. In fact, some 15% of us can recall a week of elbow pain or recurring elbow pain last year, whether or not we are employed in tasks demanding of elbow function. Some 1% to 3% of the adult population will carry the diagnosis of epicondylitis at some point during their lives, usually between ages 40 and 60. People with lateral epicondylitis have difficulty hitting a tennis ball with a top-spin backhand, but we have no clue as to why they suffer lateral epicondylitis in the first place. In fact, the vast majority of cases have no biomechanical association, let alone an association with avocation or vocation (7).

The elbow is an elegant hinge joint. For nearly all regional musculoskeletal diseases of the elbow, passive motion in flexion/extension and supination/pronation is pain free and unimpaired. The exception is osteoarthritis of the elbow, which can interfere with motion, particularly glenohumeral motion resulting in a flexion contracture. Osteoarthritis of the elbow is usually seen in the setting of calcium pyrophosphate deposition disease (CPPDD), as a consequence of overt trauma (secondary osteoarthritis), or as a consequence of exceptional arm usage such as that of baseball pitchers and pneumatic drill operators. "Primary" osteoarthritis has been described in middle-aged men, often associated with osteoarthritis of the second and third metacarpophalangeal joints, but it is rare (8).

Therefore, if glenohumeral or radioulnar motion is impeded or painful, intraarticular inflammation is the diagnosis to be excluded; the spectrum of etiologies shifts to include the inflammatory arthritides, infectious arthritis, and a hemarthrosis as a consequence of impact on the hand with an outstretched arm. Arthrocentesis is necessary to make a definitive diagnosis. The regional diseases are periarticular, involving the structures around the lateral epicondyle, the medial epicondyle, or the olecranon bursa.

Epicondylitis

It is important to recognize epicondylitis as the cause of the elbow pain and to lateralize the process. The first requires the exercise of excluding illnesses that are managed quite differently; the latter allows palliative advice.

In most instances, the patient localizes the pain to a side of the elbow. In most instances, that side is tender without other signs of inflammation. More specific signs involve the elicitation of discomfort when the lateral muscle masses are contracted against resistance. Supination of the forearm or extension of the pronated wrist against resistance elicits pain in the region of the lateral epicondyle. Flexion of the supinated wrist against resistance elicits the pain of medial epicondylitis. These signs are diagnostic; in the case of lateral epicondylitis there is some discussion (see Chapter 10) as to whether entrapment of the radial nerve in the "radial tunnel" can present in this fashion, but the arguments are not compelling.

Not only are these signs diagnostic, but they also suggest advice that can be impressively palliative. If these motions are avoided, discomfort is diminished while awaiting the likelihood of spontaneous regression of the condition. It can take weeks or months before full activities can be resumed without recrudescence—but there are few among us for whom such patience is impractical. After all, most tasks can be adjusted or accomplished in alternative fashion to avoid these particular usages. For those that can't, such as tennis in the case of lateral epicondylitis, either another avocation should be pursued for several months or the patient can "run around the backhand." This approach is the most sensible, requiring no more than patience and maturity.

Unfortunately, there is a contract between medicine and American society that thwarts "patience and maturity" and promotes the choice of unproven remedies in spite of discomfort, risk, and expense. Progressive structured exercising is often advised in America, while it is proscribed in Britain. Zeal for antiinflammatory drugs, intralesional injections, orthotics, and the last resort of surgery has primacy in the American mind. A recent double-blind comparison of intralesional corticosteroid preparations with local anesthetic documented only transient benefit of the former (9). Epicondylitis is a common experience and often provokes considerable consternation. The medical/surgical community seems resistant to disabusing the public of the need for alarm or aggressive intervention. If only common sense were more sensible.

Olecranon Bursitis

Acute olecranon bursitis as a regional musculoskeletal illness, so-called "student's elbow," is infrequent. It is suggested by the presence of frank inflammation localizing to the bursa and sparing the elbow articulation. A far more frequent explanation for such a presentation is gout or even sepsis; therefore, aspiration of the lesion is mandatory. Although acute bursitis is seldom a regional illness, chronic bursitis is more common. It is usually asymptomatic. One palpates a doughy, sometimes nodular bursa. Of course, the differential diagnosis includes the systemic rheumatic diseases, which are generally manifest elsewhere.

Treatment of acute and chronic "student's elbow" involves advice as to the avoidance of compression of the bursa and even the provision of an appropriate cushioning device. An intralesional steroid injection or a short course of a nonsteroidal antiinflammatory agent can further palliate the acute lesion.

WRIST PAIN

The wrist is a remarkable and complex joint (Fig. 8.5). The eight carpal bones can be divided into three functional components: the proximal row, the distal row, and the midcarpal row comprising the pisiform and trapezium. Nearly all flexion and extension of the wrist occurs at the articulation of the distal radius and the proximal carpal row. In deviation this holds as well, although there is some countermotion of the distal row. Axial rotation of the hand is by virtue of the range of motion of the distal radioulnar joint; the carpus contributes little if at all. Flexion is accomplished primarily by the flexor carpi ulnaris muscle inserting on the pisiform and flexor carpi radialis inserting on the base of the second metacarpal. Extension invokes the extensor carpi ulnaris, radialis, longus, and brevis, all of which insert on metacarpal heads. The second to fifth metacarpals are relatively fixed on the distal carpus. The thumb is the excep-

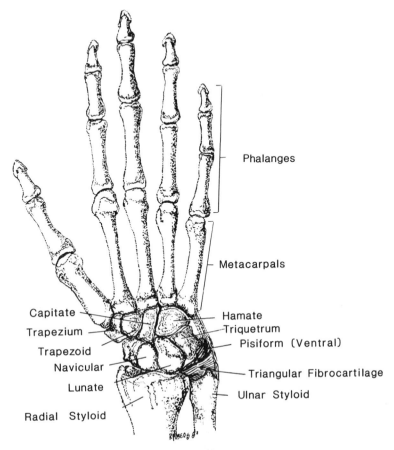

Phalanges

Metacarpals

Capitate
Trapezium
Trapezoid
Navicular
Lunate
Radial Styloid

Hamate
Triquetrum
Pisiform (Ventral)
Triangular Fibrocartilage
Ulnar Styloid

FIG. 8.5. The carpal bones are usefully divided into groups: the proximal carpal row articulates with the distal radius, and the distal carpal row with the proximal metacarpals.

tion; its articulation with the trapezium allows a considerable range of motion. With the notable exception of the abductor pollicis longus and extensor pollicis brevis, which delineate the "anatomic snuff box," all tendons crossing the wrist are embedded in fibrous retinacula, emerging in compartments defined by the fascial planes of the hand itself.

Tenosynovitis

Discomfort about the wrist is an extremely common experience; well over 25% of us can be brought to a level of awareness that facilitates recall of prolonged or recurrent episodes. Almost always there is no sign of inflammation: no redness, synovitis, crepitus, etc. There is discomfort, localized to one or another compartment, usually of the dorsal wrist, and exacerbation when that compartment is stressed. An appropriate diagnostic label for this presentation might be simply "benign localized discomfort," since the prognosis is so favorable. Unfortunately, it is customary to extrapolate from rare instances of localized pain with overt inflammation to assume that the discomfort is a forme fruste of frank tenosynovitis. There is no justification for perpetuating this fallacy and the anxiety it provokes.

Benign localized discomfort at the wrist is common. Soreness can be experienced by as many as 30% of us, particularly those of us who perform tasks involving demands on upper extremity function. However, if the elements of the tasks are themselves customary and comfortable, we need not fear damaging consequences. Fortunately, with growing awareness of the challenges faced by people involved in such tasks, attempts have been initiated to provide a more ergonomically adaptable work environment. In doing so, motion is not to be proscribed; tendon motion is prerequisite to the health of this tissue. Rather, increased awareness of individual differences in symptoms over time is the goal for management not blessed with such intuition.

One form of wrist tenosynovitis deserves special attention, de Quervain's disease. It is not clear that this is the most common "benign localized discomfort" of the wrist, but it is the most recognized in the literature. This may reflect the eponymous nature of the diagnosis, or the challenge it presents for pathophysiologic inferences and empirical surgical remedies. The discomfort involves the tendons of the extensor pollicis brevis and abductor pollicis longus as they course over the radial styloid in the most lateral extensor compartment of the wrist. These tendons comprise the dorsal and ventral walls of the anatomic snuffbox, respectively (Fig. 8.6). Clinically, the patient experiences pain and tenderness in the region of the base of the thumb and the radial styloid exacerbated by attempts to abduct and extend the thumb. Ulnar deviation of the wrist with the thumb flexed also elicits pain and is the basis of the Finkelstein test (Fig. 8.7). This association also underlies the pathophysiologic inference that repetitive motion involving such patterns of usage are causal (e.g., the "washerwoman's sprain" of past generations of diagnosticians). However, it is still not clear that such usage is causal; it may simply make the condition manifest. Furthermore, there is a critical differential diagnostic point; osteoarthritis of the first carpometacarpal joint is exceedingly common in the postmenopausal woman and is intermittently symptomatic in a fashion that mimics de Quervain's tenosynovitis. Radiographic demonstration of underlying degenerative joint disease is neither sensitive nor specific for this discomfort. Pain with isolated active recruitment of the tendons, when "straightening the thumb" with the first metacarpal fixed (Fig. 8.8), is more specific for de Quervain's.

Frank tenosynovitis does occur. The features are inflammatory: erythema, point tenderness, and even fluctuance over the course of the tendon, with posturing so that the tendon is under least tension. Movement from this neutral position elicits pain. Such a presentation should never be assumed to be an extreme example of the "benign localized discomfort" conditions. Rather, the differential diagnosis includes purulent tenosynovitis and many rheumatic dis-

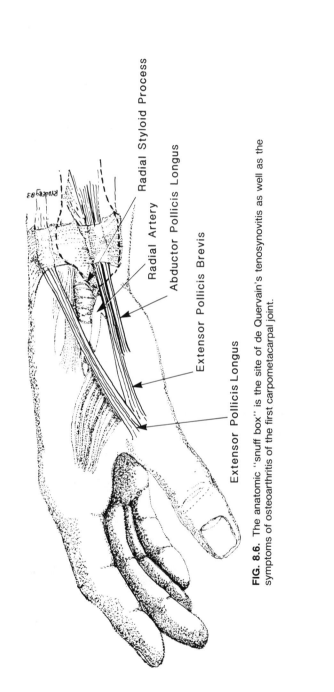

Radial Styloid Process

Radial Artery

Abductor Pollicis Longus

Extensor Pollicis Brevis

Extensor Pollicis Longus

FIG. 8.6. The anatomic "snuff box" is the site of de Quervain's tenosynovitis as well as the symptoms of osteoarthritis of the first carpometacarpal joint.

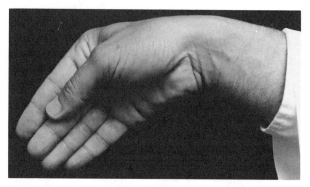

FIG. 8.7. Adduction of the thumb with ulnar deviation of the wrist is the modified Finkelstein's maneuver. It is positive if it elicits pain near the radial styloid. Disorders of the tendons of the anatomic snuff box and of the first carpometacarpal joint cause a positive Finkelstein's test.

eases, notably Löfgren's syndrome, disseminated gonococcal infection, Reiter's disease, and systemic lupus erythematosus. There are also instances of regional musculoskeletal disease of the tendons with this intensity. These are very rare, are diagnosed by exclusion, and only arguably represent an extreme of a spectrum.

The treatment of "benign localized discomfort," even in the distribution of de Quervain's, is conservative: proscribe the exacerbating usage, perhaps assist

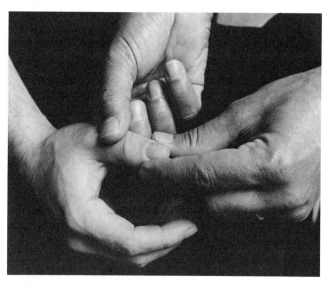

FIG. 8.8. If the first carpometacarpal joint is restrained and the thumb extended against resistance, pain in the region of the snuff box suggests a tendon disorder rather than underlying osteoarthritis.

the proscription with a splint, and occasionally inject a corticosteroid preparation into the involved tendon sheath. Coupled with reassurance and patience, these will nearly always suffice. Only anecdotes suggest sequelae in terms of restriction in motion, but most are confounded by coincidental osteoarthritis of the first carpometacarpal joint. However, patience is seldom the therapeutic posture of the American clinician or the therapeutic expectation of the American patient. Accepted practice is early recourse to injection of the tendon sheath with a long-acting corticosteroid preparation (10). Over 90% of patients whose persistent de Quervain's tenosynovitis (average duration of over 4 mo) resulted in referral to the Medical Orthopedic Clinic of Northwest Kaiser Permanente were markedly improved, if not well, 1 mo after such an injection coupled with advice to avoid usage (11). Unfortunately, there was no appropriate control intervention; fortunately, there were no complications, which, in expert hands, are exceedingly rare. I remain skeptical. I am even more skeptical regarding surgical intervention for benign localized tendon discomfort, even of the de Quervain's localization. There are no controlled trials, the rationale is tenuous, and results are uneven in spite of prolonged postoperative rehabilitation.

Ganglion

The most common "lump" or "bump" of the hand is a ganglion. Some 50% of ganglia appear over the dorsum of the wrist, particularly over the greater-lesser multangular or the scapholunate joints. Less common sites are the volar wrist, particularly between the flexor carpi radialis and brachioradialis tendons and between finger extensor and palmar flexor tendons at the metacarpophalangeal (MCP) joints. These are soft, round structures tethered to underlying tissue. They are more likely to be fluctuant on the extensor surfaces. Generally, they are asymptomatic. Most are hollow fibrous structures containing amorphous necrotic material with some connection to underlying joints or tendons. The pathogenesis is uncertain. The only indication for extirpation is cosmetic, except in the rare case where there is functional impingement on adjacent structures. Spontaneous regression is well described but not predictable.

HAND DISORDERS

The hand is simply a marvel. It serves us well throughout our lives. In spite of the continuous demands we make on the structure and its vulnerability in terms of exposure, the hand remains useful, comfortable, reliable, and dexterous as long as we avoid frank trauma. Aside from systemic diseases and localized infectious processes, there are few regional musculoskeletal afflictions of the hand that cause one to seek medical guidance.

Trigger Finger

Trigger finger is a relatively common entity. Clinical experience suggests that it is most common in midlife, but there are no formal epidemiologic studies. The cause is a fibrous thickening in a tendon and/or its associated sheath, which impedes movement. Characteristically, when the nodule interfaces with one of the fibrous tethers that anchor the tendon in its sheath, motion ceases until the nodule pops through the constraint. This sudden "give" or "unlocking" is the triggering and may be uncomfortable. The nodule is palpable, most commonly moving with a flexor tendon near the metacarpal head or distal palmar crease. Triggering is also palpable.

Most frequently, the flexor tendons of the third and fourth digits are involved, although triggering of all flexor and extensor tendons in the hand has been described and even anecdotally at the wrist. The tendon of the flexor digitorum profundus is most commonly involved, particularly as it exits its synovial sheath in the distal palm and enters the fibrous flexor sheath of the digit. The clinical literature offers up such terms as *tendovaginitis, stenosing tenosynovitis,* and the like to account for the surgeon's causal inferences. These are tenuous insights, and the terminology tends to obfuscate; *trigger finger* will suffice.

Most trigger fingers slowly improve spontaneously. Perhaps the nodule resorbs or the fibrous impedance gains laxity. If patience will not prevail or if the finger is hung up, steroid injections into the sheath or nodule are a reasonable alternative (9). Whether such injections shrink the nodule or relax the fibrous impedance is unclear. Nonetheless, the injection is often effective, and tendon rupture is exceedingly rare, even with repeated infiltration (12,13). However, surgery offers a more definitive avenue in the occasional patient.

Tendon nodules can be a sign of systemic disease and are more likely to be such if they are multiple or bilateral. Rheumatoid arthritis often produces trigger fingers as a consequence of rheumatoid nodules in and around tendons (14). Diabetes mellitus has been associated with fibrous nodules, occurring in some 5% of insulin-dependent diabetics younger than 40 (15).

Dupuytren's Contracture

Dupuytren's contractures are at least as common as trigger fingers. Furthermore, the processes are easily confused in their early stages. Judging from clinical experience, both peak in midlife, although the former are more likely in white men and more frequent during the later decades of life. Dupuytren's contractures are a consequence of hyperplasia and hypertrophy of the palmar fascia, with fibrotic nodule formation. The early presentation is with a painless nodule in the palm. This can progress to a disfiguring tight band in the palm interfering with finger extension. The fourth and fifth digits are most frequently involved.

Unlike the case with a trigger finger, palpation reveals a nontender, nodular thickening and retraction of the palmar fascia often extending across the MCP joint. If the process extends into the superficial fascia of the digits, the contracture can involve the proximal interphalangeal (PIP) and even distal interphalangeal (DIP) joints. Rarely the process extends proximally across the wrist and never onto the dorsum (although it is associated with "knuckle pads," fibrous thickening over the PIP joints). Treatment is expectant observation in the majority, as progression is predictably slow. For limiting functional compromise or cosmetic considerations, there is surgical recourse.

Osteoarthritis of the Hand

We are all at risk for osteoarthritis of the hand. In fact, this fate is nearly obligate for women in the late decades of life. Osteoarthritis of the hand is a form of degenerative joint disease with a characteristic distribution. There is loss of articular cartilage and exuberant marginal osteophyte formation. The result is progressive restriction in the range of motion and often progressive malalignment accompanied by hard excrescences at the joint margin representing the cartilage-covered osteophytes. The process targets the distal interphalangeal joints and the first carpometacarpal joint at the base of the thumb (Fig. 8.5) first and then the proximal interphalangeal joints. Occasionally, there is involvement of the second and third metacarpophalangeal joints, but this is unusual and should raise the possibility of hemochromatosis, which has a predilection for these joints and leads to osteoarthritis. The lumps about the distal interphalangeal joints are called *Heberden's nodes;* those about the proximal interphalangeal joints are called *Bouchard's nodes.* Cosmetic concerns will bring some patients to medical attention.

Osteoarthritis of the hand provokes intermittent discomfort and some functional compromise, particularly in precision and power pinch. The latter often reflects damage to the first carpometacarpal joint; power pinch provokes pain at the base of the thumb, often with some tenderness at that site, which is within the anatomic snuffbox (Fig. 8.6). This is not to be confused with tendinitis at the same site. The mainstay of therapy for symptomatic osteoarthritis of the hand is the perspective and adaptive devices provided by occupational therapists experienced with the condition. For example, power pinch is often compromised in the pincer motion because of pain at the base of the thumb. Prolonged writing can be impeded by pain at this site. The intervention is to adjust the dimensions of the object to be held so that a pincer movement with the fingertips is replaced by a pincer movement that utilizes the extent of the digits (Fig. 8.9). Providing a pen with a large diameter facilitates this movement. There are similar adaptations for pushing car door buttons, etc. Antiinflammatory drugs and injections have little role in management. Surgery is an exceptional option.

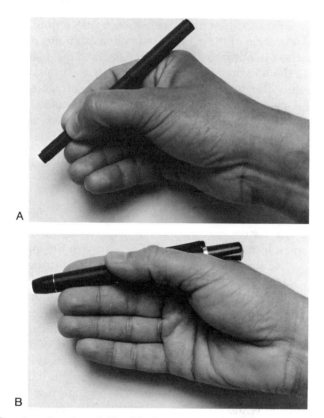

FIG. 8.9. Symptomatic osteoarthritis of the first carpometacarpal joint is exacerbated by force-ful pinching (**A**). However, if the object can be cradled the length of the opposing digits, motion of the first carpometacarpal joint is not necessary and the function is less painful (**B**).

The pathogenesis of osteoarthritis of the hand is multifactorial. More severe involvement tends to run in families. There is some association with osteoarthritis of the hip (16), suggesting that hand osteoarthritis is part of a more generalized diathesis. Interestingly, it is difficult to demonstrate an association with osteoarthritis of joints other than the hip. There is also evidence that the pattern of usage determines the pattern of osteoarthritis of the hands (17). However, this is not to say that stereotyped or repetitive usage damages hand joints. In fact, individuals so employed may be spared the magnitude of hand osteoarthritis so common in the population at large (18).

Compromise in hand function in the elderly is a marker of more global functional compromise. Compromise in hand function is perhaps the best predictor of loss of the ability to maintain an independent lifestyle (19). However, hand osteoarthritis cannot be discerned as responsible for the dependency (20). Rather, the compromised dexterity probably provides a window into other aspects of cognition.

REFERENCES

1. Mavrikakis ME, Drimis S, Kontoyannis DA, Rasidakis A, Moulopoulou ES, Kontoyannis S. Calcific shoulder periarthritis (tendinitis) in adult onset diabetes mellitus: a controlled study. *Ann Rheum Dis* 1989;48:211–4.
2. Petri M, Dobrow R, Neiman R, Whiting-O'Keefe Q, Seaman WE. Randomized, double-blind, placebo-controlled study of the treatment of the painful shoulder. *Arthritis Rheum* 1987;30:1040–5.
3. Chard MD. Diagnosis and management of algodystrophy. *Ann Rheum Dis* 1991;50:727–30.
4. Laukaitis JP, Varma VM, Borenstein DG. Reflex sympathetic dystrophy localized to a single digit. *J Rheumatol* 1989;16:402–5.
5. Atkins RM, Kanis JA. The use of dolorimetry in the assessment of post-traumatic algodystrophy of the hand. *Br J Rheumatol* 1989;28:404–8.
6. Cooke ED, Glick EN, Bowcock SA, Smith RE, Ward C, Almond NE, Beacham JA. Reflex sympathetic dystrophy (algoneurodystrophy): temperature studies in the upper limb. *Br J Rheumatol* 1989;28:399–403.
7. Binder AI, Hazleman BL. Lateral humeral epicondylitis—a study of natural history and the effect of conservative therapy. *Br J Rheumatol* 1983;22:73–6.
8. Doherty M, Preston B. Primary osteoarthritis of the elbow. *Ann Rheum Dis* 1989;48:743–7.
9. Price R, Sinclair H, Heinrich I, Gibson T. Local injection treatment of tennis elbow—hydrocortisone, triamcinolone and lignocaine compared. *Br J Rheumatol* 1991;30:39–44.
10. Neustadt DH. Local corticosteroid injection therapy in soft tissue rheumatic conditions of the hand and wrist. *Arthritis Rheum* 1991;34:923–6.
11. Anderson BC, Manthey R, Brouns MC. Treatment of de Quervain's tenosynovitis with corticosteroids. *Arthritis Rheum* 1991;34:793–8.
12. Marks MR, Gunther SF. Efficacy of cortisone injection in treatment of trigger fingers and thumbs. *J Hand Surg [Am]* 1989;14A:722–7.
13. Fauno P, Andersen HJ, Simonsen O. A long-term follow-up of the effect of repeated injections for stenosing tenosynovitis. *J Hand Surg [Br]* 1989;14B:242–3.
14. Gottlieb NL. Digital flexor tenosynovitis: diagnosis and clinical significance. *J Rheumatol* 1991;18:954–5.
15. Yosipovitch G, Yosipovitch Z, Karp M, Mukamel M. Trigger finger in young patients with insulin dependent diabetes. *J Rheumatol* 1990;17:951–2.
16. McGoldrick F, O'Brien TM. Osteoarthritis of the hip and Heberden's nodes. *Ann Rheum Dis* 1989;48:53–5.
17. Hadler NM, Gillings DB, Imbus HR, Levitin PM, Makuc D, Utsinger PD, Yount WJ, Slusser D, Moskovitz N. Hand structure and function in an industrial setting: influence of three patterns of stereotyped repetitive usage. *Arthritis Rheum* 1978;21:210–20.
18. Lawrence JS. Rheumatism in cotton operatives. *Br J Ind Med* 1961;18:270–6.
19. Williams ME, Hadler NM, Earp JAL. Manual ability as a marker of dependency in geriatric women. *J Chron Dis* 1982;35:115–22.
20. Pattrick M, Aldridge S, Hamilton E, Manhire A, Doherty M. A controlled study of hand function in nodal erosive osteoarthritis. *Ann Rheum Dis* 1989;48:978–82.

9

Lower Extremity Regional Musculoskeletal Illness

Hip, Knee, Ankle, and Foot

HIP PAIN IN THE ADULT

Pain in the hip and buttock is a challenge for the diagnostician. A number of the axial syndromes discussed in Chapter 7 can present this way, as can vascular and visceral disorders. Furthermore, pain that can be ascribed to diseases of the hip need not be perceived as hip pain. The innervation of the hip joint derives from three nerves: the obturator, femoral, and sciatic. As a result, hip pain can refer medially, anteriorly, or posteriorly. It can also present or extend distally along the course of these nerves to the knee, where hip pain can be manifest as discomfort in the medial margin. Likewise, disease of the medial compartment of the knee can refer proximally to be manifest as hip discomfort. Fortunately, the physical examination is exquisitely sensitive to disease of the hip, even more so than plane radiography. Therefore, a normal examination can exclude the hip as etiologic with considerable validity. An abnormal examination initiates a diagnostic algorithm that may well focus on hip pathoanatomy.

Anatomy

Only the shoulder exceeds the hip in range of motion. However, the hip is inherently stable; the musculature stabilizes the shoulder. The femoral head is trapped in the acetabulum by the acetabular labrum. This fibrocartilaginous lip is completed inferiorly by the transverse ligament of the acetabulum. The articulation is enclosed by a thick, fibrous capsule encompassing the labrum, the head, and the femoral neck. This capsule attaches anteriorly along the intertrochanteric line and posteriorly at the base of the neck of the femur. During development the capsule encompasses the epiphyseal plates of the femoral head and the greater trochanter.

In this way the femoral head is held tightly in the acetabulum so that weight bearing does not diminish the radiographic joint space (roughly equivalent to the thickness of the juxtaposed cartilage surfaces.) The iliofemoral ligament maintains contiguity when the hip is unloaded. In contrast, the radiographic joint spaces of both the knee and the shoulder are diminished by compressive force, implying less contiguity when the extremity is dependent. The extensive range of motion of the hip is limited by the surrounding ligaments and muscles: the hip flexors and the iliofemoral ligament limit extension to 20° to 30°, and the musculature limits hip flexion after the first 100° or so, abduction after 70°, and adduction after 25° to 30°. Internal and external rotation are limited by the pubofemoral and ischiofemoral ligaments, respectively; rotations increase in flexion where these ligaments relax.

Physical Examination

A wealth of insight is forthcoming from observing the posturing and gait of any patient with any musculoskeletal symptoms. With axial and lower extremity symptoms, this is mandatory. Patients with hip disease as the cause of their hip pain have an antalgic gait; they move slowly on the asymptomatic side and shorten the stance phase on the symptomatic side. Furthermore, internal rotation in extension is the arc most likely to be compromised by any intraarticular disease of the hip. Since internal rotation in extension is necessary to swing one's pelvis about the pivot provided by the weight-bearing hip, hip disease provokes a gait rendered less flowing by the need to hold the pelvis fixed on the compromised pivoting hip. If extension is compromised as well, the swing and forward thrust of the pelvis is further abbreviated. Increasing flexion contracture leads to compensatory posturing at the low back and knee in an attempt to maintain balance but at a price of further compromise in biomechanical stability. The experienced clinician can often spot severe hip disease as the patient walks into the office.

Destruction of the femoral head can lead to true leg length discrepancies. However, minor asymmetry, as much as 1 to 2 cm, is a normal variant with neither diagnostic specificity nor prognostic import.

Effusions of the hip cannot be detected on examination. Palpation has little localizing value; focal tenderness is nonspecific. However, determination of range of motion is exceedingly valuable. Figures 9.1 and 9.2 illustrate this portion of the examination. Normal, symmetric, pain-free arcs of motion, particularly in rotation, exclude intraarticular disease of the hip as an explanation for the hip pain, and the diagnostic evaluation is redirected (Table 9.1). Compromise in motion is not totally specific; psoas irritation can be provoked with internal rotation in extension, and femoral and sciatic stretch signs can confound this examination (though with care such stretching is avoidable in discerning hip motion—as illustrated in Fig. 9.2). With such provisos, compromised range of motion strongly suggests intraarticular disease.

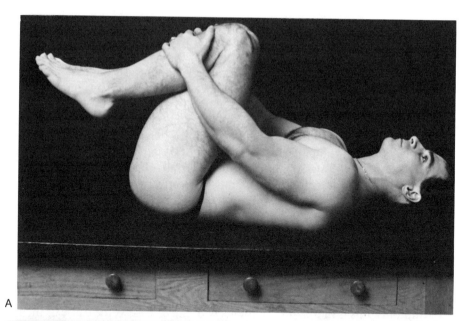

A

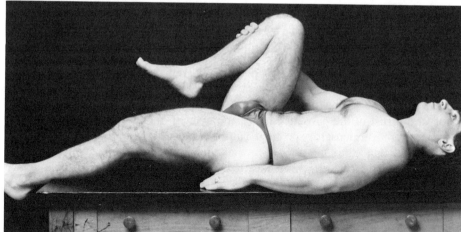

B

FIG. 9.1. The detection of a flexion contracture of the hip. The knees are drawn up to the knee-chest position as tolerated (**A**). Then one leg at a time is extended while the contralateral knee-chest position is maintained (**B**). The knee-chest position flattens the lumbar lordosis. The ability to extend the leg so that it is flat on the table requires some 30° of extension at the hip. Extension as limited as demonstrated would indicate a 30° flexion contracture.

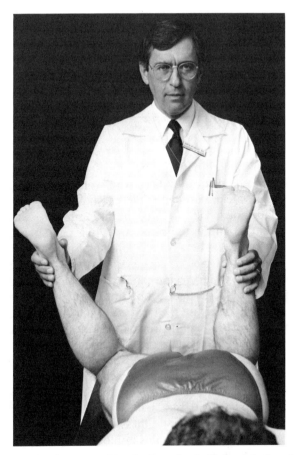

FIG. 9.2. Rotations of the hip are traditionally determined with the patient supine. However, the illustrated maneuver is more sensitive to subtle abnormalities and more specific for intraarticular pathology. With the patient prone and the knee flexed, the hip is rotated in extension. One is seeking asymmetry in range of motion. If the patient can tolerate the prone position, restricted rotations suggest intraarticular pathology as rotation in extension is less likely to be confounded by the stretch signs of radiculopathy.

Bursitis

There are at least 18 bursae periarticular to the hip. Ascribing hip pain to "bursitis" is a venerable assertion, although generally tenuous at best. Of all of these bursae, three are invoked as the cause of hip pain with localized tenderness: the ischiogluteal, iliopectineal, and trochanteric. Ischiogluteal bursitis is "weaver's bottom"; there is said to be pain and tenderness over the ischial prominence, reflecting inflammation in this bursa. However, as is true for all of

TABLE 9.1. *Differential diagnosis of referred "hip" pain*

Hernias: Richter's, femoral
Abscesses: psoas, pelvic
Radiculopathy: T-12, L-1, L-2
Entrapment neuropathy: meralgia, obturator
Knee disease
Ureteral colic

these bursitides, frank inflammation is not a feature. Furthermore, the condition is rarely diagnosed, even in cyclists, who would seem at particular risk. Contemporary diagnosticians are more likely to be impressed that the tenderness is near the sciatic notch and to ascribe the discomfort to sciatica rather than bursitis. In any event, attention to posture usually is palliative.

The trochanteric bursa lies between the tendon of the gluteus maximus and the posterolateral prominence of the greater trochanter. Trochanteric bursitis is a common label affixed to hip region pain with peritrochanteric tenderness. Usually, the tenderness is restricted to a point that is posterior and superior to the trochanter, quite distant from the location of the bursa, which is 3 to 4 cm deep to the skin posterolateral to the trochanter. Injecting local anesthetic and corticosteroid into the tender tissue is common practice and is associated with transient relief. However, transient benefit from empirical injection therapy is far from convincing support of the pathogenetic inference; such experimental support is long overdue. Until then, trochanteric bursitis is no more than a descriptive label for hip pain with focal tenderness. As we have learned for other examples of regional musculoskeletal illness, many regional diseases, such as subtle radiculopathies, can present in this fashion, requiring only explanations and patience and not multiple injections and trials of analgesic and antiinflammatory drugs.

My skepticism heightens for the concept of iliopectineal bursitis. This bursa is contiguous with the capsule of the hip and separates the iliopsoas muscle from the iliopectineal eminence. It occasionally communicates with the synovial cavity of the hip. Since it lies medially in Scarpa's triangle, it is said to cause pain in the anterior pelvis, groin, and thigh exacerbated with movement. However, the diagnosis eludes all contemporary modalities for confirmation, and the number of viable competing explanations remains overwhelming. Iliopectineal bursitis is a heuristic label—as may be many of the regional musculoskeletal illnesses ascribed to "bursitis."

Intraarticular and Periarticular Diseases of the Hip

Osteoarthritis is the most common disease of the hip and, probably, the explanation for most hip pain. However, there is a differential diagnosis.

Infection

Most individuals with septic hip or with osteomyelitis of the femur or pelvis will not be misdiagnosed with a regional disease. Fever, rest pain, or pain at night will provide compelling clues to direct the diagnostician to appropriate imaging studies and diagnostic aspirations. There is a pitfall in that all of these infections can be quite insidious in onset and progression. This is particularly true for tuberculous arthritis. Any systemic symptom or suggestion of night/rest pain should place the diagnostician on guard.

Primary Neoplasms of the Hip Joint

There are primary tumors of the synovium and metaplastic conditions such as pigmented villonodular synovitis. These present with the picture of arthritis with pain and restriction of motion. The diagnosis requires a high index of suspicion; usually there is a degree of destruction on plane radiographs and increased activity on scintiscanning. Pigmented villonodular synovitis is suspected when synovialysis reveals bloody fluid and synovial biopsy documents infiltration with hemosiderin-laden macrophages. Fortunately, both primary tumors and pigmented villonodular synovitis are rare lesions and are particularly rare at the hip; more accessible joints such as the knee (1) are targeted. It is also true that cancer rarely metastasizes to any synovial bed, an observation that suggests insights into the pathogenesis of metastasis that still elude investigators. In fact, of all neoplasms, only lymphoproliferative diseases, multiple myeloma, and leukemia (particularly in childhood) infiltrate the synovium with any regularity. While intraarticular neoplasms are not much of a worry, periarticular neoplasms are an important consideration.

Malignant Primary Bone Tumors

Malignant primary bone tumors about the hip are rare in the adult. Chondrosarcoma has a predilection for the femur and pelvis and a peak incidence in the fifth and sixth decades. Giant cell tumors usually present in the third or fourth decade, with a propensity for the end of a long bone. Ewing's sarcoma also has a predilection for the femur and occurs even earlier. With all of these primary tumors, the presenting symptom is pain in the region of the lesion, often with nocturnal exacerbation. Each produces radiographically discernible bony destruction and can lead to pathologic fractures. However, past midlife, primary tumors are far less frequent than metastatic lesions to the hip and pelvis. Again, the clue is pain that is prominent at rest and at night. Imaging techniques are localizing, and biopsy is diagnostic.

Osteoid Osteoma

Osteoid osteoma is a benign focus of dysplasia consisting of an osteoid nidus surrounded by an osteosclerotic zone. The lesion is unifocal and can occur throughout the appendicular skeleton. However, 20% of osteoid osteomas occur in the proximal femur and another 10% occur in the pelvis. The typical patient presents in the second decade of life, although the onset of symptoms in the third and even fourth decade is well described. The symptoms are characteristic: dull aching pain prominent at rest and at night and relieved by activity or nonsteroidal antiinflammatory drugs, classically aspirin. With hip region involvement there may be an antalgic gait but rarely signs of intraarticular inflammation. The osteoma can often be discerned on plane radiographs as a small, round lesion with a lucent center. It is hypervascular and therefore readily detected by scintigraphy. Surgery is a reasonable option with persistent or severe symptoms; however, the natural history is one of spontaneous regression in symptoms after 4 to 6 yr of illness.

Transient Osteoporosis and Avascular Necrosis

Transient osteoporosis of the hip is a form of reflex sympathetic dystrophy. This process is far more common in the upper extremity and was discussed in the previous chapter. Osteonecrosis, also termed aseptic or avascular necrosis (AVN), is far more common in the lower extremity and particularly at the femoral head. The etiology is unclear; there appears to be a compromise in the maintenance of the structural integrity of the subchondral bone of the femoral head. Microfracturing, progressive collapse, and ineffective repair result. In all likelihood, judging from the clinical settings in which AVN is most prevalent (Table 9.2), the initiating factors are diverse, but there may be a final common pathway to collapse of the femoral head and secondary osteoarthritis of the hip. For example, fracture of the neck of the femur can directly compromise blood

TABLE 9.2. *Clinical settings in which avascular necrosis of bone is most prevalent*

Established associations
    Fracture of the femoral neck
    Hypercorticism
    Systemic lupus erythematosus
    Irradiation
    Gaucher's disease
    Decompression sickness
Suggested associations
    Alcoholism
    Some congenital malformations
    Pancreatitis

supply to the head. However, the explanation for systemic lupus erythematosus or hypercorticism is less facile. There is some suggestion of venous hypertension in the femoral neck and a further suggestion that early "core decompression" can halt what is otherwise inexorable progression. However, the experience with this procedure is far from uniform, suggesting either that the theory is flawed or that there are alternative explanations in some cases. It is also important to realize that transient osteoporosis of the hip can mimic early AVN in symptoms and by all imaging techniques including MR (2); however, the former is self-limited without destructive potential. The symptoms of AVN are pain at rest and with weight bearing accompanied by signs on examination of intraarticular inflammation. Early on, plane radiographs are normal; one must resort to scintiscanning or, more definitively, to magnetic resonance imaging for diagnosis.

Osteoarthritis of the Hip

Osteoarthritis is the major intraarticular disease of the hip in the adult. Table 9.3 documents the age-dependent prevalence of severe osteoarthritis in the United States based on a household survey performed 20 yr ago.

By age 80, some 2% of Americans will have severe osteoarthritis of a hip. Another 2% will have less severe involvement. These are small but impressive numbers. However, they pale in comparison to the number of Americans who experience pain in the hip region in any given month. The distinction between a pathologic condition in a musculoskeletal region (the disease) and symptoms in the same region (the illness) is critical to understanding all regional musculoskeletal disorders. The discordance between disease and illness is far more striking than the concordance. For example, over 40% of the individuals whose hip osteoarthritis was detected in the NHANES I survey (Table 9.3) could recall no symptoms of hip illness in the previous month. A similar degree of sensitivity to illness pertains to physical signs on examination. This concept of disease-illness discordance will be developed shortly when we consider knee pain. Here we will focus on the hip joint and its disease.

TABLE 9.3. *Prevalence of Grade 3–4 osteoarthritis of the hip*

Age (yr)	Number examined	Prevalence (%) in men	Prevalence (%) in women
25–34	672	0.2	—
35–44	528	—	—
45–54	746	0.1	—
55–64	1,288	0.7	1.6
65–74	1,233	2.3	1.2

From Maurer, ref. 9.

The Definition of Osteoarthritis as a Disease

Osteoarthritis is defined as a form of pathologic condition. For the clinician, the diagnosis conjures up compromised joint motion and radiographic abnormality (and an ill-conceived assumption that there will be associated symptoms). Defining the limits of normal, including the radiographic limits, is difficult. Even grading the magnitude of established disease is difficult; interobserver reliability does not reach 50%. That is because of the wide variation in the width of the normal joint space and in the willingness to label irregularities of bone at the joint margin as osteophytes.

The normal hip joint is incongruous; with weight bearing a lateral rim of the cartilage of the femoral head is brought into contact with a restricted weight-bearing region of the acetabular dome. The weight-bearing cartilage is thicker with sparser chondrocytes. With aging, the joint becomes more congruous, bringing the more atrophic cartilage into contact and accounting for the difference in angulation. This alteration in femoral head tilt has been held to be pathogenetic for osteoarthritis but is more likely a benign consequence of aging (3).

Osteoarthritis is the process of loss of articulating cartilage accompanied by ineffective repair by the remaining cartilage and adjacent bone. The dominant theory pivots on biomechanical insult. Sheering forces interrupt the collagen network such that the articular cartilage loses the ability to restrain the swelling pressure of the glycosaminoglycans and imbibes water. This swollen cartilage seems further vulnerable to disruption by sheering forces. However, there is an alternative hypothesis based on the fact that cartilage biology is highly dynamic. After all, cartilage is a living tissue with turnover rates measured in weeks. One could argue that osteoarthritis is a disease of ineffective repair rather than biomechanical insult. This perspective suggests that influences that support connective tissue repair, such as repetitive motion, would retard the process. It also suggests that osteoarthritis might be a target for pharmacologic reversal rather than interventional resignation until it is time for salvage. For now, clinicians have little to offer other than to document the progressive loss of cartilage, the reactive formation of bony spurs (osteophytes), which are cartilage covered and form at the joint margins, and the degradation of the elegant subchondral bony plate into an irregular, coarse structure riddled with cysts. Such is osteoarthritis, a sclerotic, damaged joint whose only redeeming feature is a diminished likelihood of fracture (4).

Fortunately, and inexplicably, osteoarthritis targets very few joints in an individual. There is some tendency to symmetry, but little to multifocality. Patients with osteoarthritis of the hip are no more likely to suffer osteoarthritis of any other joint than are sex- and age-matched individuals whose hips are spared. Furthermore, obesity does not predispose to hip osteoarthritis. There are some data to the contrary, but they are neither impressive nor reproducible. The inferences that derive from these observations have important ramifications regarding the pathogenesis of osteoarthritis in general and of the hip in particular; usage cannot be a primary or even a major precipitating influence. Otherwise the same individual whose hip is afflicted should have the knee at risk, and this is not the case. Furthermore, with or without osteoarthritis of the hip or knee, the ankle is always spared. If usage or obesity were influencing the proximal disease in an important fashion, it is hard to imagine the mechanism by which the ankle escapes the insult.

The Management of Osteoarthritis of the Hip

Total hip replacement is an extraordinary advance, certainly assuming a place of honor in the pantheon of 20th century advances. In the hands of an accomplished surgeon, the patient with regional hip disease who is otherwise well has every reason to anticipate pain-free ambulation with a normal gait within a month of surgery. No other joint has yielded to the onslaught of reconstructive surgery in such a gratifying fashion. This probably reflects the inherent stability of the normal hip and of its prosthetic replacements; other joints depend to a greater extent on extraarticular supporting structures for stability and function. Because the outcome is so favorable, appropriate advice is more demanding of the wisdom of the physician and the quality of patient-doctor rapport. Total hip replacement is an elective procedure that should be postponed until the risk/benefit ratio becomes compelling. More than one patient tolerates crutch walking rather than assume the risks; others seek the surgical solution early on. There are features that tend to dissuade one from electing total hip replacement for osteoarthritis of the hip.

If pain with weight bearing or intermittent painful locking (probably reflecting loose bodies or osteophytic encroachment of the arc of motion) are the principal indication for surgery, palliation with drugs is likely and intermittency of symptoms is possible. Pain is well managed only if perspective is maintained.

If restriction in motion is the issue, adaptation is possible mainly by altering behavior. A handicap in golf is a tenuous surgical indication. Discussions of perceived disabilities can often lead to recommendations regarding mobility that are palliative and postpone the need to elect surgery, sometimes for years.

Although the patient has every right to anticipate a favorable outcome, catastrophic postoperative risks are measurable. There is a risk of death from any of a number of complications, most of which are related to diseases of the cardiovascular system. The procedure is lengthy, fluid shifts are considerable, and a degree of hypothermia is employed. This risk is low, less than 0.01%, in major series—although one must realize that the experience of "major series" may not generalize to surgeons or surgical groups with less experience.

There is a risk of infection of the prosthesis, which may respond to prolonged antibiotic therapy but may not, in which case removal of the prosthesis without substitution is the standard of therapy, the Girdlestone procedure. Gait is supported by the gluteal muscles rather than the hip; the outcome is less compromise than one might imagine—but still catastrophic. This risk is also low, less than 0.1%, in major series and clearly is dependent on the experience and technique of the surgical team.

There is a risk of viral transmission from transfusions. This risk is eliminated with autochthonous transfusions; patients store their own blood in anticipation of the procedure. Otherwise, the risk of non-A, non-B hepatitis and HIV transmission persists even though it has been dramatically reduced by appropriate blood bank screening.

There is a likelihood of thrombophlebitis, approaching 50%. However, with any one of a number of local measures and/or anticoagulation schemes, the risk of sequelae, including pulmonary emboli or chronic thrombophlebitis, is low.

Not all outcomes are favorable. Pain can return for any of several reasons. The prosthesis can loosen. Traditionally, the metallic components are seated in bone with methyl methacrylate glue. Recently, surgeons have also been utilizing porous metals that permit bony ingrowth for anchoring. Failure rates vary, although all are acceptably low once the decision is made for surgery.

There are soft-tissue pain syndromes, many of which occur in the setting of heterotopic bone formation, particularly myositis ossificans. This complication has been minimized by surgical approaches that do not require exposure by virtue of elevating the greater trochanter. Nonetheless, some ossification is often apparent, although it is usually asymptomatic. The exception is in patients with ankylosing spondylitis, where this complication can be clinically significant in as many as 10% of patients. The current solution utilizes low-dose, postoperative external radiation; this maneuver and/or improved surgical technique seems to have decreased the complication substantially.

The prosthesis has a finite life expectancy. Furthermore, since inherent repair is impossible, the longevity is inversely dependent on the quantity of use/abuse. Weight-bearing exercises are to be avoided and non–weight-bearing usage encouraged. If the patient is seeking surgery to permit a return to jogging, for example, he or she should be disabused. Cycling makes more sense and is better advice preoperatively. With care, a successful prosthesis has a life expectancy measured in decades.

The management of the patient with hip osteoarthritis is a process of compromise until the specter of postoperative catastrophe, albeit remote, becomes tolerable. Even if the risk is only 1 in 1,000, the physician should have exercised sufficient forethought to be able to look the patient or the patient's family in the eye should catastrophe eventuate. The path to this decision is not one of benign neglect. It is important that thigh musculature be maintained for optimal function during the years of conservative management and for optimal postoperative function. Exercise regimens with little weight bearing should be emphasized: cycling, swimming, quadriceps setting, etc. Although there are reservations (which have been brought to realizations for the knee), nonsteroidal antiinflammatory agents are traditionally offered in this setting. The patients with hip osteoarthritis tend to be younger than patients with knee pain in the setting of knee osteoarthritis and perhaps that is why drug toxicity is not as associated with the treatment of hip pain as with the treatment of knee pain.

KNEE PAIN

Knee pain is remarkably common. Based on a national household survey, 10% of Americans experience at least 1 mo of significant daily knee pain each year. This frequency increases as we age, from 6% in the third decade of life to 18% in the seventh, with a slight preponderance of female sufferers. The individual who feels compelled to seek medical attention should be greeted with diagnostic wariness. After all, seldom is this their first experience with knee pain; something about its quality and/or duration has precipitated the choice to be a patient. Fortunately, since the knee is so accessible, most diagnostic uncertainty can be dispelled with a thorough initial history and physical examination. Clues to systemic disease and for arthritis elsewhere are sought. Then the painful knee is examined closely. Overt inflammation, whether from trauma, some form of synovitis (including infected or crystal induced), or hemarthrosis, is usually obvious; there may be warmth, even erythema, obvious effusion, and spontaneous posturing in 30° of flexion to diminish intraarticular pressure. However, it behooves the clinician to learn to identify subtle inflammation of the knee. It is possible to detect small synovial effusions if one learns to elicit a "bulge sign" (Fig. 9.3). One can demonstrate a bulge sign in some asymptomatic knees; for example, in as many as 10% of women beyond midlife who are overweight. However, the bulge sign in the symptomatic patient leads to one of the most useful diagnostic maneuvers in clinical medicine—the diagnostic arthrocentesis. Clinicians should be accomplished in aspirating several milliliters of fluid for synovialysis. Synovialysis offers a wealth of diagnostic information (Table 9.4).

The patient who has mechanical knee pain without effusion or with a noninflammatory effusion has regional knee pain. This knee pain is quite discordant from radiographic abnormalities of the knee. This holds even in the seventh decade but is the rule earlier in life. Ascribing knee pain to pathoanatomic aberrations in and about the knee is a tenuous exercise (5). However, it is the traditional exercise and contains some nubbins of truth.

The Patellofemoral Pain Syndrome

The quality of knee pain experienced in the earlier decades of adult life and echoed again by some in the later decades is distinctive. The description is of the insidious onset of pain localizing anteriorly or anteromedially. It is occasionally

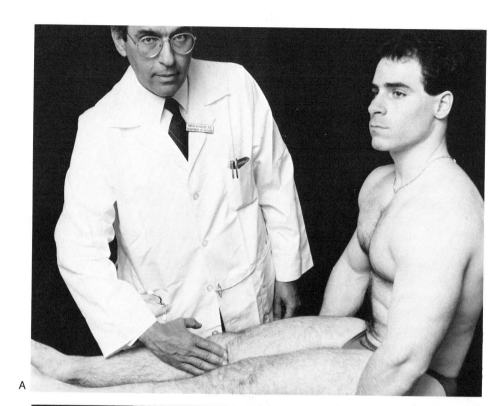

A

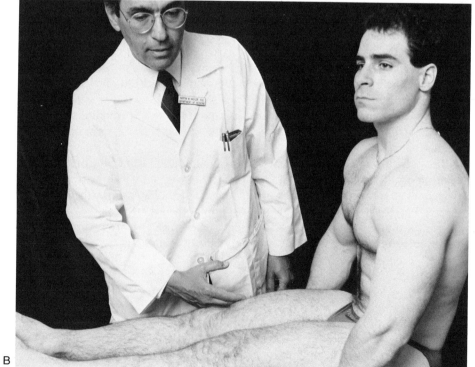

B

FIG. 9.3.

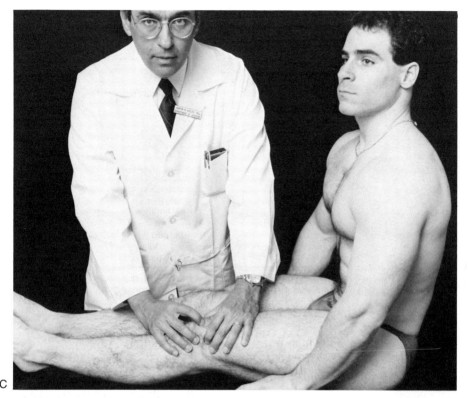

C

FIG. 9.3. The detection of a subtle synovial effusion. The most subtle sign that there is sufficient fluid to render arthrocentesis productive is called the "bulge sign." With the knee extended and relaxed, the medial aspect is stroked with a cephalad motion (**A**). Then the lateral aspect is stroked with a caudad motion (**B**) and the medial aspect is observed for outpouching, or the bulge. With a larger effusion, the patella can be made to float by simultaneously compressing medial and lateral aspects; the floating is detected by a "click" when the patella is depressed onto the condyles (**C**).

bilateral. Women are more likely to bring this discomfort to medical attention. The discomfort is exacerbated by activity, especially going up and down stairs, as opposed to most other forms of knee pain, where descending is more difficult. Prolonged sitting ("the movie sign") aggravates the discomfort. Other symptoms such as joint noise or a sense of momentary "catching" over the final arc of extension are less specific. On examination, there is often tenderness elicited by maneuvering the patellofemoral articulation.

Attempts to ascribe this presentation to pathoanatomy of the patellofemoral joint are unconvincing. Data addressing the reliability, specificity, and validity of differences in patellofemoral biomechanics, including forces, alignment, and tracking, is unconvincing short of frank dislocations. Chondromalacia patellae is an age-dependent surface degeneration targeting the central and medial part

TABLE 9.4. *Interpretation of synovialysis*

Type of effusion	Hallmark	Disease association	Special feature
Noninflammatory	Mononuclear cell predominence, usually 100s/mm³	Normal fluid Trauma Osteoarthritis SLE	
Inflammatory	Granulocyte predominence	Inflammatory arthritides (*RA*, etc.)	
		Infection	+ cultures
		Gout	Urate crystals
		Pseudogout	CPPD crystals
		Parainfection (DGI, SBE)	Appropriate cultures +
Bloody	Grossly blood tinged	Intraarticular fracture	Bone spicules or fat droplets
		Pigmented villonodular synovitis	+ synovial biopsy

SLE, systemic lupus erythematosus; RA, rheumatoid arthritis; DGI, disseminated gonococcal infection; SBE, subacute bacterial endocarditis; CPPD, calcium pyrophosphate dihydrate.

of the transverse ridge, which progresses to central and lateral denudation of bone, sparing the odd facet. However, the process is demonstrable in 50% of the young adult population and ubiquitous in the elderly. Ascribing symptoms to such pathologic conditions is an insurmountable biostatistical challenge.

Given these limitations to current pathogenetic hypotheses for patellofemoral pain, surgical interventions remain purely empirical. One is well advised to take recourse in the benignity of the natural history, which has long been documented.

Synovial Plicae

Plicae are folds of synovium that are remnants of the embryologic development of the synovial sac. The ontogeny of the knee is a process of fusion of three cavities, the suprapatellar, medial, and lateral. Frequently, a fold of synovium remains in four characteristic locations: suprapatellar, medial, lateral, and infrapatellar (the "ligamentum mucosum"). From cadaveric studies, 50% of knees have plicae.

Plicae have been recognized for generations and long held to be individual differences to which no symptoms were ascribable. This has changed with the use of arthroscopy to evaluate unexplained knee pain in the United States. Visualizing the cause of knee pain in many younger patients is an exercise in inferential leaping; visualizing the unexpected commandeers logic. As the zeal tempers, only the medial plica is generally implicated in the minds of arthroscopists. During flexion, the medial plica crosses the femoral condyle. It is thought that trauma, including the trauma of repetitive motion, perhaps in the setting of subtle malalignment, is a stressor that elicits inflammation. The symptom ascribed to this process is the patellofemoral pain syndrome with the addition of a sensation of medial snapping or popping. The medial joint line is tender and the plica can be palpated, particularly if the knee is examined in 20° of flexion. Arthroscopic excision is performed in the absence of a controlled trial—but against my advice in the case of my patients.

Internal Derangements

For stability the knee is totally dependent on extra- and intraarticular ligaments. These structures are best viewed as an integrated restraining continuum; they have considerable effect on more global knee function. The menisci serve major functions in knee joint biology: They contribute to stability by increasing the congruence between tibial and femoral surfaces. They absorb the shock of weight bearing and contribute to distributing the load; even in the standing posture menisci bear as much as 50% of the load. The lateral menisci bear the entire force of the load on the lateral compartment; the medial menisci share half the load with the cartilage of the medial plateau. Menisci enhance distribution of fluid and contribute to the low coefficient of friction within the joint. Finally, menisci function as spacers in preventing the impingement of adjacent structures during joint apposition.

Internal derangement is the term used to describe abnormalities in intraarticular structures. The collateral ligaments are susceptible to strain, and the menisci are susceptible to disruption, even in the absence of discrete and forceful trauma. The classic symptoms of meniscal disease include locking, instability, effusions, and pain at the joint line. Locking occurs more often in anterior tears. Instability, "giving way," occurs more often in posterior tears but is described with many internal derangements. These symptoms and the various orthopedic signs used to detect internal derangements have severely limited sensitivity and specificity; one study documented a 22% false-negative and a 33% false-positive rate for the clinical assessment of medial meniscal tears. Furthermore, even in the orthopedic setting, with its overt accrual bias, 20% of patients diagnosed with "a probable meniscal tear" experience spontaneous remission of their symptoms. If these data are not enough cause for diagnostic and therapeutic circumspection, the experience with surgical meniscectomy is further daunting. One decade after the procedure, 70% of the operated knees remain symptomatic; by two decades, 40% manifest degenerative joint disease. Of course, this may reflect primary cartilage damage that occurred coincident with the meniscal damage and which would have progressed without the meniscectomy. However, there are no data supporting such an assertion. The contemporary arthroscopic meniscectomy is a major advance in surgical technology and in operative and perioperative morbidity. Long-term results must await long-term follow-up. We may learn that arthroscopic meniscectomy offers far more advantage to the surgeon in terms of technical facility and income than it offers advantage to the patient with knee pain. Furthermore, we may learn this lesson from the potentially bitter long-term experience of the many thousands of Americans who submit to the intervention unaware that it is an unproven remedy. Unproven or not, it ranks among the most frequent surgical procedures performed in the United States and has been the most frequent in several recent years.

Osteoarthritis of the Knee

Osteoarthritis is a well-defined pathoanatomic entity readily demonstrable by modern imaging techniques. For a century the pathologic condition that is this disease has been ingrained in the mind of every medical student: inexorable progression from subtle biochemical alterations in articular cartilage through cartilage loss and reactive bone formation to the end-stage of eburnated bone and exuberant osteophytosis. We all shudder at the image of the patient suffering with end-stage osteoarthritis, bedeviled by a deformed, unstable, incapacitating, and painful knee. What physician can listen to the complaint of knee pain without conjuring up the image of such an outcome? What physician can see an osteophyte on x-ray without inferring that it reflects the process that is causing the knee to hurt? How many patients with knee pain have learned that an end-stage knee is to be their fate? How many have come to understand that all we can offer is empathy and antiinflammatory drugs until, some day, they must limp before a surgeon seeking relief?

Osteoarthritis is indeed a well-defined pathoanatomic entity. However, the traditional clinical construct, *osteoarthritis,* is a paralogism. There is a body of information that allows a far more reasonable and useful approach to the patient with knee pain. Recent papers examining the benefit of structured exercise programs and weight reduction (6,7) contribute to this enlightenment.

The epidemiology of osteoarthritis and the epidemiology of knee pain have little in common—not nothing in common but surprisingly little in common (8). Multiple surveys in several countries bear witness to this fact. The relevant data from one such survey are presented in Table 9.5. This was a household survey undertaken by the National Center for Health Statistics in the 1970s (9) with follow-up of the patients with osteoarthritis 10 yr later (10). Clearly, at all ages, more of us suffer knee pain than bear radiographic stigmata of osteoarthritis of the knee. True, those with more severe radiographic disease are somewhat more likely to experience difficulty with activities requiring mobility (9) . However, progression of radiographic osteoarthritis of the knee is slow and not predictable, whereas symptoms can exacerbate or regress regardless of radiographic progression (11). This dissonance between the disease, osteoarthritis, and the illness, "osteoarthritis," may be counterintuitive, but it is incontrovertible.

TABLE 9.5. *Percentage of the U.S. population that recalls experiencing at least 1 month of daily knee pain in the past year contrasted with the prevalence of any radiographically demonstrable knee osteoarthritis*

Age (yr)	Symptoms of knee pain (%)		Radiographic osteoarthritis (%)	
	Men	Women	Men	Women
25–34	5.7	5.2		
35–44	7.4	8.1		
45–54	12.0	11.5	2.3	3.6
55–64	11.5	15.0	4.0	7.2
65–74	14.9	19.7	8.4	17.9
25–74	9.5	10.9		

From Maurer, ref. 9.

The NHANES data (Table 9.5) do more than make this point. They raise a telling corollary issue. How can nearly 10% of the adult population cope with a month or more of knee pain each year without the benefit of diagnostic imaging or prescription drugs or surgical intervention? If you think it is because they have less extensive pathoanatomy, reread the previous paragraph. Rather, there must be personal resources that permit all of these people with knee pain to persevere until the symptoms subside. Those who choose to be patients do so because they have exhausted their reserves. What shakes their confidence? Certainly, the unstable, diseased knee might. But not always. In fact, if one examines several influences that might account for the perception of severity of knee pain, the magnitude of osteoarthritis pales in comparison to psychosocial variables (12). To some important extent, the complaint of pain in the knee, with or without incapacity, is a surrogate for difficulty coping with pain in the knee. Without awareness of this phenomenon, the physician is all too wont to seek nothing but osteoarthritis and to reach for a prescription pad or a scalpel. With awareness of the degree to which knee pain may be a surrogate complaint, other options become apparent.

This is the context in which a study of the role of weight-bearing exercise for incapacitating knee pain (6) was conducted and the possibility that weight reduction might be palliative (7) was explored. Both hypotheses would seem doomed if one is wedded to the teaching that osteoarthritis is inexorable and the end-stage joint is its legacy. But both groups of investigators were able to demonstrate benefit with interventions that provide a biomechanically more favorable knee and a psychologically more favorable milieu in which to cope.

Is there more to do for knee pain? Antiinflammatory agents offer less benefit (13) than their potential for toxicity (14). In fact, acetaminophen probably offers as much palliation as any nonsteroidal antiinflammatory drug (15). Reconstructive surgery for the knee remains a salvage option mainly for the elderly. In younger decades (Table 9.5) surgical interventions are too often unproven remedies foisted on those who carry the anxiety and uncertainty associated with such inane labels as chondromalacia patellae or synovial plicae, both incidental findings. It is also an unproven remedy for all those who ambulate with reasonable comfort in spite of the detection of anterior cruciate ligament damage or other internal derangements. Imaging, "repair," and "rehabilitation," medicalize what others find within their range of coping. To whose benefit?

Some day, we hope, there will be interventions that can be shown to impede the progression of osteoarthritis and obviate the need to contend with the end-stage knee. But even these interventions are unlikely to obviate the need to cope with knee pain. There will never be a substitute for perspective, insight, and sound advice.

FOOT PAIN

The foot is a remarkable structure. Just consider that, when we run, each foot distributes some 6 times our body weight in a gliding and stable fashion with each step and seldom with symptoms. To accomplish this, an intact and healthy integument is necessary, as is an integrated spring-like musculoskeletal array. There are many disorders of the integument and many systemic diseases that can present as foot pain and/or compromise this function. Here we will touch on diseases of the integument and focus on the musculoskeletal array and its derangements, which underlie regional musculoskeletal illness of the foot.

The Principle Diseases of the Integument of the Foot

Corns and calluses are the banes of the existence of so many people that their management is the bread and butter of a free-standing profession, chiropody or podiatry. That podiatry thrives is a testament to the effectiveness of their therapeutics as well as a reproach to rheumatology and to orthopedics, which disciplines traditionally downplay these diseases of the integument in their training programs and practices.

Both calluses and corns form where pressure or friction is repetitively applied to the foot in gait. Both are hyperkeratotic responses of the epidermis. The soles of the feet, particularly the heel and over the metatarsal heads, are normally callused. However, thickly callused feet are at risk for painful fissures and, possibly, compromise in the comfort of gait if the callusing is extreme. Attention to skin hydration and to footwear is prophylactic and palliative. Rarely should paring of the calluses or the application of keratolytic agents be necessary.

Corns are painful lesions. They are most common on the dorsolateral aspect of the fifth metatarsal, suggesting that this is an epidermal response to chronic abrasion from ill-fitting footwear. A corn is a sharply demarcated hyperkeratotic lesion. Paring of a corn, unlike that of a callus, will remove a discrete, avascular, translucent, central core.

Diseases of the nails rival calluses and corns in prevalence and nuisance. Ingrown toenails are painful, may lead to paronychia, and require skilled attention. Onychomycosis is the other blight of nails notable for nuisance. This is a fungal infestation of keratin by species of *Trichophyton* and occasionally *Candida albicans,* often associated with infestation of intertriginous skin between the toes. The initial infestation is an asymptomatic white and then brown patch on top of one or two nails, which may remain stable for years in spite of the rapid turnover of the nail itself. However, the process can progress so that the nail becomes thickened and friable. Extension to the base is common, as is involvement of the nail plate itself. Then the nail becomes cracked, is destroyed, and separates from the plate. Occasionally, there is mild discomfort; more severe discomfort suggests a complicating paronychia. Invasion of the deeper tissues or metastasis is exceedingly rare. The only reliable treatment is systemic antibiotic therapy with griseofulvin, but seldom is even the relatively low risk of toxicity (mainly hypersensitivity reactions) justifiable, and recurrence is common. Hygiene should be advised; topical antifungal agents may be tried, but seldom is the effort rewarded.

Regional Musculoskeletal Diseases of the Foot

The array of the midfoot creates a longitudinal arch running along the medial border from the first metatarsophalangeal (MTP) joint to the tuberosity of the calcaneus (Fig. 9.4). The forefoot is arrayed as a transverse arch between the first and fifth MTP joints, with an axis that transects the necks of the second, third, and fourth metatarsals (Fig. 9.5). Gait involves first heel strike, then planting and stabilizing or "stance" on the first and fifth metatarsal heads, and push-off from the first MTP and hallux. The arches are the springs that dissipate

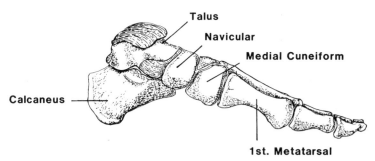

FIG. 9.4. The medial aspect of the bony array of the foot. Gait involves heel strike, then stance on the first and fifth distal metatarsals, followed by push-off at the first metatarsophalangeal joint. The arch serves as a spring to dissipate some of the considerable forces involved.

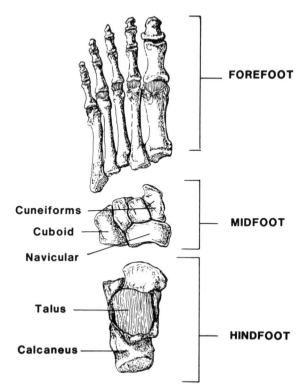

FOREFOOT

Cuneiforms

Cuboid   MIDFOOT

Navicular

Talus

HINDFOOT

Calcaneus

FIG. 9.5. The bony array of the foot is conveniently categorized as forefoot, midfoot, and hind-foot. Each region has characteristic pathologic and symptom complexes.

the force. Close observation of a patient's gait can greatly enhance diagnostic inferences regarding disorders of the feet. There are many individual differences in the normal foot; the most common is pes planus, often associated with increased valgus of more proximal structures. It is remarkable how seldom such individuals suffer foot pain. Yet, those who do are greeted with a wealth of orthotic devices attempting to adjust gait with undocumented success. Likewise, the common finding of leg length discrepancy, even in terms of an inch, seems to elicit the prescription of a lifting device in spite of the inability to demonstrate correlative symptoms in systematic studies. Fortunately, society is demanding control over the form and function of footwear by virtue of consumer demand and choice. The purveyor is required to attend to comfort in the face of individual differences.

Heel Pain

Most regional musculoskeletal illness of the foot localizes to the heel or the transverse arch. As for the heel, the differential diagnosis is limited to entities some of which are patent on examination: plantaris rupture, retrocalcaneal bursitis, "pump bumps" (granulomas at the site of chronic irritation from footwear, usually the distal Achilles tendon). Usually, the discomfort is with heel strike and the examination localizes tenderness to the tuberosity of the calcaneus (Fig. 9.6). There is no reason to x-ray such a patient; the finding of an exostosis (a "spur") is nonspecific. Furthermore, injection therapy with anesthetic or corticosteroid is counterintuitive and unsupported by trial. The intuitively appealing intervention is to unload the heel by utilizing orthotics that disperse the pain until the process heals.

Metatarsalgia

Metatarsalgia describes a series of conditions presenting as pain in some part of the transverse arch. Often there is no overt explanation, rendering palliation by gait adjustment with footwear or a metatarsal bar a reasonable empirical trial. There may be focal tenderness in the sesamoids associated with the first MTP joint or in the neck of a metatarsal, often the fourth. These structures are susceptible to insufficiency fractures ("stress" or "march" fractures). Treatment is reassurance and advice as to gait adjustment.

Morton's neuroma is a neurofibroma or angioneurofibroma involving the large superficial branch of the external plantar nerve as it courses between metatarsal heads, usually in the more lateral web spaces. The presentation is with paresthesias or cramplike pain, usually near the fourth metatarsal head and usually exacerbated when shoes are worn. Hyperesthesias are present in the involved web space. The management is gait adjustment in an attempt to reduce impingement. Surgical exploration is an option if symptoms persist.

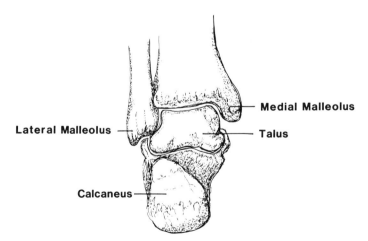

FIG. 9.6. The calcaneus suffers the impact of heel strike transduced through the talus. Reactive bone formation, "heel spurs," are common at the site of impact. However, degenerative changes of the articulating surfaces of the hindfoot are rare.

Hallux Rigidus

Hallux rigidus and hallux valgus are deformities that usually occur as a consequence of degenerative disease of the first MTP joint. The latter is part of the bunion complex, usually seen in the later decades of life. Hallux rigidus can occur much earlier, leading to speculations as to etiology, such as osteochondritis desiccans of the first metatarsal head or congenital malalignment. Both conditions impede gait by interfering with push off at the hallux. Furthermore, both are associated with osteophytosis, which, when exuberant, can interfere with the effectiveness of footwear. The range of interventions commences with adaptive footwear and moves on to a menu of inventive surgical empiricisms.

REFERENCES

1. Gumpel JM, Shawe DJ. Diffuse pigmented villonodular synovitis: non-surgical management. *Ann Rheum Dis* 1991;50:531–3.
2. Hauzeur J-P, Hanquinet S, Genenois P-A, Appelboom T, Bentin J, Perlmutter N. Study of magnetic resonance imaging in transient osteoporosis of the hip. *J Rheumatol* 1991;18:1211–7.
3. Croft P, Cooper C, Wickham C, Coggon D. Osteoarthritis of the hip and acetabular dysplasia. *Ann Rheum Dis* 1991;50:308–10.
4. Cooper C, Cook PI, Osmond C, Fisher L, Cawley MID. Osteoarthritis of the hip and osteoporosis of the proximal femur. *Ann Rheum Dis* 1991;50:540–2.
5. Hadler NM. Knee pain is the malady—not osteoarthritis. *Ann Intern Med* 1992;116:598–9.
6. Kovar PA, Allegrante JP, MacKenzie CR, Peterson MGE, Gutin B, Charlson ME. Supervised fitness walking in patients with osteoarthritis of the knee: a randomized, controlled trial. *Ann Intern Med* 1992;116:529–34.
7. Felson DT, Zhang Y, Anthony JM, Naimark A, Anderson JJ. Weight loss reduces the risk for symptomatic knee osteoarthritis in women: the Framingham study. *Ann Intern Med* 1992;116:535–9.
8. Hadler NM. Osteoarthritis as a public health problem. *Clin Rheum Dis* 1985;11:175–85.
9. Maurer K. Knee, hip, sacroiliac joints in adults age 25–74: United States 1971–1975. In: National Center for Health Statistics. *Basic Data on Arthritis.* Department of Health, Education and Welfare Publication Number (PHS)79-1661. Vital and Health Statistics Series 11, No. 213, 1979.
10. Davis MA, Ettinger WH, Neuhous JM, Mallon KP. Knee osteoarthritis and physical functioning: evidence from the NHANES I epidemiologic follow-up study. *J Rheumatol* 1991;18:591–8.
11. Massardo L, Watt I, Cushnaghan J, Dieppe P. Osteoarthritis of the knee joint: an eight year prospective study. *Ann Rheum Dis* 1989;48:893–7.
12. Salaffi F, Cavalieri F, Nolli M, Gerraccioli G. Analysis of disability in knee osteoarthritis: relationship with age and psychological variables but not with radiographic score. *J Rheumatol* 1991;18:1581–6.
13. McAlindon T, Dieppe P. The medical management of osteoarthritis of the knee: an inflammatory issue? *Br J Rheumatol* 1990;29:471–3.
14. Hadler NM. There's the forest: the object lesson of NSAID "gastropathy." *J Rheumatol* 1990;17:280–2.
15. Bradley JD, Brandt KD, Katz BP, Kalasinski LA, Ryan SI. Comparison of an antiinflammatory dose of ibuprofen, an analgesic dose of ibuprofen, and acetaminophen in the treatment of patients with osteoarthritis of the knee. *N Engl J Med* 1991;325:87–91.

10

The Entrapment Neuropathies

The major peripheral nerves of the upper and lower extremities are at risk for compression and consequent physiologic compromise at particular sites in their course. Most such entrapment neuropathies are "idiopathic"; they occur without a discrete precipitant and are not associated with any underlying disease process. However, the nerves are at risk at these same points and some others for traumatic disruption in the setting of major tissue damage or even with major blunt trauma. The current discussion is designed to provide a clinically relevant foundation of information. However, the reader is urged to turn to a recently published treatise on the topic for further discussion (1).

Rheumatoid synovitis can also impinge on the peripheral nerves as they traverse foci of inflammation, generally at the same points of susceptibility as seen in idiopathic entrapments. Other systemic diseases either wreak havoc at specific sites or, in the case of infection or neoplasm, in the presence of pathologic tissue. We will mention some of these as we discuss particular entrapments.

Features of the clinical presentation are common to all entrapment neuropathies.

- Dysesthesias characteristically localize to the sensory distribution of the nerve.
- Discomfort and paresthesias are more prominent at rest than with usage.
- There is greater susceptibility of sensory fibers than motor fibers to the insult.
- A Tinel's sign is frequently present, meaning that percussion of the nerve at the site of entrapment elicits dysesthesias in the sensory distribution of the nerve.
- Electrodiagnostic studies provide the gold standard for all entrapment neuropathies.

The reliability of all of these features, including electrodiagnostic findings, varies from site to site and as a function of the pathogenesis, particularly in patients whose entrapment is a consequence of systemic disease.

The pathogenesis of the idiopathic entrapment neuropathies is under intensive study. Normally, peripheral nerves withstand the impressive microvascular changes that can be induced with relatively low pressures. However, with prolonged and/or increased pressure and deformation, the zone between the compressed and the free nerve suffers a permeability change, leading to interfascicular edema, a steeper pressure gradient, and more pronounced impedance to conductivity. Large diameter fibers are more susceptible to compression than are smaller fibers. Nerves that have suffered from other processes, such as the microcirculatory disease of diabetes, are particularly at risk for prolonged and even permanent damage. These principles are illustrated by consideration of the major entrapment syndromes.

THE THORACIC OUTLET SYNDROME

Thoracic outlet syndrome is a concept with a colorful history (2). Near the turn of the century it was suggested that the neurovascular structures that comprise the brachial plexus and associated vessels could be compromised as they exit the thoracic cavity. Ever since, generations of surgeons have tried to expound on this pathogenetic inference. Many have taken on the challenge of defining the clinical consequence and inventing the appropriate surgical intervention. They leave in their wake untenable hypotheses and nonspecific signs that should be discarded: associations with pendulous breasts, cervical ribs, or drooping shoulders or with any of the variations of Adson's sign. Adson's sign, the ability to occlude the brachial artery by some forceful vector in posturing of the neck, can be shown to be positive in nearly all of us. It is totally nonspecific, regardless of the posture employed. Furthermore, almost every imaginable form of pectoral girdle pain has been ascribed to thoracic outlet syndrome in spite of the overt lack of specificity.

Nonetheless, there is such an entity. However, the diagnosis should be reserved for two presentations: the vasculopathic and the axonopathic (3). In the former, often associated with the extremes of usage (such as the case of a professional baseball pitcher), there is occlusion of the brachial artery and/or vein resulting in ischemic symptoms. In the latter, the entrapment is manifest by a painful extremity notable for the stigmata of axonal degeneration. Given the anatomy at risk, the presentation reflects compression of the lowest part of the brachial plexus, leading to motor compromise and atrophy first in the thenar eminence (median nerve) and then in the muscles innervated by the ulnar nerve. Reflexes are spared. There is ulnar sensory loss with median sparing. Documenting this pathophysiology with electrodiagnostic testing is straightforward, as is recourse to the judgment of a surgeon. Short of these two dramatic presentations, thoracic outlet syndrome is a tenuous diagnosis at best. Short of these two presentations, surgical intervention is without basis in theory or in clinical trial. Until the latter is available, the procedure is to be decried.

ULNAR ENTRAPMENTS

Entrapment neuropathy of the ulnar nerve usually presents with dysesthesias in the sensory distribution of the nerve, often lancinating in quality (Fig. 10.1). Hypesthesia can follow, again in the ulnar distribution. Finally, weakness of ulnar-innervated muscles is a prodrome to atrophy. The latter, in the hand, can lead to the classic claw deformity. However, the clinical presentation of ulnar nerve entrapment is notoriously variable. Insidiously progressive atrophy can occur with little discomfort and even little sensory loss, the so-called *tardy ulnar palsy*. More typically, there is neuritic discomfort.

The ulnar nerve is at risk for entrapment at two sites distal to the shoulder: at the elbow and at the wrist. In the former site it is superficial at the condylar groove (in the vernacular, the "funny bone") and further at risk as it passes around the ulna deep to the flexor carpi ulnaris in the "cubital tunnel." The

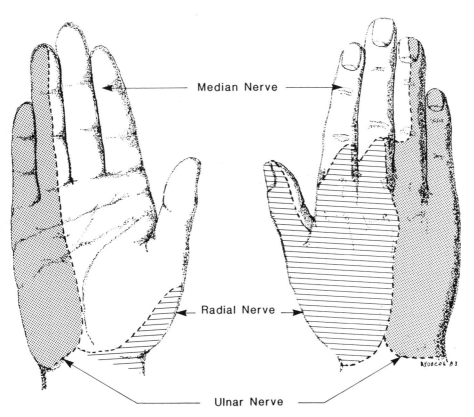

FIG. 10.1. The sensory distribution of the three nerves that innervate the hand.

orientation of the nerve in this tunnel is dynamic; it flattens and stretches with elbow flexion to accommodate the 1-cm increase in the circumference of the posterior elbow capsule. Tinel's sign can help one gain confidence that the neuritic symptoms in the distribution of the ulnar nerve actually reflect entrapment about the elbow. Electrodiagnostic studies at this site are highly variable and often not convincing. However, if one can eliminate the two other sites that can mimic this presentation, cervical radiculopathy or entrapment at the wrist, then conservative therapy at the elbow is the treatment of choice. Padded splints that buffer the elbow and impede full flexion are commonly employed. Nearly all patients experience complete, long-lived remission without recourse to surgery.

At the wrist the ulnar nerve is superficial to the flexor retinaculum between

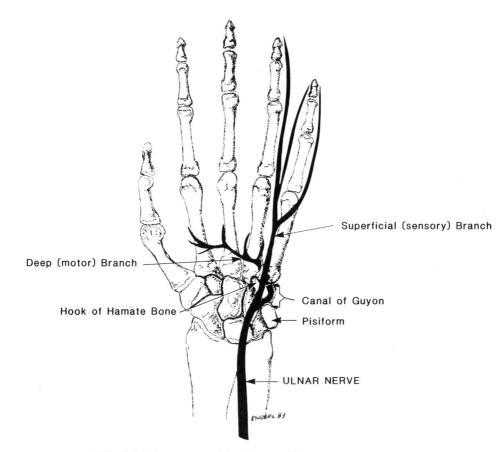

FIG. 10.2. The anatomy of the ulnar nerve as it courses into the hand.

the pisiform and the hook of the hamate deep to the superficial volar carpal ligament in a 4-cm conduit called Guyon's canal (Fig. 10.2). Aside from such systemic diseases as rheumatoid arthritis, the most common cause of ulnar entrapment in Guyon's canal is a ganglion. Lipomas, anomalous muscles, and fractures are other causes. Occupational syndromes involving the ulnar nerve at the wrist are rare. Cyclists often experience ulnar dysesthesias, presumably because of their prolonged posturing. However, they rapidly recover when a normal posture is assumed. The "hypothenar hammer syndrome" is a consequence of repetitive blunt trauma to the hypothenar eminence, usually from using the hand as a hatchet. However, thrombosis and ischemia of the ulnar side of the hand are of greater concern than is ulnar neuropathy (4).

MEDIAN NERVE ENTRAPMENTS

The median nerve is susceptible to entrapment as it enters the forearm lying between the two heads of the pronator teres. The diagnosis is suspected when symptoms suggest the carpal tunnel syndrome yet Tinel's sign localizes proximally and, late, there is compromise in the power of the long finger flexors. The

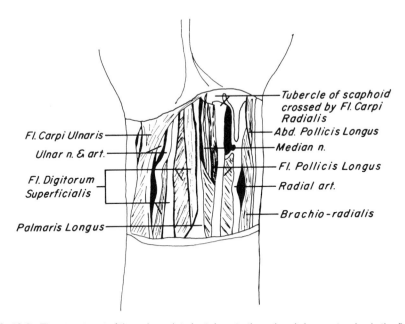

FIG. 10.3. The structures of the volar wrist. Just deep to the palmaris longus tendon is the flexor retinaculum, which defines the floor of the carpal tunnel. The median nerve is the only neural structure in the tunnel, accompanied by a number of flexor tendons. *Fl.,* flexor; *n.,* nerve; *art.,* artery; *Abd.,* abductor.

diagnosis is occasionally confirmed electrodiagnostically but with considerable difficulty. Rather, carpal tunnel syndrome is excluded electrodiagnostically. The diagnosis is aided if pronation against resistance leads to symptoms. This is a rare cause of median neuropathy; the last patient I saw was a bass player who experienced the symptoms when he played by picking the strings rather than bowing. Treatment is to restrain forceful pronation so that the pronator muscle involutes.

The median nerve is more susceptible to entrapment as it traverses the wrist deep to the flexor retinaculum (Fig. 10.3). In fact, carpal tunnel syndrome is the most frequently encountered entrapment neuropathy. The experience of the Mayo Clinic in caring for its Olmstead County catchment area suggests that the prevalence approximates 99/100,000 person-years (5). In other words, if you observe 1,000 adults for 1 yr, you would anticipate that one would develop carpal tunnel syndrome. And even that one may not come to surgery. As we will discuss in Section III, idiopathic carpal tunnel syndrome is not increased in prevalence as a function of upper extremity usage as long as the elements of usage are comfortable and customary. It is also not a predictable consequence of vibration exposure, as for jackhammer or chain saw operators. It can follow forceful impact of the volar wrist, but this is a rare presentation.

TABLE 10.1. *Clinical features of the patients diagnosed as having carpal tunnel syndrome at the Mayo Clinic between 1961 and 1980*

Parameter	Finding
Total number of patients	1,016
Female	798
Male	218
Symmetry	
Unilateral	42%
Right	29%
Left	13%
Mean age at diagnosis	
Men	50
Women	51
Electrodiagnostic studies	
Number studied	505
% positive	73
Symptoms	
Median paresthesias	100%
Nocturnal paresthesias	71%
Proximal radiation	38%
Percentage with signs	Right/left
Positive Tinel's	55/44
Positive Phalen's	55/52
Decreased hand sensation	30/26
Thenar atrophy	20/15

From Stevens et al., ref. 5.

An appreciation of the clinical syndrome of carpal tunnel syndrome (i.e., the form in which it is recognizable by leading clinicians among their patients) is forthcoming from the Mayo Clinic experience (5). The characteristics of the patients in whom carpal tunnel syndrome was diagnosed between 1961 and 1980 are presented in Table 10.1. Idiopathic carpal tunnel syndrome is bilateral in nearly 50% of patients. The clinical presentation is the prototype for an entrapment neuropathy. The presentation initially is of dysesthesias, even lancinating pain in the radial side of the hand. If the thumb is involved, the discomfort can extend its length; angina seldom passes the interphalangeal joint. Occasionally, the discomfort radiates proximally toward the elbow but seldom further. The dysesthetic sensation often awakens the patient, causing the patient to leave the bed and shake the hand. There may be a perception of swelling, even of clumsiness early on, without objective correlates. However, with progression, weakness in pinch and even atrophy of the abductor pollicis brevis (Fig. 10.4) are apparent. Further denervation leads to more thenar atrophy and more overt thumb weakness.

Carpal tunnel syndrome is well described as a complication of late pregnancy, hypothyroidism, rheumatoid arthritis, amyloidosis, and acromegaly. The nerve can be impinged upon with fractures of the wrist or intraarticular inflammatory processes such as tuberculosis. The peripheral neuropathies associated with diabetes, amyloidosis, and renal failure have some predilection for the median nerve in the tunnel, rendering these patients at greater risk for carpal tunnel syndrome but less likely to respond to traditional medical or surgical approaches to this entrapment neuropathy. This syndrome is not a

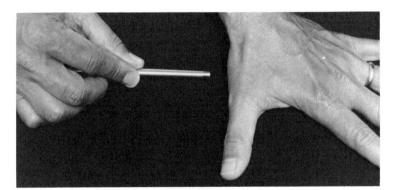

FIG. 10.4. The abductor pollicis brevis muscle forms the most lateral aspect of the thenar eminence (*pointer*). This muscle is innervated only by the median nerve. Therefore, atrophy of the abductor pollicis brevis is diagnostic of median neuropathy and an indication for electrodiagnostic studies to diagnose carpal tunnel syndrome. If one demonstrates delayed median conduction at the wrist, as well as denervation of the abductor pollicis brevis, surgical division of the flexor retinaculum is advisable.

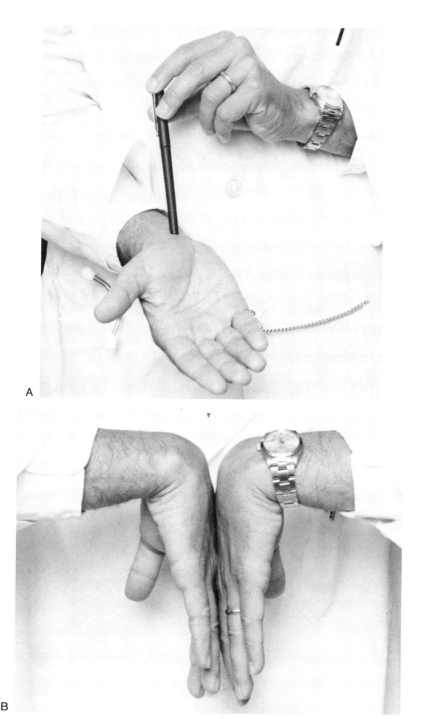

A

B

FIG. 10.5. Tinel's sign for median entrapment at the wrist is elicited by tapping the palmaris longus tendon over the flexor retinaculum (*pointer*) (**A**). If the tap elicits discomfort or dysesthesias that radiate into the thumb, Tinel's sign is considered positive. Local tenderness at the site of percussion is nonspecific. Phalen's sign is the reproduction of symptoms when the posture illustrated (**B**) is maintained for at least a minute. It has a marginal predictive value.

manifestation of pyridoxine deficiency; prescribing pyridoxine has an unfavorable risk/benefit ratio (6).

In idiopathic carpal tunnel syndrome, impedance to conduction is associated with dramatic increases in the hydrostatic pressure measurable in the carpal tunnel (7). However, this observation lends itself only to intraoperative diagnosis and only if one takes great pains to avoid the myriad of artifacts that awaits the uninitiated. It is far more customary to rely on electrodiagnostic testing to gain confidence in one's clinical impression. Nerve conduction velocities are sensitive perhaps at the 90% level at least. However, it is easy to do these studies poorly and even more easy to overinterpret borderline results. Prerequisite to surgery, the electrodiagnostic abnormalities should be unequivocal.

If one takes electrodiagnostic abnormalities as the gold standard for diagnostic confirmation, as one should, it is possible to test the specificity and sensitivity of the classic signs and symptoms. This was the design of a study performed at the Brigham and Women's Hospital based on patients referred for electrodiagnostic studies for any reason (8). Only Tinel's sign (Fig. 10.5) and drawings by the patient of the distribution of pain in the hand have sufficient sensitivity and specificity to be diagnostically informative. These signs have a positive predictive value of 0.71. However, to discern the value of these signs, one needs a referral population where some 40% have carpal tunnel syndrome by electrodiagnostic criteria. If fewer actually had the disease, the sensitivity and specificity of even Tinel's sign and the drawing would be inadequate for clinical utility. For screening in such a population, even these signs are unreliable and invalid.

The majority of patients respond to conservative management, including splinting and corticosteroid injections. Even those patients referred to surgical subspecialists can be treated with injection and splinting with the expectation that some 25% will experience total regression (9). With persistent pain or any indication of thenar atrophy, surgical recourse is reasonable.

RADIAL NERVE ENTRAPMENTS

The radial nerve is remarkably buffeted from compression. It is at risk as it courses around the humerus but usually as a result of prolonged improper positioning during anesthesia or sleeping on the arm, particularly when inebriated ("Saturday night palsy"). The result is wrist-drop; sensory impairment is variable.

At the elbow the radial nerve divides into two branches. The deep branch, the posterior interosseous nerve, passes into the supinator muscle through the arcade of Frohse and courses within the muscle in the supinator canal. Near the elbow, the posterior interosseous nerve is at risk of entrapment, particularly by the synovial proliferation of rheumatoid arthritis. The result is weakness in dorsiflexion of the wrist, even wrist-drop. In the setting of rheumatoid arthritis, the differential diagnosis for wrist-drop is rupture of the extensor tendons near the radial styloid, by far the more likely cause.

There is a longstanding argument as to whether entrapment of the posterior interosseous nerve in the arcade of Frohse is painful, presenting as much as does lateral epicondylitis. I am not convinced. I am also not convinced that the sensory branch of the radial nerve is often spontaneously compressed, provoking lancinating thumb pain, which is exacerbated with the Finkelstein maneuver, thereby mimicking de Quervain's tenosynovitis (10). This has been ascribed to specialized exposures in "wristwatch neuropathy" or even "handcuff neuropathy," but the concept remains tenuous .

LOWER EXTREMITY ENTRAPMENTS

Entrapment of peripheral nerves in the lower extremity is far less frequent than in the upper extremity and has been subjected to far less extensive investigation. Clinically, to diagnose and treat these neuropathies one must know the sensory and motor innervation of the major nerves of the lower extremities.

The Femoral Nerve

The femoral nerve branches at the inguinal ligament into several motor branches to the quadriceps complex. It also continues into the leg as the saphenous nerve, which provides cutaneous innervation. The femoral nerve and its branches are rarely compromised in the absence of trauma and/or hematomas. Weakness of the knee extensors may be caused by trauma to the femoral nerve, although L-4 radiculopathy is a far more likely cause. Electrodiagnostic studies can be useful if the diagnosis is in doubt.

The Lateral Cutaneous Nerve

The lateral cutaneous nerve of the thigh exits the pelvis through or beneath the inguinal ligament. This is a purely sensory nerve. Compression causes hyperpathia and paresthesia in the lateral thigh, Bernhardt's disease, or meralgia paresthetica (Fig. 10.6). The symptoms are worsened by abduction of the leg or prolonged standing. The pathogenesis has been ascribed to either entrapment at the inguinal ligament or as the nerve pierces the fascia to reach the skin. The differential diagnosis includes L-3 radiculopathy. Treatment is aimed at relieving any pressure of garments to the course of the nerve. Electrodiagnostic studies are unreliable and surgical decompression, even at the inguinal ligament, is often disappointing.

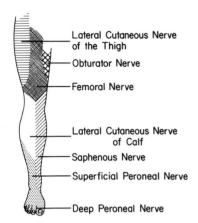

Lateral Cutaneous Nerve of the Thigh

Obturator Nerve

Femoral Nerve

Lateral Cutaneous Nerve of Calf

Saphenous Nerve

Superficial Peroneal Nerve

Deep Peroneal Nerve

FIG. 10.6. The sensory innervation of the leg.

The Obturator Nerve

Compressive obturator neuropathies are very rare. They present as medial thigh pain and paresthesias and occasionally as weakness in the thigh adductors. Usually, the cause of the compression is overt: obturator hernia, extrusion of cement from a total hip replacement, or abscess. Electrodiagnostic studies are useful.

The Sciatic Nerve

The sciatic nerve is well cushioned throughout its course. It may be at some risk in the pyriform fossa, particularly with prolonged sitting. This assertion, called the *pyriformis syndrome* by its proponents, is difficult to establish in the face of the high prevalence of sciatica. In the popliteal fossa the sciatic nerve divides into the common peroneal nerve and the tibial nerve. The common peroneal nerve courses around the lateral aspect of the proximal fibula to pass through the superficial head of the peroneus longus muscle in the "fibular tunnel." It is in this portion of its course that it is particularly susceptible to external compression, resulting in foot-drop and some sensory compromise. Common peroneal palsy is the most common of the lower extremity neuropathies. The common peroneal nerve divides on emerging from the fibular tunnel into the deep and superficial peroneal nerves. The latter runs in the anterior compartment of the leg. With trauma or even excessive exercise, this compartment can become inflamed to the point of tissue compromise, provoking a surgical emergency. Lesions or insults that affect the common peroneal nerve cause paralysis of the peroneal muscles (ankle eversion) as well as paralysis of the anterior compartment muscles (ankle and toe extension). Any sensory loss

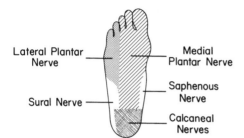

Lateral Plantar Nerve

Sural Nerve

Medial Plantar Nerve

Saphenous Nerve

Calcaneal Nerves

FIG. 10.7. The sensory innervation of the sole.

is confined to the dorsum of the foot and is of little functional significance. With partial injuries to the common peroneal nerve, the deep division seems more vulnerable, compromising hallux and ankle dorsiflexion. The resulting gait disorder requires attention to orthotics so some functional gait can be regained.

The tibial nerve gives off the sural nerve in the popliteal fossa and continues on into the leg deep to the gastrocnemius. At this point it is vulnerable as part of a compartment syndrome. In this setting the palsy is usually partial and temporary and is often manifest as painful paresthesias of the foot. A Tinel's sign is often present in the calf. The tibial nerve emerges at the medial aspect of the Achilles tendon and then passes deep to the flexor retinaculum at the medial malleolus to enter the sole and serve sensation as the medial plantar nerve (Fig. 10.7). This retinaculum forms the roof of the tarsal tunnel. Tarsal tunnel syndrome is analogous to carpal tunnel syndrome except that symptoms are even more variable and electrodiagnostic standards less definitive. Usually, the symptoms are prominent with weight bearing, although nocturnal dysesthesias are well described. Tarsal tunnel syndrome is suspected if there is tenderness and a positive Tinel's sign just behind the medial malleolus. Although even more variable, electrodiagnostic studies are useful. Treatment of the tarsal tunnel syndrome is conservative: orthotics and occasional steroid injections. Surgical success is highly uncertain.

Interdigital Neuroma

Morton's neuroma is probably a form of compression neuropathy. The patient presents with pain in a web space, often the third or fourth, with dysesthesias to the sides of the adjacent toes. The cause is a fibroma, usually a neurofibroma or an angioneurofibroma. It is thought that the pathoanatomy is in response to microtrauma to the common digital nerve at the web space, perhaps from compression in push-off. Treatment is conservative; orthotics and even steroid injection may be of value. Neurectomy is the last resort.

REFERENCES

1. Gelberman RH (ed.) *Operative Nerve Repair and Reconstruction.* Volumes 1 and 2. Philadelphia, JB Lippincott, 1991.
2. Hadler NM. Work-related disorders of the upper extremity. In: Hadler NM, Bunn WB (eds.) *Occupational Problems in Medical Practice.* New York, DellaCorte, 1990:234–6.
3. Hall CD. Neurovascular syndromes at the thoracic outlet. In: Hadler NM (ed.) *Clinical Concepts in Regional Musculoskeletal Illness.* Orlando, Grune & Stratton, 1987:227–44.
4. Foster DR, Cameron DC. Hypothenar hammer syndrome. *Br J Radiol* 1981;54:995–6.
5. Stevens JC, Sun S, Beard CM, O'Fallon WM, Kurland LT. Carpal tunnel syndrome in Rochester, Minnesota, 1961 to 1980. *Neurology* 1988;38:134–8.
6. Amadio PC. Pyridoxine as an adjunct in the treatment of carpal tunnel syndrome. *J Hand Surg [Am]* 1985;10A:237–41.
7. Gelberman RH, Rydevik BL, Pess GM, Szabo RM, Lundborg G. Carpal tunnel syndrome: a scientific basis for clinical care. *Orthop Clin North Am* 1988;19:115–24.
8. Katz JN, Larson MG, Sabra A, Krarup C, Stirrat CR, Sethi R, Eaton HM, Fossel AH, Liang MH. The carpal tunnel syndrome: diagnostic utility of the history and physical examination findings. *Ann Intern Med* 1990;112:321–7.
9. Gelberman RH, Aronson D, Weisman MH. Carpal tunnel syndrome: results of a prospective trial of steroid injection and splinting. *J Bone Joint Surg [Am]* 1980;62A:1181–4.
10. Saplys R, Mackinnon SE, Dellon AL. The relationship between nerve entrapment versus neuroma: complications and the misdiagnosis of de Quervain's disease. *Contemp Orthop* 1987;15:51–7.

SECTION III

The Claimant with Musculoskeletal Disability

By definition, regional backache interferes with function. Attempts to lean forward, even while seated, exacerbate the pain. Lifting is problematic and more so when the object cannot be held close to the body. All of this follows from an understanding of the biomechanics of the lumbar spine. Figure III.1 depicts the results of studies performed over 20 yr ago by Nachemson and his colleagues (1) in Gothenburg, Sweden. Clearly, dramatic increases in intradiscal pressure are associated with minor shifts in posture, shifts that are part of daily living. Leaning forward while seated places as much stress on the lumbar spine as would modest materials handling. Furthermore, only total recumbency unloads the lumbar spine. Active posturing while recumbent (2) entails impressive increments in force (Fig. III.2). Even passive flexion while recumbent, such as propping one's head on pillows to read or watch television, entails major increments in force. No wonder we hear from patients that their backache is worse even when they do no more than write at their desk. And we hear that bed rest was neither restful nor palliative. Biomechanical considerations alone would predict such. And biomechanical considerations alone suggest motions and postures to be avoided.

The challenge is not just to the worker faced with materials handling; the housewife vacuuming or lifting her child is faced with a dilemma, as is the physician hunched over a desk or operating table. All of us face the potential for the illness of work incapacity. Most of us, apparently, meet the challenge because we can adapt our task to the incapacity. Sometimes this involves postponing vacuuming, raising the height of our desk relative to the chair, or taking advantage of the empathy of our supervisors or co-workers. These are some of the homeostatic mechanisms available to most of us in coping. However, if

154

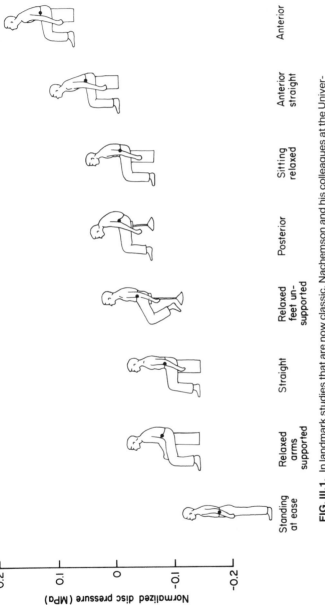

FIG. III.1. In landmark studies that are now classic, Nachemson and his colleagues at the University of Gothenburg in Sweden determined actual intradiscal pressures as a function of posture. A pressure transducer was inserted into the spine, and pressures were recorded during various activities. The subjects were healthy young female physical therapists, and the disc space studied, for convenience, was L-3. These aspects of the investigation limit our ability to generalize to other populations, particularly the elderly and particularly since a good deal of the pathology of the lumbar spine is more caudad. Nonetheless, the results are illuminating. When we stand, the intradiscal pressure reflects the weight of the upper half of our body. Clearly, sitting postures, particularly slouching postures, add to the stress on the disc space. Whatever is hurting the patient with regional backache, sitting, particularly anterior sitting, is likely to make it hurt more. There is no mystery. (Adapted from Andersson et al., ref. 1.)

155

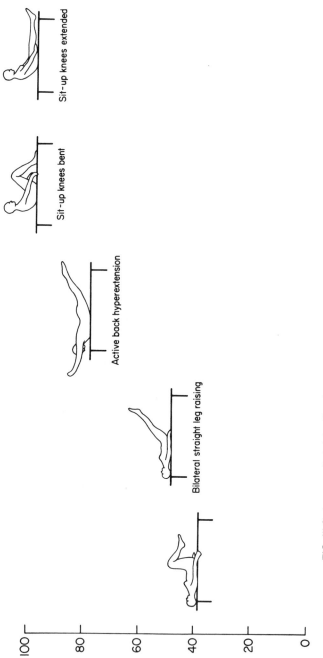

FIG. III.2. Increments in intradiscal pressure as a function of variations in recumbent postures. The research methods and the laboratory are the same as noted in Fig. III.1. Lying perfectly flat unloads the lumbosacral spine, thereby unloading whatever abnormality is hurting the patient with regional backache. However, lying perfectly flat is boring and incompatible with nearly every vocation or avocation. Variations in posture in bed, including propping one's head up on pillows, can produce more force than standing erect. No wonder patients are noncompliant with prescribed bed rest. This noncompliance is homeostatic! (Adapted from Nachemson and Elfstrom, ref. 2.)

such mechanisms fail us because either they are inadequate or they are exhausted by the duration of our illness, what then?

America provides access to one of three avenues of recourse for any of us who no longer can cope with an illness of work incapacity and who are willing to apply: All avenues are gauntlets operated in the belief that, without a gauntlet, no system could distinguish deserving from undeserving applicants. Two of the programs demand an element of culpability; the illness of work incapacity must be a consequence of some harm that befalls you as a result of the actions of another. If such actions did not occur in the context of your employment, the mechanism of recourse is the legal remedy known as a tort. A tort is a suit brought to right a wrong whether you suffered a discrete forceful insult or were damaged by a manufactured product. Relevant to our considerations are product liability ("toxic tort") suits that have been pursued when women with silicone breast implants or workers exposed to solvents or consumers of L-tryptophan have developed rheumatic symptoms.

If your injury arose out of and in the course of your employment, you are solely indemnified by your Workers' Compensation Insurance policy. Workers' Compensation Insurance programs are administered on a state-by-state basis and are particularly relevant to regional backache and other regional musculoskeletal illness. If the backache is deemed to be an "injury" that arose out of and in the course of employment and occurred by accident, the sufferer is entitled to coverage under Workers' Compensation Insurance. These policies not only provide all medical care, but also supplement income until the employee is as well as he or she is going to get. Then the policy provides fiscal compensation for compromised wage-earning capacity or for the actual decrement in wages earned as a consequence of any persisting disability. The Workers' Compensation model is "no fault" in design and has largess that far outstrips the disability program administered by the Social Security Administration. Workers' Compensation programs are efficient in providing benefits (and potentially efficient in monitoring safety) in response to injuries that are a consequence of discrete traumatic events involving external forces. These make up over 80% of the claims. The bulk of the remainder of claims relate to regional backache and, recently, to regional arm pain. These are responsible for over 80% of the cost of this system.

America also provides a program of recourse when no individual or other agent can be held culpable. This is administered by the Social Security Administration as Social Security Disability Insurance (SSDI) for those of us who have had considerable employment experience and as Supplemental Security Insurance (SSI) for the rest of us. The intent is to insure Americans against poverty as a consequence of the illness of work incapacity (whatever its cause). To qualify one must no longer be employed and must be deemed incapable of any employment that can earn even minimum wage. The intent, albeit limited, is noble.

The criteria for awards are stringent and stated. Nonetheless, implementation has proven difficult since the program was formulated in the 1950s.

The roles of the treating physician as regards the administration of these three avenues for redress and recourse are different. For SSDI/SSI the treating physician provides a data base which, when adequate, is the basis for an award by the staff employed on behalf of the Secretary of Health and Human Services. For Workers' Compensation programs, the role of the treating physician is less passive. In treating any patient under such coverage, the physician or surgeon is tacitly certifying that the regional backache is a compensable injury. If the patient doesn't return to full health rapidly, the policy encourages and indemnifies attempts on the part of the treating physicians and surgeons to intervene aggressively. This accounts for intervention rates that, while they vary from place to place in the United States, far outstrip the experience with the management of regional backache in circumstances other than that covered by Workers' Compensation. Furthermore, the surgical intervention rate in the United States far outstrips that for compensable backache in other industrialized nations. If the patient still is not well, the treating physician will participate in a determination regarding the likelihood of further improvement and the advisability of further intervention; the patient/claimant is far less active and controlling in this process than if he or she were a patient rather than a Workers' Compensation Insurance claimant.

Torts, SSDI/SSI, and Workers' Compensation algorithms relentlessly converge on disability determination, the decision that the illness/injury renders the worker less competent to work. In America, more than elsewhere, this determination pivots on the quantity of documented and demonstrable abnormality—the concept of impairment-based disability determination. This precept holds that the more pathology, the more damage, the more likely the claimant will be ill and that, if there is sufficient pathology, the illness will include the illness of work incapacity. The precept has administrative appeal. However, for regional backache (and almost every other disorder short of global catastrophe), the measurement of impairment is of limited reliability and abysmal validity! As discussed in Section II, the demonstration of pathologic conditions at the axial skeleton is almost totally nonspecific. Therefore, as many people who are disabled by backache will lack putatively determinative pathology as will people in whom such is demonstrable. Nonetheless, the SSDI/SSI algorithm procures nearly 300,000 "contracted examinations" annually and the Workers' Compensation algorithm procures at least as many "independent medical examinations" in quest of pathologic documentation. Claimants are beleaguered if not demoralized in a Kafka-esque demand that they prove that they are ill. All too often the outcome is escalating illness behavior, a litigious contest, and an inexorable degradation of the humanity of the claimant, resulting in recourse to America's "pain clinics" for redress (3). This section is designed to explore the interaction between patient/claimant and physician/expert in all three of these circumstances.

REFERENCES

1. Andersson BJG, Ortengren R, Nachemson A, Elfstrom G. Lumbar disc pressure and myoelectric back muscle activity during sitting. IV. Studies on a car driver's seat. *Scand J Rehabil Med* 1974;6:104–14.
2. Nachemson A, Elfstrom G. Intravital dynamic pressure measurements in lumbar discs: a study of common movements, maneuvers and exercises. *Scand J Rehabil Med* 1970;2:[Suppl 1]:1–40.
3. Hadler NM. Back pain and the vortex of disability determination. *Semin Spine Surg* 1992;4:35–41.

11

Torts and Musculoskeletal Disease

A tort is a suit brought to right a wrong. All that is required is that a plaintiff prove that the defendant's conduct was the cause-in-fact of his or her injury (1). If one person does violence to the tissues of another, causality is not at issue, only damages. This would be the case in an automobile accident where a plaintiff incurred traumatic dissolution of the integrity of a joint so that secondary osteoarthritis is a consequence. Causality is not at issue. Establishing the form and magnitude of compensation is a convoluted and often contentious process. For example, if a finger joint is injured and its structure distorted, the consequences are far less than if the involved joint had been a knee, unless the injured party is a pianist or a surgeon. These are the considerations that fuel the disability determination industry and are the subject of Chapter 15. In this chapter we shall consider two circumstances where the question of causality is at issue for musculoskeletal diseases. In these two circumstances, a specific event is documented to coincide with the onset of musculoskeletal disease. Neither the specific event nor the outcome is the issue; the issue is how society can determine whether the event and the outcome are other than happenstance. Unlike the remainder of this book, this chapter does not consider the regional musculoskeletal diseases. Rather, the subject is the systemic rheumatic diseases. These are sick individuals, often afflicted in multiple organ systems and often facing the illness of work incapacity. I am taking this license because the issue of causality has colored the care of many of these patients and is a topic of considerable interest in the lay press. Therefore, it perturbs common sense. We will consider two categories of causal issue.

Toxicopathic Rheumatic Disease. The pneumoconioses are chronic pulmonary diseases that result from exposure to environmental toxins. When the perpetrator of the exposure can be identified (e.g., a mining company), that party can be held accountable for the clinical consequences. The legal mechanism for redress is commonly termed *toxic tort litigation.* During the past decade it has become clear that there are rheumatic diseases that result from toxic exposures.

The Traumatic Precipitation of Systemic Rheumatic Disease. Many rheumatic diseases have discrete points of onset. Sometimes a chronic rheumatic disease can become manifest or be observed to flare coincident with a discrete physically and/or psychologically traumatic event. Certainly, most traumatic events of this nature have no such outcome. But the etiology and pathogenesis of most rheumatic diseases are incompletely understood at best. Therefore, it is possible that the discrete event is etiopathic. How does one establish cause? If cause can be established, can culpability be assigned and a legal remedy pursued?

THE MEDICOLEGAL CONUNDRUM

Both of these issues of causation are fascinating and hold scientific promise. At first glance, they suggest hypotheses that should be testable. In the spirit of John Stuart Mill, any hypothesis that withstands the onslaught of such testing holds sway until the next round of testing, based on new technology or new insights, causes it to topple. Such is the nature of scientific truth. To be testable, each hypothesis must be limited in scope; no hypothesis is to be considered so "important" that one can freely generalize from it. We accumulate the surviving hypotheses to draw the important inference. However, not all scientific hypotheses are testable! An untestable hypothesis must be recognized as such, as little more than abstraction. Some are untestable because we lack the technical wherewithal, others because there is no feasible experimental design. Furthermore, attempting to test such hypotheses is worse than futile; any result would more likely be a chance event rather than a reflection of biology. Scientific insights must wait for someone to come up with a testable format. Until then, the questions are indeterminate and science would best move on to other issues.

However, neither law nor clinical medicine is afforded the luxury of such forbearance. A best-guess determination is demanded of both: of the law in the context of litigation and of the clinician in the context of advising an individual patient. Although scientific truth is welcomed in the legal process and valued in the clinical process, it does not subsume legal truth or, for that matter, clinical truth. The contrary is the case. Legal truth, in the context of the usual issues of causation, is that which sways the "finder of fact": judge, jury, or empowered administrator. When the science is incontrovertible, it can carry the day (as may be the case in one instance when we turn to toxicopathic rheumatic disease). If the science is less persuasive, the law is expected to discern and rely on the "preponderance of evidence." For questions of causation the "preponderance of evidence" is an exercise in biostatistics. It is feasible to assign such an exercise to an appropriately constituted academic body or government agency to create and keep current a series of epidemiologic evidentiary standards (2). Personal injury attorneys, insurers, and policy makers would then be in a position to advise litigants so that any legal action would proceed efficiently with a view toward a more predictable outcome. However, for too many issues of causality the evidentiary standards would be based on the statistics of co-variance, and no single causal variable is likely to predominate. The "evidentiary standard" would be a consensus drawing on the prejudices of and interpretations by the members of the body charged with standard-making. Our legal system is designed to handle such a circumstance on a case-by-case basis.

The system turns to the "expert witness" in its quest for the "preponderance of evidence." It is expected that the experts for the plaintiff and for the defense can argue for their respective inferences having performed an adequate statistical assessment of the available data (3). However, a review of scientific evidence presented in the courtroom reveals that the reasoning process displayed is far less persuasive than the credibility and deportment of the expert (4). This must be so for experts rendering opinions about most examples of systemic rheumatic diseases; given the utter dearth of substantive scientific evidence regarding most litigious issues, any "expert" should recuse himself. However, we are now accruing some information of a substantive nature that relates to the two categories of causality.

TOXICOPATHIC RHEUMATIC DISEASES

There are rheumatic diseases that result from acute and chronic toxic exposures (5). Any doubts have faded in the face of the rapid unfolding of the story of the tryptophan-associated eosinophilia-myalgia syndrome. The syndrome was first recognized in endemic form in New Mexico in 1989 (6). Clinical investigation in rheumatology is no stranger to serendipity. Silver et al. (7) were quick to realize that both cutaneous sclerosis and fasciitis were part of the illness, as was aberrant tryptophan metabolism. Sternberg et al. (8) first piqued our interest in the role of tryptophan metabolism in the pathogenesis of scleroderma a decade ago when they observed the development of a scleroderma-like illness during therapy with L-5-hydroxytryptophan and carbidopa. Now Crofford et al. (9) at the National Institutes of Health (NIH), FDA, and Centers for Disease Control (CDC) have collaborated to develop a rat model that offers great insight into the pathogenesis of the tryptophan-associated eosinophilia-myalgia syndrome. The epidemiology of the syndrome suggests that a particular preparation of L-tryptophan is noxious (10). Only when this preparation is fed to Lewis rats do they develop histopathologically demonstrable fasciitis and perimyositis. The toxic moiety in the implicated tryptophan preparation has been identified as a modified tryptophan dimer that is produced as a byproduct of the manufacturing process. That such a happenstance, a seemingly innocuous amino acid congener introduced into our environment, can provoke the dramatic subacute to chronic illness we recognize as eosinophilic fasciitis (11,12) is daunting. That the illness can persist and perhaps progress when the patient is no longer ingesting the toxin (2,7,13) is more than daunting. Finally, those individuals whose eosinophilic fasciitis is unassociated with L-tryptophan are clinically indistinguishable from those who had ingested L-tryptophan (14), suggesting that a similar toxic moiety lurks in the environment.

This is not the only instance of a scleroderma-like illness resulting from toxic exposure. Chronic occupational exposure to vinyl chloride and polyvinyl chloride places the worker at risk for acrosclerosis, acroosteolysis (15), Raynaud's phenomenon, and hemangiosarcoma of the liver (16). The risk is not great, but the association is readily demonstrable and the causal inference cogent (17). Furthermore, the disease seems to result from direct, prolonged, and intense exposure to the polymerization reactants. However, the reactive nature of vinyl chloride may not be prerequisite; a similar yet relatively inert agent, the solvent perchlorethylene, is also associated with this syndrome (18). If we had an animal model or if there was some way to distinguish the exposed worker who would be afflicted from those spared, a decade of progress beyond hypothesis generation would have ensued. The "toxic-oil syndrome" seems destined for similar doldrums. This was a new illness that occurred in epidemic form in Spain in 1981. The manifestations were protean, including catastrophic neurologic involvement on occasion and frequent musculoskeletal involvement with many features of scleroderma (19,20). It is thought that contaminated rapeseed oil, denatured with 2% aniline and intended for industrial use, illicitly found its way into distribution as a foodstuff (21). The epidemic nature of the illness facilitated identification of this toxic exposure, but understanding of its role in the pathogenesis of the illness remains elusive.

Other toxicologic associations with scleroderma-like illness are less convincing (22). Generally, they suffer from various forms of accrual bias. Berkson's paradox, simply stated, is the observation that complicated, confounded disease is more likely to be referred to a specialist or a specialized center and subsequently be described in the literature than is less confounded disease. That could explain why the number of patients with coincident pneumoconiosis and scleroderma is more impressive in the experience of Rodnan et al. (23) than in a case-control study (24). Berkson's paradox could also explain the association of connective tissue disease, mainly scleroderma-like illness, with cosmetic surgery utilizing silicone implants (25) and even with organic solvents such as trichloroethylene (26) and perchloroethylene (9). Most of these observations involve limited series of patients or single case reports. The absence of systematic data and wariness about Berkson's paradox were the reasons offered by the FDA Advisory Panel for hedging on recommendations regarding the systemic risks, if any, of silicone gel breast implants. After all, the published American experience with unequivocal scleroderma occurring in women with implants numbers less than 40 cases. Over 2 million American women have undergone silicone breast augmentation. However, women in general and women of the age likely to undergo silicone implantation are at greatest risk for developing scleroderma. A lower limit estimate of the prevalence of scleroderma based on a study in Tennessee would be 30 cases per million women (27). The prevalence in England is somewhat higher, and that in Germany and Denmark at least 3 times as high (28). To demonstrate that the association of silicone breast implants and scleroderma is more than coincidence would require a prospective randomized study. Even a well-done extensive case-control study would be useful. Clearly, if there is systemic risk from the implants, it is not an overwhelming risk; sensitivity to the plight of these women and reassurance for nearly all is in order. But all we have today is Berkson's paradox and the level of alarm that forces women with these implants to enter into some of the clinical contracts discussed in Chapter 3.

The reporting of single cases is a longstanding tradition in medicine which still has a place, and a service to perform, for a sophisticated readership. Attempting to define and perturb the cause of a patient's disease is the clinician's role. The lack of an explanation seems to render our patient's clinical quandary all the more diabolic. For the many diseases of unknown pathogenesis, attempting to deduce the cause is a seductive exercise. Often the exercise is initiated by the patient; more often the patient is a participant in our quest to deduce the cause. When we with our patient achieve insight, our conclusion can take on the incontrovertibility of prescience—Berkson's paradox be damned. Some of us, sometimes, feel compelled to share our insight with our colleagues, even to weather the gauntlet that is the clinical literature and to withstand the arrogance of the ultimate derogatory, "That is but a mere clinical anecdote!" For those of you who persevere, we, the clinical readership, applaud. Berkson's paradox compromises our level of confidence in the validity of the causal inference implicit in your association, but it doesn't mean that it is invalid. Besides, it is often interesting, hypothesis generating if you will; it causes clinicians to consider their own experience and investigators to broaden their perspective. But the clinical anecdote has little to offer any other arena.

Berkson's paradox is not solely the purview of the epidemiologist; it can shadow a patient into the office. For example, I recently consulted on the case of a 42-yr-old computer engineer referred by the medical director of the large telecommunications firm for which he worked. Some 4 mo earlier the equipment in his poorly ventilated office had been cleaned with solvents so that fumes lingered for some days. Analysis of the cleaning solvents revealed chemicals similar to some noted above. Shortly thereafter, he noted Raynaud's phenomenon and some proximal weakness. By the time of my evaluation he had acrosclerosis, periungual telangiectasias, esophageal dysmotility, and mild myositis. The working diagnosis of early scleroderma, perhaps with overlap with polymyositis, was reasonable and offered. The patient was absolutely convinced that the solvent exposure was responsible for his illness. Based on the literature reviewed above his conviction cannot be dismissed casually.

Such a happenstance tests the mettle of our social conscience. For a century the industrial West has attempted, with uneven success, to provide redress for workplace injuries. The American solution is directly relevant to this patient. If he is right, he has suffered an accidental personal injury in the course of employment that qualifies for benefits under Workers' Compensation Insurance in all 58 American jurisdictions. As we shall discuss in Chapter 12, all of his medical care should be paid for and any compromise in wage-earning capacity should be compensated by one of the many approximations the Workers' Compensation system has evolved in its extraordinarily inventive administrative machinations. In testimony to our national ethic, this largess is meant to be forthcoming expeditiously and without contest. In exchange for such insurance, the American worker has forgone his right to sue his employer for exposing him to the hazard (this "tort immunity" for the employer is the feature that renders Workers' Compensation Insurance the prototype exclusive of no-fault remedy). He can sue the manufacturer of the toxin to which he was exposed and may recover damages even if the toxic potential of the substance had not previously been appreciated; this is a product liability suit or "toxic tort." Furthermore, the recognition of the toxic exposure should engender prophylactic task and workplace redesign. The Occupational Safety and Health Administration (OSHA) is empowered to monitor and enforce such activity. And the Workers' Compensation insurer can raise the premium ("experience rating") paid by the employer and passed on to the consumer if such a hazard is allowed to persist and claims continue.

This is a patchwork for redress and remediation. But that isn't its most serious drawback. There is a pitfall in this convoluted algorithm that awaits any unaware patient and the treating physician. The entire sequence is dormant until the patient chooses to be a claimant; he must seek, demand, and secure his entitlement. And then the system is designed to be adversarial. First the patient will enter a contest regarding causation (29). At the same time, he will have to prove that he is ill and that his injuries have compromised his function and/or quality of life. This is the exercise of disability determination (30), which will occupy us in Chapter 15.

For my patient, the argument for causation is based on precedent coupled with a stochastic assault on Berkson's paradox. He and his attorney are mounting such an assault against the Workers' Compensation insurer who currently fails to appreciate the connection between the solvent exposure and scleroderma, for understandable reasons. For all claimants, the exercise of disability determination is a gauntlet based more on administrative tradition than on reason (31). Therein lies the pitfall; both the contest of causation and the vortex of disability determination are iatrogenic. The former fuels resentment into anger. The latter is clinically counterproductive if not contraindicated; you can't get well if you have to prove that you are sick. Even in instances where causation is less contentious (e.g., patients exposed to the toxic tryptophan preparation or to vinyl chloride), the vortex of disability determination looms. I will not defend our system. There are alternatives that serve other countries in their quest to provide a safe workplace and redress for their injured worker with varying success (32,33). But for now, we are stuck with the American system. It behooves every treating physician whose patient is considering a Workers' Compensation claim or a toxic tort to be cognizant of the forces that will be brought to bear on the patient/claimant and of the sociopolitical constraints that will be imposed on clinical judgments (34).

Seeking redress based on the clinical literature for the rheumatologic consequences of exposure to toxic tryptophan preparations, to vinyl chloride, or to solvents is a trying exercise at best. Seeking redress by extrapolating from the experimental literature to argue for such toxicologic possibilities as erosive arthritis from sulfa drugs (35) or ciprofloxacin (36,37) or lupus from dietary constituents (38) can prove excruciating. The claimant must remain someone's patient and that someone needs to be above the fray, with the perspective and wisdom to counsel effectively. We will return to this contention.

THE TRAUMATIC PRECIPITATION OF SYSTEMIC RHEUMATIC DISEASE

In 1959 Gelfand and Merliss (39) introduced their paper on "Trauma and Rheumatism" as follows:

> The relationship between a specific injury and the subsequent appearance of arthritis, or the aggravation of a preexisting arthritis, is a problem that grows more important as the number of automobile accidents increases and as the percentage of older people with painful or diseased joints increases among the general population. This relationship forms the basis of thousands of suits brought before American courts each year.
> Yet there is surprisingly little literature on this subject.

The same introduction pertains today. That the literature remains scant, and largely the exercise of Berkson's paradox, is a reflection of the untestability of the hypothesis. Nonetheless, we will review what little there is of it by diagnosis.

Traumatic Influences on Rheumatoid Arthritis

By 1959 it was realized that rheumatoid arthritis was not simply a more inflammatory and polyarticular variant of osteoarthritis. The very fact that it was a systemic disease rendered trauma an unappealing pathogenetic mechanism (40). Yet the near concurrence of major trauma and severe rheumatoid arthritis has perplexed more than one observer, has caused several to publish their befuddlement, and has encouraged many more to assert the meaningfulness of the association in their teachings and in the courts. In some editions of some of the standard treatises on rheumatic diseases, authorities contributed to these undercurrents (41,42). Some of the more tantalizing anecdotes are those where a single traumatized joint remains inflamed and heralds the onset of inflammatory polyarthritis (43).

In addition to this background noise, there is an interesting study from Finland. Julkunen et al. (44) mailed a questionnaire to 270 consecutive patients 1 to 2 yr after discharge from an intensive care unit for multiple trauma; 204 responded. A control population was selected from the Helsinki City Census List of 40- to 45-yr-old adults; 150 questionnaires were mailed and 103 responses were received. All respondents who reported morning stiffness, tenderness, or swelling in joints were invited to a clinical, radiographic, and serologic rheumatologic examination. The major results are presented in Table 11.1. A remarkable aspect of this study is that a sizable majority of those to whom questionnaires were mailed responded and nearly all who had rheumatic symptoms attended the examination. What is truly extraordinary is the incidence of rheumatoid arthritis in the multiple trauma patients in the 2 yr following discharge, over 1% per year. One would expect the finding observed in the controls over that period, almost none. This is not a perfect study, nor is any other. Here there is evidence of accrual bias, issues in recall, inadequate matching of patients and controls, inadequate statistical analysis in the publication, and much more. But the investigators were convinced that, of their 247 patients with multiple trauma and with no prior history of RA, at least 3 developed RA within 2 yr of discharge. That is interesting, indeed. The Helsinki study would be easy to reproduce with more exacting design, including a greatly expanded study population. Such confirmation is 26 yr overdue.

TABLE 11.1. *Results of the 1974 Helsinki study of the incidence of rheumatoid arthritis in the 2 years following multiple trauma*

Parameter	Trauma patients	Controls
Number of respondents	204	103
Percent female	26	32
Age (yr)	31.3	41.1
RA[a] in close relatives (%)	8.8	20.4
Morning stiffness (%)	48	32
Joint swelling (%)	42.2	30.1
Number examined	96	25
RA verified (%)	5.4	2.9
Old cases (%)	2.5	2.9
New cases (%)	2.9	0

From Julkunen et al., ref. 44.
[a] RA, rheumatoid arthritis.

Traumatic Influences on Psoriatic Arthritis

Over a century ago, Koebner described the phenomenon that still bears his name. In many patients with psoriasis, traumatizing normal skin provokes a psoriatic lesion at the site (45). Could it be that traumatizing the joint of a patient with psoriasis can lead to a "deep Koebner" of that joint? Several clinical observers are convinced they have witnessed such a phenomenon (39,46,47) manifest as the chronic mono- or oligoarthritis so typical of psoriatic arthropathy. Others have witnessed acroosteolysis, another rheumatic manifestation of psoriasis, following discrete trauma. For example, Miller et al. (48) described resorption of the tuft of the terminal phalanx in a psoriatic patient after a needle puncture of a single nail. To further sweep us up in this line of reasoning, one can wonder if the prototype of psoriatic arthropathy, symmetric inflammation and destruction in and about the distal interphalangeal joints, represents a "deep Koebner." After all, there is reason to postulate that these joints in the hands are subjected to more trauma in everyday usage than are other hand joints (49,50). All of this is intriguing. But is it insightful and prescient, or simply Berkson's paradox?

Traumatic Influences on the Spondyloarthropathies

There is no particular reason to postulate a role for trauma in the pathogenesis of any of the spondyloarthropathies. After all, there is a wealth of data suggesting an infectious trigger in a genetically susceptible host. However, clinical experience (51) still bolsters expert testimony regarding trauma. For that reason, Jacoby et al. (52) attempted to settle the issue with something of a case-control study. They surveyed by questionnaire 126 patients with ankylosing spondylitis and 51 with mechanical back pain seen in their clinic. All of the latter and 90% of the former completed the questionnaire. There was no discernible difference between the groups in the association of the onset of their disease or in flares of their disease with major or minor traumatic events. Again, the study is seriously flawed. But, unlike the Helsinki study (40), the result is neither surprising nor tantalizing. I would favor laying this causal inference to rest.

THE SYSYPHEAN TASK OF DEFINING THE TOXIC OR TRAUMATIC CAUSALITY OF SYSTEMIC RHEUMATIC DISEASE

In more than one moment of consternation, I have decried epidemiology as the science that promulgates the "scare of the week." In spite of the odds, epidemiology seems drawn to tackle the two issues for which it is most ill equipped: (a) The outcome is rare but does not cluster. (b) The outcome and the potential causal inferences are ubiquitous. In the both instances, "associations" are so likely to reflect chance events that the advisability of initiating epidemiologic studies should be called into question. That is not true when the rare outcome clusters; witness the ramifications of the initial observation in New Mexico of the eosinophilia-myalgia syndrome. It is not true when the "ubiquitous" variable can be constrained and defined, as in Table 11.1. But exploratory epidemiology, seeking correlations in the population at large, is fraught with pitfalls. The same holds for clinical investigations. Clinical investigations are forms of epidemiologic investigation where the population studied comprises patients, not people. In patient populations, exploratory epidemiology is similarly susceptible and constrained epidemiology, constrained to a particular subset of the population of patients, must first contend with Berkson's paradox.

These impediments are well known. We know how to design studies that are a match for them. We also know how to predict whether a study is a match. If we demand the latter calculation, an assessment of the power of the study to test a given hypothesis, then the literature of the future will be less littered with the detritus of uninterpretable data as is the literature of the past.

REFERENCES

1. Keeton WP. *Prosser and Keaton on the Law of Torts.* New York, West, 1984:263.
2. Muscat JE, Huncharek MS. Causation and disease: biomedical science in toxic tort litigation. *J Occup Med* 1989;31:997–1002.
3. Bunn WB, Stave G. Atraumatic compensable occupational diseases—the physician and expert testimony. In: Hadler NM, Bunn WB (eds.) *Occupational Problems in Medical Practice.* New York, DellaCorte, 1990:67–80.
4. Black B. Evolving legal standards for the admissibility of scientific evidence. *Science* 1988;239:1508–12.
5. Hadler NM. Managing toxicopathic rheumatic diseases in the current legal climate. *Arthritis Rheum* 1991;34:634–7.
6. Centers for Disease Control. Eosinophilia-myalgia syndrome: New Mexico. *MMWR Morb Mortal Wkly Rep* 1989;38:765–7.
7. Silver RM, Heyes MP, Maize JC, Quearry B, Vionnet-Fuasset M, Sternberg EM. Scleroderma, fasciitis and eosinophilia associated with the ingestion of tryptophan. *N Engl J Med* 1990;322:874–81.
8. Sternberg EM, VanWoert MH, Young SN, Magnussen I, Baker H, Gauthier S, Osterland CK. Development of a scleroderma-like illness during therapy with L-5-hydroxytryptophan and carbidopa. *N Engl J Med* 1980;303:782–7.
9. Crofford LJ, Rader JI, Dalakas MC, Hill RH, Page SW, Needham LL, Brady LS, Heyes MP, Wilder RL, Gold PW, Illa I, Smith C, Sternberg EM. L-Tryptophan implicated in human eosinophilia-myalgia syndrome causes fasciitis and perimyositis in the Lewis rat. *J Clin Invest* 1990;86:1757–63.
10. Belongia EA, Hedberg CW, Gleich GJ, White KE, Mayeno AN, Loegering DA, Dunette SL, Pirie PL, MacDonald KL, Osterholm MT. An investigation of the cause of the eosinophilia-myalgia syndrome associated with tryptophan use. *N Engl J Med* 1990;323:358–65.
11. Freundlich B, Werth VP, Rook AH, O'Connor CR, Schumacher HR, Leyden JJ, Stolley PD. L-Tryptophan ingestion associated with eosinophilic fasciitis but not progressive systemic sclerosis. *Ann Intern Med* 1990;112:758–62.
12. Varga J, Uitto J, Jimenez SA. The cause and pathogenesis of the eosinophilia-myalgia syndrome. *Ann Intern Med* 1992;116:140–7.

13. Culpepper RC, Williams RG, Mease PJ, Koepsell TD, Kobayashi JM. Natural history of the eosinophilia-myalgia syndrome. *Ann Intern Med* 1991;115:437–42.
14. Martin RW, Duffy J, Lie TJ. Eosinophilic fasciitis associated with use of L-tryptophan: a case-control study and comparison of clinical and histopathologic features. *Mayo Clin Proc* 1991;66:892–8.
15. Wilson RH, McCormick WE, Tatum CF, Creech JL. Occupational acroosteolysis. *JAMA* 1967;201:577–81.
16. Lilis R, Anderson H, Nicholson WJ, Daum S, Fischbein AS, Selikoff IJ. Prevalence of disease among vinyl chloride and polyvinyl chloride workers. *Ann NY Acad Sci* 1975;246:22–41.
17. Dinman BD, Cook WA, Whitehouse WM, Magnuson HJ. Occupational acroosteolysis. I. An epidemiological study. *Arch Environ Health* 1971;22:61–73.
18. Sparrow GP. A connective tissue disorder similar to vinyl chloride disease in a patient exposed to perchlorethylene. *Clin Exp Dermatol* 1977;2:17–22.
19. Mateo IM, Izquierdo M, Fernandez-Dapica MP, Navas J, Cabello A, Gomez-Reino JJ. Toxic epidemic syndrome: musculoskeletal manifestations. *J Rheumatol* 1984;11:333–8.
20. Alonso-Ruiz A, Zea-Mendoza AC, Salazar-Vallinas JM, Rocamora-Ripoli A, Beltran-Gutierrez J. Toxic oil syndrome: a syndrome with features overlapping those of various forms of scleroderma. *Semin Arthritis Rheum* 1986;15:200–12.
21. Kilbourne EM, Rigau-Perez JG, Heath CW, Zack MM, Falk H, Martin-Marcos M, de Carlos A. Clinical epidemiology of toxic-oil syndrome. *N Engl J Med* 1983;309:1408–14.
22. Haustein UF, Ziegler V. Environmentally induced systemic sclerosis-like disorders. *Int J Dermatol* 1985;24:147–51.
23. Rodnan GP, Benedek TG, Medsger TA, Cammarata RJ. The association of progressive systemic sclerosis (scleroderma) with coal miners' pneumoconiosis and other forms of silicosis. *Ann Intern Med* 1967;66:323–34.
24. Sluis-Cremer GK, Hessel PA, Nizdo EH, Churchill AR, Zeiss EA. Silica, silicosis, and progressive systemic sclerosis. *Br J Ind Med* 1985;42:838–43.
25. Kumagai Y, Shiokawa Y, Medsger TA, Rodnan GP. Clinical spectrum of connective tissue disease after cosmetic surgery. *Arthritis Rheum* 1984;27:1–12.
26. Walder BK. Do solvents cause scleroderma? *Int J Dermatol* 1983;22:157–8.
27. Medsger TA, Masi AT. Epidemiology of systemic sclerosis (scleroderma). *Ann Intern Med* 1971;74:714–9.
28. Steen VD. Systemic sclerosis. *Rheum Dis Clin North Am* 1990;16:641–54.
29. Hadler NM. Occupational illness: the issue of causality. *J Occup Med* 1984;26:587–93.
30. Carey TS, Hadler NM. The role of the primary physician in disability determination for Social Security Insurance and Workers' Compensation. *Ann Intern Med* 1986;104:706–10.
31. Hadler NM. Who should determine disability? *Semin Arthritis Rheum* 1984;14:45–51.
32. Hadler NM. Disabling backache in France, Switzerland, and the Netherlands: contrasting sociopolitical constraints on clinical judgment. *J Occup Med* 1989;31:823–31.
33. Hadler NM. Impairment rating in disability determination for low back pain: placing the AMA Guides and the Quebec Institute Report into perspective. *John Burton's Workers' Compensation Monitor* 1990;3(2):4–7,13–4.
34. Bunn WB, Berté F. Role of the physician in the Workers' Compensation process. In: Hadler NM, Bunn WB (eds.) *Occupational Problems in Medical Practice.* New York, DellaCorte, 1990:133–44.
35. Miller ML, Ward JR, Cole BC, Swinyard EA. 6-Sulfanilamidoindazole induced arthritis and periarthritis in rats. *Arthritis Rheum* 1970;13:222–35.
36. Schlüter G. Toxicology of ciprofloxacin. In: *First International Ciprofloxacin Workshop, 1985, Leverkusen.* Amsterdam, Excerpta Medica, 1985:61–7.
37. Alfaham M, Holt ME, Goodchild MC. Arthropathy in a patient with cystic fibrosis taking ciprofloxacin. *Br Med J* 1987;295:699.
38. Malinow MR, Bardana EJ, Pirofsky B, Craig S, McLaughlin P. Systemic lupus erythematosus-like syndrome in monkeys fed alfalfa sprouts: role of a nonprotein amino acid. *Science* 1982;216:415–7.
39. Gelfand L, Merliss R. Trauma and rheumatism. *Ann Intern Med* 1959;50:999–1009.
40. Jonsson E, Berglund K. Trauma and rheumatoid arthritis. *Acta Med Scand* 1949;135:255–61.
41. Duthie JJR. Rheumatoid arthritis. In: Copeman WSC (ed.) *Textbook of Rheumatic Diseases.* 4th ed. London, Livingstone, 1970:264.

42. Pinals RS. Traumatic arthritis and allied conditions. In: McCarty DJ (ed.) *Arthritis and Allied Conditions.* 9th ed. Philadelphia, Lea & Febiger, 1979:989.
43. Williams KA, Scott JT. Influence of trauma on the development of chronic inflammatory polyarthritis. *Ann Rheum Dis* 1967;26:532-7.
44. Julkunen H, Räsänen JA, Kataja J. Severe trauma as an etiologic factor in rheumatoid arthritis. *Scand J Rheumatol* 1974;3:97-102.
45. Melski JW, Bernard JD, Stern RS. The Koebner (isomorphic) response in psoriasis: associations with early age of onset and multiple previous therapies. *Arch Dermatol* 1983;19:655-9.
46. Wright V. Psoriatic arthritis. In: Scott JT (ed.) *Copeman's Textbook of the Rheumatic Diseases.* 5th ed. New York: Churchill Livingstone, 1978:537-45.
47. Langevitz P, Buskila D, Gladman DD. Psoriatic arthritis precipitated by physical trauma. *J Rheumatol* 1990;17:695-7.
48. Miller JL, Soltani K, Tourtellotte CD. Psoriatic acro-osteolysis without arthritis: a case study. *J Bone Joint Surg* 1971;53:371-4.
49. Radin EL, Parker HG, Paul IL. Pattern of degenerative arthritis: preferential involvement of distal finger-joints. *Lancet* 1971;i:377-9.
50. Hadler NM, Gillings DB, Imbus HR, Levitin PM, Makuc D, Utsinger PD, Yount WJ, Slusser D, Moskovitz N. Hand structure and function in an industrial setting. *Arthritis Rheum* 1978;21:210-20.
51. Wisnieski JJ. Trauma and Reiter's syndrome: development of reactive arthropathy in two patients following musculoskeletal injury. *Ann Rheum Dis* 1984;43:829-32.
52. Jacoby RK, Newell RLM, Hickling P. Ankylosing spondylitis and trauma: the medicolegal implications. A comparative study of patients with non-specific back pain. *Ann Rheum Dis* 1985;44:307-11.

12

Workers' Compensation and Regional Backache

The Industrial Revolution was not a cataclysmic event. Rather, it wrought its change over the course of decades. Nonetheless, the West was seldom proactive regarding the human consequences of abandoning a semifeudal agrarian economy for industrialism and capitalism. In particular, considerations of worker health and safety always lagged behind considerations of profitability and do so even today. We should know better. Perhaps some would grant the leadership and the establishment of the mid-19th century a modicum of leniency for abandoning compassion and empathy; after all, they were witnessing a new phenomenon. Never before had so many ordinary people abandoned their serfdom to take employment for "the man." This is a relationship that is inherently uneasy; it is a window on human nature unfettered by noblesse oblige. I suppose there have always been caring, cautious, and empathic employers. By the end of the 19th century, however, some of the human costs of industrialization were already all too apparent. For one, workers who had suffered major, catastrophic injury were too numerous to ignore. Attempts to abandon them to the uneven beneficence and obscurity of charity no longer were met with dutiful acquiescence. Injured workers were demanding more. The response of the establishment, embodied in common law, was to block uniform or litigated redress. America chose the British precedents in this regard. Injured workers lost their rights according to common law on any or all of the following grounds: (a) No one made workers take their jobs. If one took a job, one assumed all responsibility for any untoward consequence. (b) If workers were injured on the job, workers had to prove that their actions were not contributory. (c) The third tenet of common law was most effective in blocking redress. It held that the employer was responsible for any untoward outcome on the job only if the employer directly demanded the noxious activity. If the employer was represented by an agent, your supervisor, for example, then the employer was exonerated and the supervisor was culpable.

This last is the "fellow servant" notion. It was first articulated by Lord Abinger in England in 1837 and was adopted by Judge Shaw in Boston in 1842. It places culpability on the fiscally feeble shoulders of a fellow employee. Even if an injured employee could marshal the personal and financial resources to seek redress by litigation, suing the supervisor offered no more than the potential for a moral victory.

THE PRUSSIAN MODEL FOR WORKER HEALTH AND SAFETY LEGISLATION

Social reform took root in Europe just a century ago. It was driven to some extent by social conscience. It was driven to some extent by the likelihood that litigation would erode the three "unholy sisters" listed above. It was driven to a greater extent by political exigencies. The fledgling unions championed the plight of the worker, gave voice to liberal thought, and held military expansionism hostage. The right wing was forced to yield. This was a time of empire. It was Otto von Bismarck who strut the European continent and who was held at bay. German social legislation was passed in 1884. Lord Cecil, the Marquess of Salisbury and the last of the larger-than-life Victorian prime ministers, shepherded similar social legislation through Parliament in 1897. The Prussian precedent took hold and came to be accepted as inviolate, if not sacred, in the Western mind as the century unfolded. There are several tenets of the Prussian precedent that beg inspection. Two are particularly germane to our considerations at this point: (a) If the illness of work incapacity was a consequence of an injury that was related to work, it deserved special consideration. All useful medical care should be forthcoming, and the injured should not be fiscally penalized. (b) If, however, the pathogenesis of the illness of work incapacity could not be ascribed to the employment but only to fate, then the individual was entitled to less largesse.

Almost every industrialized Western state remains wedded to this distinction: Suffering an accident in the workplace is special, and the injured is indemnified to a far greater degree than someone with an illness. Furthermore, the injured worker is entitled to some form of wage replacement; the ill are entitled to far less. The injured worker is indemnified by Workers' Compensation Insurance; the ill by programs that traditionally were labeled "Invalid Pensions" in Europe and Social Security programs in the United States. These latter will be discussed in detail in Chapter 14. In this chapter we will focus on Workers' Compensation Insurance, particularly in the context of backache. I should point out that not all countries remain wedded to the Prussian model. Some, such as Holland and several Scandinavian countries, have discarded the "accident" distinction and indemnify for the illness of work incapacity regardless of its cause. Others, such as Switzerland and New Zealand, have taken the "accident" distinction to the extreme of indemnifying all against accidental injury and its disabling consequences, whether or not the injury is work related (1,2).

WORKERS' COMPENSATION INSURANCE IN THE UNITED STATES

Social legislation did not cross the Atlantic with lightning speed. In fact, the American versions of Invalid Pension took over 50 yr in the crossing (see Chapter 14). However, the injured worker in America, in parallel with events in Europe, was gaining power in the courts and a union voice. The only effective political pressure was for Workers' Compensation statutes. Driving the movement were the same interests that operated in Europe. However, legislating insurance somehow seemed unconstitutional, a form of taxation beyond constitutional limits. For that reason, the American program took some unique twists.

Multiple Jurisdictions

The program was not to be a national program. Rather, each state, several territories, and federal entities developed their own programs—some 58 American jurisdictions.

The Workers' Compensation Insurance Industry

Furthermore, each of the states except eight placed the burden on the employer to purchase insurance for employees from a private-sector purveyor. There came into existence a new private-sector insurance industry including such giants as Liberty Mutual, Cigna, INA, etc. Eight of the states (e.g., Ohio) still retain the insurance function within their own administration with varying degrees of autonomy. Furthermore, many states allow employers to "self-insure" as long as the employer meets standards in terms of size, capitalization, and administration. These insurance enterprises rapidly adopted the principle of actuarial based underwriting; their premiums are calculated so that they have in hand the funds to cover the entirety of any award. If an employee is deemed totally and permanently disabled, the company puts aside sufficient funds to pay the lifetime of pension. The companies also have the right to "experience rate" employers and industries; if any are singled out for extraordinary numbers or magnitude of claims, the premiums rise accordingly. Today, Workers' Compensation Insurance premiums exceed 2% of payroll nationwide, but there is tremendous variability from jurisdiction to jurisdiction and from industry to industry (3). The result is that these insurance companies have amassed fortunes that they invest and dispense with relatively little government oversight. Their recent pleas of poverty reflect intemperance, bad judgment, and lack of oversight in the 1980s.

Less than Universal Coverage

Most states demand that only larger employers provide Workers' Compensation Insurance for their employees. The law might stipulate a cut-off of 25 or more employees, for example. That means that the self-employed (including the small farmer), the part-time employee, the migrant, and the employees of small firms often have no coverage. Furthermore, a few states have even greater loopholes; for example, states like Texas do not mandate Workers' Compensation coverage at all. Worker's Compensation in America is not a universal program.

Consumer Costs

The burden for providing insurance is placed on the employer. But the cost is not transferred to the insured worker; it is placed on the consumer as part of the cost of goods. This is the aspect that was thought to be de facto taxation. The first American statute was passed into law in New York State in 1910 and was immediately contested on these grounds. The U.S. Supreme Court found the paradigm constitutional. Between 1910 and 1949 (Mississippi), all states passed Workers' Compensation statutes.

Tort Immunity

One of the pressures brought upon management to provide Workers' Compensation Insurance was the threat of tort by injured workers. The trade-off for establishing the program is a feature that is unique to the American statutes. In exchange for indemnification under Workers' Compensation, workers give up their constitutional right to sue their employers for the harm suffered. Workers' Compensation Insurance is the prototype "no-fault" or "exclusive remedy" insurance. Workers do not have to contend with concepts such as contributory negligence or the fellow servant rule; if they suffer workplace injury, they are insured. However, employers have "tort immunity." In recent years the inventive plaintiff's bar has devised a number of so-called end-runs around tort immunity. For example, if employers manifest malfeasance, the employers are liable (an "intentional tort"). Or if employers have a dual capacity, when their own product is utilized by their own employees, and the product is defective or dangerous, the employers are liable in terms of "product liability." However, generally, employers enjoy the tort immunity built into the American system.

Medical Care

All statutes stipulate that the injured worker is to receive all necessary medical care and often rehabilitation until the worker is as well as possible. This end point is variously termed "maximal medical improvement," "fixed and stable," and, in Europe, "consolidation." The principle is to spare no expense. The assumption is that the care will be cost-effective and reasonable. In many jurisdictions, employees are free to chose their providers. In some, the employer and/or insurer provides a list of acceptable providers or even chooses and makes the referral. However, little control is exerted on the interventions provided or the charges submitted. Medical care represents over a third of the cost of these Workers' Compensation programs. Furthermore, medical care indemnified by Workers' Compensation is escalating in cost more rapidly than medical care in any other segment of the American health-care enterprise (4). It is becoming clear that the charges billed Workers' Compensation carriers for medical care related to a given diagnosis (e.g., backache) greatly exceed those submitted to other insurers, both public and private, for the same diagnosis (5). It is also becoming clear that the likelihood of interventions is increased for the same diagnosis if the patient is insured by Workers' Compensation (6). We shall return to these issues.

DEFINING THE WORKPLACE BACK INJURY

Nearly all American Workers' Compensation statutes define the indemnified as someone who has suffered a "personal injury . . . arising out of and in the course of employment." Many stipulate that the injury occur "by accident," which is often further defined as an "unlooked-for mishap or an untoward event which is not expected or designed." Clearly, the legislators were envisioning a discrete event that could be identified in time and one that involved an element of violence. Little did they realize how rapidly the jurisdictions would be embroiled in debate over the scope of these definitions.

Early in the century every jurisdiction had to contend with the concept of an "occupational disease." Clearly, exposure to beryllium, silica, asbestos, lead, and other toxins can injure the worker. But the definition of an "injury" suggested some specific noxious event that was temporally discrete. The solution was to enact separate legislation to cover these occupational diseases.

The jurisdictions were also forced to contend with the concept of a discrete pathologic outcome in the absence of a violent precipitant. The issue was raised by claimants seeking redress for their inguinal hernias. The date that the hernia was first noted was discrete. Furthermore, it is often rendered more noticeable with a Valsalva maneuver such as most employ during materials handling. Does that mean that materials handling caused the herniation? Many jurisdictions decided in the affirmative. It was this exercise in semiotics that gave birth to the term *rupture,* which all of use to apply to inguinal herniation with impunity. The implication is of a violent outcome, rather than a manifestation of a congenital difference. If the outcome is so violent, the precipitant must be sufficient and the injury compensable.

This was the medicolegal framework that greeted the landmark paper of Mixter and Barr (7) in 1934. William Jason Mixter was a senior neurosurgeon on the staff of the Massachusetts General Hospital in Boston with a particular interest in spinal tumors. Joseph S. Barr was his junior colleague in orthopedics. Barr was aware of the writings of the pathologist Schmorl and his associates in Heidelberg, which questioned the teaching that enchondromas, cordomas, and other tumors were common in the lumbosacral spine; their interpretation was that the tissue represented extrusion of nucleus pulposus through the annulus fibrosus. Mixter and Barr proceeded to reproduce the pathologic observations and then to subject a series of 19 patients, most with cauda equina syndrome and with myelographic evidence of encroachment, to laminectomy and fusion. The 1934 paper described their results as highly positive; the pathologic concept was real and the cause of back pain in the setting of the cauda equina syndrome. A year later Mixter expanded the clinical correlate to backache without cauda equina syndrome (8). These papers came to capture the thinking of the American neurosurgical and orthopedic communities; elsewhere they held sway but never to the same degree. They would do so in part because the clinicopathologic correlation seems incontrovertible. (It is nearly totally flawed, as discussed in Chapter 7). But there was a more compelling force.

The precept caught fire in America because of the choice of terminology in the series of papers. The process responsible for the backache was a "rupture" of the disc; the term appears in the titles of the papers. *Rupture* is a highly emotive term. It implies a tearing apart or rendering asunder of the disc. The implication is of horrible anatomic damage. The label has had far greater effect on the plight of those afflicted with backache than the occasional pathogenic event it is meant to describe or the surgical remediation it engendered. In 1934, Americans, in particular, rapidly came to perceive regional backache as a dire illness mandating diagnosis with the promise of surgical cure (9). Concomitantly, the Workers' Compensation establishment adopted the backache as an injury even in the absence of an insult involving external force. Particularly if the diagnosis is "ruptured disc," it was argued, the clinicopathologic result is such devastation that an injury must be considered causal. If the diagnostic inference of ruptured disc is putatively validated by a scar, there is little argument regarding causation to this date (10).

After World War II, the incidence of compensable backache began to escalate around the industrial world. Furthermore, surgery, indemnified by Workers' Compensation insurers, began to escalate (although no other country managed to stay apace the American zeal). In spite of these machinations, the numbers of chronically disabled and the cost of their compensation are nothing short of astonishing (11,12). Claimants with work disability from backache or back injuries face a convoluted gauntlet in their quest for recourse and redress (13). The gauntlet itself represents another enterprise laboring in the sphere of health care and health policy, not only in America but throughout the industrial world. The costs here too are staggering. We shall return to the plight of these permanently disabled in Chapter 15.

There is another ramification of this watershed in diagnostic labeling and its rapid adoption by the Workers' Compensation paradigm. After World War II, no one could suffer a backache again without wondering what they did to cause it. No physician could examine a patient with a backache, let alone a claimant, without making the inquiry, "What were you doing when it started?" And no person could suffer a twinge in the back without contending with the self-diagnosis of a "ruptured disc" or "slipped disc" and the anxiety that surgery and disability might be their fate. Our language and our common sense has changed. We can blithely talk about our "back injury" or say "I injured my back" or "I did in (or pulled out) my back" in the absence of a violent precipitant. Before 1934 we did not have the intellectual construct to support such language; it would be as if we considered a headache a "head injury" or we talked about our pneumonia as a "lung injury." Such descriptors remain incongruous. Yet "back injury" is comfortable and so is the medical-surgical algorithm that has evolved, underwritten by Workers' Compensation, to become the "standard of care." There is a mandate by most patients and all claimants to define the cause of the pain and, particularly if a "ruptured disc" is present, to fix it. Because of data, arguments (Chapter 7), and, most persuasively, the salubrious spillover from malpractice suits, some segments of the surgical community have tempered their zeal for this "standard of care." Most segments have not. And it is still the expectation of the American patient and the demand of the American claimant. This country has been so medicalized regarding their backache that reeducation represents a far more pressing public health need than adequate access to imaging studies.

THE CONTEST OF CONSOLIDATION

The array of diagnostic procedures and of remedies offered the patient with backache in all Western countries is a testimony to the inventiveness of medical and nonmedical practitioners. Much of this enterprise is underwritten by Workers' Compensation Insurance. As detailed in Chapter 7, most of the diagnoses are unprovable, most of the remedies are unproven, and some are even proven to be without benefit (14). Yet the enterprise thrives. Why?

If you have acquired the illness of work incapacity in the context of a backache, Workers' Compensation is the most appealing recourse generally available in our society. Not only is your medical care underwritten, but you will not suffer income loss while you are healing. Too many working Americans, perhaps a third, have no other coverage. The majority have some form of health insurance. But nearly every health insurance policy places limits on the quantity of medical care it covers, and few, if any, indemnify wage loss. For the latter, one usually has "sick leave" to fall back on until it runs out. No wonder any ill worker should consider whether the illness qualifies for coverage under Workers' Compensation Insurance. No wonder regional backache found a niche in Workers' Compensation coverage and occupies this niche with the greatest of tenacity on the part of labor and of the providers of care.

Thanks to Mixter and Barr, establishing this niche was not difficult. However, occupying it is. Becoming a Workers' Compensation claimant with a regional backache is to expose oneself to a gauntlet. You are not forewarned. Most claimants regain health rapidly and escape unscathed. But a few sink into the contest. These few represent less than 10% of all Workers' Compensation claimants, yet the contest and its consequences consume some 90% of the direct costs of the entire Workers' Compensation program. The total cost for all *compensable* back pain in the United States in 1986 exceeded $11 billion (15).

There are two fronts to this contest. To have entered, the backache must have been deemed an injury. This is the Contest of Causation, to which we will turn shortly. However, there is a more insidious contest that plays out between the provider of care and the claimant. This contest plays out under the banner of getting well as soon as possible and therefore deludes all of the participants. Workers' Compensation Insurance is designed to pay for all interventions that will get the patient well enough to return to work as rapidly as possible. This is the engine that drives contest. It is coupled to the presumptions that the cause of the back injury can be defined and, once defined, cured.

Whenever a patient with acute low back pain is accepted for treatment as a claimant with an acute back injury, both the claimant and the practitioner commence the hunt for the cause. The history of this "event" and prior episodes is detailed. Physical examinations are undertaken, often in exhaustive detail, to define the extent of instability, the presence of radiculopathy, the compromise in mobility, and other "signs" thought to be interpretable. And always there is the recommendation for imaging: plane films, CT scans, and MR are accepted as routine by physicians, claimants, and insurers. The "great technological advance" of imaging the American back by MR is estimated to have added about $1 billion (16) to the cost of diagnosis and treatment in 1991, mainly to the cost of the compensable backache. And, while these tests and others are under way, the claimant is exposed to the potpourri of interventions discussed in Chapter 7. Of course, "the culprit" is proscribed. After all, since usage on the job is held to be the cause of the accident, it must be avoided. From the outset, and by contract, the evaluation is disabling.

Unfortunately, too few individuals have normal imaging studies. Unconscionably, too few physicians and chiropractors are willing to discount a "finding." Rather, the findings are interpreted as consistent with the practitioner's preconceived notions of pathogenesis. If it appears manipulable, the claimant and the insurer is informed. If it appears operable, likewise. Furthermore, the implicit or explicit advice is that the claimant would be unlikely to heal without the intervention purveyed. Hence, Workers' Compensation is expected to underwrite the extraordinary enterprise that awaits the American back injury. And it does.

As was made clear in Chapters 2, 5, and 7, for all but a rare claimant with regional backache, this represents treatment by sophistry. The history (17), details of the physical examination (18), imaging techniques (19), even specialized electrodiagnostic studies to assess muscle recruitment (20) are all of limited utility. They are fraught with inadequacies in specificity, sensitivity, predictive value, and accuracy. They are so fraught that they probably offer more obfuscation than enlightenment and clearly generate more anxiety than they are worth. Besides, whoever is orchestrating the "diagnostic work-up" generally has a limited therapeutic armamentarium in hand, if not in mind. (When you have a hammer, all the world seems a nail. [*sic!*]) In the hands of the surgeon, surgery is all too ready an option. In the hands of the chiropractor, manipulation seems appropriate. Others advocate drugs, still others rest, and others various forms of exercise. Woe be to the claimant who doesn't get well. If one modality doesn't work, another will be tried. In fact, each practitioner will exercise his or her trade until it is exhausted and then, if the claimant is not back to work, blame the claimant. This is the implication of such terms as *the failed back,* utilized by surgeons to impugn the personality of the claimant rather than their own judgments (21).

The "failed surgical back" is the most dramatic example of the enormous disadvantage claimants bring to the Contest of Consolidation (Fig. 12.1). However, the disadvantage pertains to nearly every therapeutic setting. The only way for claimants to win this contest is to perceive themselves well enough to return to prior work. If symptoms persist in the face of whatever modalities are "customary" for a particular purveyor, the contest continues. There are very few purveyors in the American medical world who don't take recourse to surgery at some point in their algorithm. There are a few, even some who have published their experience. In the uncontrolled experience from single centers, surgery has little to recommend it over conservative management for backache with (22,23) or without (24) radiculopathy. The patients arrive at maximum medical improvement with the same likelihood. The expense incurred involves multiple trade-offs such as the high cost of aggressive interventions versus the lower cost of less dramatic interventions applied repeatedly. The upshot is that the moneys expended, the cost, to reach this plateau is the same for surgical and conservative algorithms (25).

Even in the world of conservative management, the menu is extensive. Advocates and zealots are common, and the claimant is a passive subject for whatever modalities happen to be practiced with the goal of "maximal medical improvement." There are controlled trials to bolster the advocates for intensive exercise programs (26), for more gentle manual and physiotherapy regimens (27), for extension exercises (28), for the chiropractic (29), and for "back schools" (30). Perhaps all of these modalities work in the special hands of their advocates. Maybe none of them work; rather, the "control" intervention in their hands is detrimental. It is possible to "control" many of these interventions but nearly impossible to avoid the introduction of overt bias. After all, these interventions involve highly personal interactions with claimants and always perturb the interpersonal dynamics of the workplace. The challenge is to approach the "control" with the same interpersonal dynamic as the experimental group receives. That is indeed a challenge, since most of these interventions are studied by individuals with conviction and vested interest.

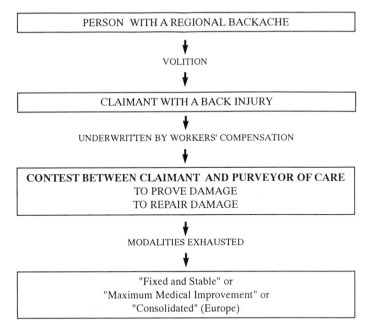

FIG. 12.1. The Contest of Consolidation awaits any person with low back pain who chooses to be a Workers' Compensation claimant with a low back injury and who doesn't get well in a hurry. Claimants are insured for all necessary interventions until they are as well as they are going to get. That status is variously termed "maximum medical improvement," "fixed and stable," or "consolidation" (the European term). The purveyor of interventions is paid for any intervention that he or she deems necessary; neither the indication nor the charge is routinely questioned. Since the treating contract is based on injury to the back, it seems reasonable to all concerned to define the damage and attempt to fix it. The subliminal analogy is to a fracture or the like. This is an exercise in sophistry that awaits nearly all claimants. Furthermore, "consolidation" is a euphemism for exhaustion of interventions, after which the validity of the claimant's illness is more likely to be impugned than the clinical judgment that drove the contest.

It is also important to realize that the outcome measure, the mystical plateau of "fixed and stable" (Fig. 12.1), is a moving target. It is declared when the physician or other provider calls a halt. That need not be at a plateau of physiologic stability. More usually, treatment is stopped because the modalities that the particular purveyor provides are exhausted. It is difficult for the claimant to call a halt short of becoming asymptomatic or at least disclaiming all disability; short of that, calling a halt is likely to be interpreted as noncompliance with appropriate therapeutic advice and further interpreted to suggest that the claimant is motivated to persist in the injured role by some form of secondary gain.

Further affecting studies that take "consolidation" as their end point is the fact that there are several levels of consolidation, including outcomes that fall short of regaining the level of health that permits you to return to your previous employment. The state of consolidation runs quite a gamut: it may mean return to being fully well, or return to work as before, or return to work with a partial disability, or persisting total disability. As will become clear when we consider the Contest of Causation, there is every reason to think that all of these outcomes relate more to the process of the claim and the experience in the Contest of Consolidation than to any particular pathogenetic mechanism or treatment modality. Further, there is every reason to believe that the Contests that are inherent to the administration of Workers' Compensation Insurance impede healing and confound illness. Certainly, the experience of low back pain for those who seek care as patients is far more benign than for those who seek care in the Contest of Consolidation (31).

THE CONTEST OF CAUSATION

There are some truths about the incidence of backache that emerge from multiple surveys in multiple settings (32,33). Backache colors the lives of all and does so often (Section I). Furthermore, by definition, regional backache hurts more if the low back is biomechanically stressed. Furthermore, materials handling is not necessary; even anterior sitting can cause backache to be excruciating. Given the association of the intensity of pain with posture, it is no surprise that few workplaces are configured to avoid all postures that might exacerbate pain (and none could be). What is remarkable is that most people can find a way to carry on, even in the workplace, in the face of most episodes of low back pain. The few who can't may have a more painful illness. But there are two other possibilities: the task content may be too demanding, or the task context may thwart tolerance. In either case, the choice to seek care under Workers' Compensation is not phrased in this fashion. To the contrary, the insurance hinges on the assertion that the task was causal; rendering the pain less tolerable is a far more contentious rationale.

Accepting a claimant for treatment under a Workers' Compensation policy is tantamount to certifying the claimant to be "injured." This de facto certification commences at the work site with the completion of a "First Report of Injury" document and, as required by law, recording of the event on an OSHA 200 log. This certification underlies the contract between the claimant and anyone to whom he or she turns for treatment. After all, most treatment is indemnified by Workers' Compensation for the injury. The contest is not enjoined until the claimant does not recover rapidly. Then the Contest of Causation takes its place alongside the ongoing Contest of Consolidation. The Contest of Causation relates to the definition of injury; it assumes that there must be something demonstrably different and pathogenetic about the claimant's interaction with his or her task.

Ergonomics and human factors have participated in the development of the world of the industrial backache almost since its inception. The state of the art 20 yr ago was described succinctly by Brown (34) in the introduction to his monograph (with its extensive annotated bibliography) published by the Ontario Ministry of Labor, "During the past 30 years a great deal of accident prevention education has been directed towards the reduction of back injuries. This has not produced any great change in the incidence of this condition and the author presents evidence that there can be no specific mandatory method for lifting all loads." Twenty years later, the same statement holds, even though clever ergonomic insights continue to come, though they are slower to go; psychophysics (35), preemployment strength testing (36), training in lifting techniques (37), and task design parameters (38,39) all have proponents, each with some attempt at generating supportive data. However, formal studies render cardiovascular fitness (40) and isometric lifting strength (41) unlikely explanations for a person with low back pain choosing to be a claimant under Workers' Compensation. Guidelines for manual lifting have been promulgated by the National Institute for Occupational Safety and Health (NIOSH) (42), but even these do not engender sufficient consensus to allow the formulation of enforceable work practices standards. Why all these false starts? For regional musculoskeletal illness of the low back, pattern of usage must be critical, if not in precipitation then in manifestation (43). Yet ergonomics has offered little relief for the incidence of atraumatic accidents.

The answer is becoming more clear thanks to a series of epidemiologic studies employing multivariate designs. There is a discordance between the experience of symptoms and the recording of accidents. Why does a person with backache choose to be a claimant with a back injury? Magora (44,45) was perhaps the first to realize that psychosocial parameters overwhelm task descriptors in most of the industries he studied. The point has now been forcefully brought home by the studies of Bigos and his colleagues (46) and confirmed by the work of others (47,48). Biomechanics is not irrelevant to the experience of backache. To the contrary. But it is a minor determinate of the decision by a person with backache to seek redress though Workers' Compensation. That decision is far more driven by the context of the task, the psychosocial setting, than the content of the task, the ergonomics!

BACKACHE AS AN INJURY

The construct that labels a regional backache an injury and the enterprise that ministers to the construct each has a life of its own and is part of the fabric of our society. However, each is an iatrogenic conspiracy. The entire system requires a person with a regional musculoskeletal illness to become a claimant with an injury for its raison d'être. The entire system depends on persistent illness for its sustenance. It was designed to offer redress to those among us who are faced with incapacitating tragedy; its history and traditions are ethical and defensible. However, it has evolved to encompass such predicaments of life as regional musculoskeletal disease, stress (49), and the like. In this circumstance, the system maintains illness and promulgates disability as an act of self-service (50).

To his credit, late in life, even Joseph Barr (51) came to this realization and publicly regretted his conscious choice to describe the "ruptured disc" in a fashion that would place the patient under the umbrella of Workers' Compensation. It is also to his credit that he realized the sociopolitical ramifications of the initial observations. An even more eminent name in the pantheon of surgery, T. Billroth (52) of Berlin, came to a similar realization a decade before the Mixter and Barr observation.

> But the state, which trains competent physicians at such great sacrifice, has a right to demand that the physicians be not too completely unprepared for the questions it may put to them . . . . The physician, as one of the most important members of the community, is expected not only to help in cases of individual sickness, but in community diseases as well. He is even expected to do his part in curing the stupidity and indifference of humanity. A beautiful task, but one that can be accomplished only by many generations of physicians and then only imperfectly! Before anyone can become interested in it, he must be filled with an almost sentimental enthusiasm for humanity in general.

Billroth embodied the spirit of German medical education, which became the model for American medical education (53). Unfortunately, these somewhat eloquent sentiments were lip service. After all, he goes on to say, "if the whole of Social Medicine must needs be part of the curriculum of the medical student, it must not take more than two hours per semester, let us say, during the last two semesters; otherwise it will surely be detrimental to his other studies." No wonder Barr took 35 yr to grasp the ramifications of his observation.

REFERENCES

1. Hadler NM. Industrial rheumatology: the Australian and New Zealand experiences with arm pain and backache in the workplace. *Med J Aust* 1986;144:191–5.
2. Hadler NM. Disabling backache in France, Switzerland, and the Netherlands: contrasting constraints on clinical judgment. *J Occup Med* 1989;31:823–31.
3. Burton JF. Workers' compensation benefits and costs: new records. *John Burton's Workers' Compensation Monitor* 1992;5(2):1–6.
4. Burton JF. Health care costs in Workers' Compensation. *John Burton's Workers' Compensation Monitor* 1990;3(3):1–5.
5. Boden L. Workers' Compensation medical costs. In: Greenwood J, Taricco A (eds.) *Perspectives on Health Care Costs in Workers' Compensation.* Horsham, Pennsylvania, LRP Publications, 1992:27–54.
6. Hadler NM. Epilogue. In: Greenwood J, Taricco A (eds.) *Perspectives on Health Care Costs in Workers' Compensation.* Horsham, Pennsylvania, LRP Publications, 1992:339–44.
7. Mixter WJ, Barr JS. Rupture of the intervertebral disc with involvement of the spinal canal. *N Engl J Med* 1934;211:210–5.
8. Mixter WJ, Ayer JB. Herniation or rupture of the intervertebral disc into the spinal canal. *N Engl J Med* 1935;213:385–95.
9. Hadler NM. Regional musculoskeletal diseases of the low back. Cumulative trauma versus single incident. *Clin Orthop* 1987;221:33–41.
10. Hadler NM. Legal ramifications of the medical definition of back disease. *Ann Intern Med* 1978;89:992–9.
11. Bombardier C, Baldwin J-A, Crull L. The epidemiology of regional musculoskeletal disorders: Canada. In: Hadler NM, Gillings DB (eds.) *Arthritis and Society.* London, Butterworths, 1985:104–18.

12. Worrall JD, Appel D. The impact of Workers' Compensation benefits on low-back claims. In: Hadler NM (ed.) *Clinical Concepts in Regional Musculoskeletal Illness.* Orlando, Grune & Stratton, 1987:281–98.
13. Hadler NM. Criteria for screening workers for the establishment of disability. *J Occup Med* 1986;28:940–5.
14. Quebec Task Force on Spinal Disorders. Scientific approach to the assessment and management of activity-related spinal disorders. *Spine* 1987;12[Suppl 1]:S1–S59.
15. Webster BS, Snook SH. The cost of compensable low back pain. *J Occup Med* 1990;32:13–5.
16. Liang MH, Modic MT, Herzog RJ. Discussion of MRI and/or CT. In: Weinstein JN (ed.) *Clinical Efficacy and Outcome in the Diagnosis and Treatment of Low Back Pain.* New York, Raven Press, 1992:91–2.
17. Biering-Sorensen F, Hilden J. Reproducibility of the history of low-back trouble. *Spine* 1984;9:280–6.
18. McCombe PF, Fairbank JCT, Cockersole BC, Pynsent PB. Reproducibility of physical signs in low-back pain. *Spine* 1989;14:908–18.
19. Deyo RA, Bigos SJ, Maravilla KR. Diagnostic imaging procedures for the lumbar spine. *Ann Intern Med* 1989;111:865–7.
20. Mirka GA. The quantification of EMG normalization error. *Ergonomics* 1991;34:343–52.
21. North RB, Campbell JN, James CS, Conover-Walker MK, Wang H, Piantadosi S, Rybock JD, Long DM. Failed back surgery syndrome: 5-year follow-up in 102 patients undergoing repeated operation. *Neurosurgery* 1991;28:685–91.
22. Alaranta H, Hurme M, Einola S, Falch B, Kallio V, Knuts L-R, Lahtela K, Torma T. A prospective study of patients with sciatica: a comparison between conservatively treated patients and patients who have undergone operation. Part II. Results after one year follow-up. *Spine* 1990;15:1345–9.
23. Saal JA, Saal JS. Nonoperative treatment of herniated lumbar intervertebral disc with radiculopathy. *Spine* 1989;14:431–7.
24. Saal JA. Dynamic muscular stabilization in the nonoperative treatment of lumbar pain syndromes. *Orthop Rev* 1990;19:691–700.
25. Shvartzman L, Weingarten E, Sherry H, Levin S, Persaud A. Cost-effectiveness analysis of extended conservative therapy versus surgical intervention in the management of herniated lumbar intervertebral disc. *Spine* 1992;17:176–82.
26. Mitchell RI, Carmen GM. Results of a multicenter trial using intensive active exercise program for the treatment of acute soft tissue and back injuries. *Spine* 1990;15:514–21.
27. Koes BW, Bouter LM, van Mameren H, Essers AHM, Verstegen GMJR, Hofhuizen DM, Houben JP, Knipschild PG. The effectiveness of manual therapy, physiotherapy, and treatment by the general practitioner for nonspecific back and neck complaints. *Spine* 1992;17:28–35.
28. Radisav S, Johnell O. Conservative treatment of acute low-back pain: a prospective randomized trial. McKenzie method of treatment versus patient education in "Mini Back School." *Spine* 1990;15:120–3.
29. Meade TW, Dyer S, Browne W, Townsend J, Frack AO. Low back pain of mechanical origin: randomised comparison of chiropractic and hospital outpatient treatment. *Br Med J* 1990;300:1431–7.
30. Versloot JM, Rozeman A, van Son AM, van Adderveeken PF. The cost-effectiveness of a back school program in industry: a longitudinal controlled field study. *Spine* 1992;17:22–7.
31. Greenough CG, Fraser RD. The effects of compensation on recovery from low-back pain. *Spine* 1989;14:947–55.
32. Cypress BK. Characteristics of physician visits for back symptoms: a national perspective. *Am J Public Health* 1983;73:389–95.
33. Heliovaara M, Sievers K, Impivaara O, Maatela J, Knekd P, Makela M, Aromaa A. Descriptive epidemiology and public health aspects of low back pain. *Ann Med* 1989;21:327–33.
34. Brown JR. *Manual Lifting and Related Fields: An Annotated Bibliography.* Ontario, Quebec, Labor Safety Council of Ontario, Ontario Ministry of Labor, 1972:1–583.
35. Snook SH. The design of manual handling tasks. *Ergonomics* 1978;21:963–85.
36. Chaffin DB, Herrin GK, Keyserling WM, Foulke JA. Pre-employment strength testing. DHEW (NIOSH) Publication No. 77-163, 1977.
37. Ayoub MA. Control of manual lifting hazards. I. Training in safe handling. *J Occup Med* 1982;24:573–7.

38. Ayoub MM, Gidcumb CF, Hafez H, Intaronont K, Jiang BC, Selan JL. *A Design Guide for Manual Lifting.* Occupational Health and Safety Administration, Department of Labor, 1983:1–438.
39. Pope MH, Wilder DG. Avoiding injury: finding an appropriate task. In: Hader NM, Gillings DB (eds.) *Arthritis and Society.* London, Butterworths, 1985:119–32.
40. Battié MC, Bigos SJ, Fisher LD, Hansson TH, Nachemson AL, Spengler DM, Wortley MD, Zeh J. A prospective study of the role of cardiovascular risk factors and fitness in industrial back pain complaints. *Spine* 1989;14:141–7.
41. Battié MC, Bigos SJ, Fisher LD, Hansson TH, Jones ME, Wortley MD. Isometric lifting strength as a predictor of industrial back pain reports. *Spine* 1989;14:851–6.
42. National Institute of Occupational Safety and Health. Work practices guide for manual lifting. DHSS (NIOSH) Publication 81-122, 1981.
43. Hadler NM. Industrial rheumatology: clinical investigations into the influence of the pattern of usage on the pattern of regional musculoskeletal disease. *Arthritis Rheum* 1977;20:1019–25.
44. Magora A. Investigation of the relation between low back pain and occupation. V. Psychological aspects. *Scand J Rehabil Med* 1973;5:191–6.
45. Magora A. Investigation of the relation between low back pain and occupation. *Scand J Rehabil Med* 1974;6:81–8.
46. Bigos SJ, Battié MC. The impact of spinal disorders in industry. In: Frymoyer JW, Ducker TB, Hadler NM, Kostuik JP, Weinstein JN, Whitecloud TS III (eds.) *The Adult Spine: Principles and Practice.* New York, Raven Press, 1991:147–54.
47. Svensson H-O, Andersson GBJ. The relationship of low-back pain, work history, work environment, and stress. *Spine* 1989;14:517–22.
48. Burton AK, Tillotson KM, Troup JDG. Prediction of low-back trouble frequency in a working population. *Spine* 1989;14:939–46.
49. Halleck SL. Mental distress in the workplace: legal and medical aspects. In: Hadler NM, Bunn WB (eds.) *Occupational Problems in Medical Practice.* New York, DellaCorte, 1990:249–60.
50. Hadler NM. The vortex of disability determination: the object lesson of impairment rating for axial pain. In: Hadler NM, Bunn WB (eds.) *Occupational Problems in Medical Practice.* New York, DellaCorte, 1990:261–6.
51. Barr JS. Lumbar disk in retrospect and prospect. *Clin Orthop* 1977;129:4–8.
52. Billroth T. *The Medical Sciences in the German Universities.* New York, Macmillan, 1924:89–90. Welch WW, translator.
53. Altschule MD. The German influence on American medical education: the Flexner report. In: *Essays on the Rise and Decline of Bedside Medicine.* Philadelphia, Lea & Febiger, 1989:375–403.

13

Coping with Arm Pain in the Workplace

> When job demands . . . repeatedly exceed the biomechanical capacity of the worker, the activities become trauma-inducing. Hence, traumatogens are workplace sources of biomechanical strain that contribute to the onset of injuries affecting the musculoskeletal system.

In 1986 this inference was drawn by the staff of the National Institute for Occupational Safety and Health from the discussions during a consensus meeting held the year before (1). It is perpetuated under the rubric, "cumulative trauma disorders (CTDs)." As an invited participant in these deliberations, I was asked to chair a committee to consider the research issues that related to arm pain in the workplace. The committee agreed that the substantive data to test the "cumulative trauma disorder" hypothesis were too meager to allow for policy statements or health initiatives. The committee also agreed that properly designed studies were feasible and overdue. I took strong exception to premature promulgation of such a construct for fear that we might recapitulate the Australian experience with repetition strain injury (RSI). Nonetheless, the inference was drawn by NIOSH officialdom and stated as unequivocal in spite of its considerable sociopolitical ramifications. To appreciate these ramifications one must realize the scope of the inference. Clearly, it is possible to impart sufficient force to musculoskeletal structures to do violence and thereby cause damage. Such events are to be avoided at all cost, regardless of the setting; such traumatic injuries arising out of or even in the course of employment are intolerable. However, does using the musculoskeletal system repetitively and in a fashion such that any element of the usage is comfortable and customary lead to damage, to "cumulative trauma disorders"? Clearly, NIOSH is a proponent of the affirmative. Theirs is a seductive hypothesis, grounded in the engineering concept of metal fatigue. If you use your back or arm or leg repetitively, shouldn't it wear out? It follows that if the arm does wear out as a consequence of work-related usage, any illness and any resulting disability should be indemnified under Workers' Compensation. Theirs may be a seductive hypothesis, even

TABLE 13.1. *Regional disorders of the upper extremity that are proposed as compensable in certain jurisdictions*

Disorder	Putative insult	"Injury"
"White finger"	Extraordinary usage: vibration in the cold	Raynaud's phenomenon dysesthesias
Kienböck's disease	Uncertain	Avascular necrosis of the lunate bone
CTDs[a]	By definition, customary usages performed repetitively	Entire spectrum of regional disorders of the upper extremity, notably carpal tunnel syndrome

[a] CTD, cumulative trauma disorder.

common sense, but it runs counter to established biology. The musculoskeletal system is not inert. It is a living organ that is constantly turning over and remodeling. From our understanding of the physiology of bone, cartilage, tendon, and muscle, usage is prerequisite to healthy tissue and optimal function. Motion is prescribed for the healing of a sutured tendon, for the recovery from a knee replacement, for the management of joints damaged by inflammatory arthritis, for the recovery from septic arthritis, and on and on. And all this prescription is based on clinical experience and supported by reasonably designed clinical trials. Usage is even taken to the extreme of "no pain, no gain," thanks to the unfounded zeal of sports enthusiasts. But in the context of occupational safety and health, usage is impugned. The legal ramifications are substantial.

With the promulgation of the "cumulative trauma disorder" concept, NIOSH has taken a century-old tradition in occupational health and safety one step further. They have expanded the pathogenetic inferences regarding trauma, and they have added the upper extremity to the traditional target, the low back. To appreciate the implications of this line of reasoning, we will consider three clinical disorders of the upper extremity: vibration injury, Kienbock's disease, and use-related arm pain. In terms of the quality of the insult and the specificity and magnitude of the pathologic outcome, these three disorders run quite a gamut (Table 13.1).

KIENBÖCK'S DISEASE AND COMPRESSION/VIBRATION INJURY

Tools used in several industries require considerable force to be maneuvered and expose the worker's hands and upper extremities to vibration. Grinding machines, jackhammers, and chain saws are examples. Using these machines is anything but "customary and comfortable"; any specific pathologic outcome would indeed qualify as a *cumulative trauma disorder,* as I have defined the term. Some individuals can manage these tasks without symptoms. For many, intermittent digital numbness and tingling is the price they pay (2). There is also a significant percentage for whom severe dysesthesias, Raynaud's phenomenon, and, rarely, arthropathy (3) are consequences (4,5). Force, vibration, and cold exposure are the insults that underlie the "white finger disease" of lumberjacks (6). All of this digital abnormality is well established and should be preventable (7).

What is less well established is whether using one's hands in forceful postures, with or without a vibratory insult and with or without thermal stress, can affect structures other than the soft tissues of the fingertips. Certainly, pattern of usage can influence the pattern of degenerative joint disease in the hands (8). But can particular usages provoke more proximal nerve injury, tendon damage, or dissolution of bony integrity? In the growing bone, when the epiphyseal growth plate is still present, it is thought that compression injury can cause microfracture into the joint and fragmentation of the bearing surface (9), resulting in such osteochondroses as Perthes', Freiberg's, or Panner's diseases or osteochondrosis dissecans. It's an appealing theory supported mainly by extrapolation from laboratory experimentation. But is adult bone similarly susceptible to compression injury? An example of this argument is the longstanding debate regarding the role of vibration and compression in the pathogenesis of Kienböck's disease (10).

Kienböck's disease is an abnormality of the lunate bone of the wrist (11). Often it is asymptomatic. However, it may be present in patients presenting with wrist pain and stiffness. The diagnosis is based on radiographic images; findings range from sclerosis with or without cystic changes to fragmentation. The pathogenesis is thought to relate to the peculiar blood supply of the lunate, which may render the bone susceptible to avascular necrosis after traumatic insult. The majority of those who present with symptoms recall a traumatic antecedent. However, while the trauma may precipitate wrist symptoms and medical consultation, the disease of the lunate may be, in fact, likely to be an asymptomatic, incidental finding. The reason for my skepticism is that, while most radiographic surveys (12,13) demonstrate impressive cystic changes about the proximal carpal row in workers exposed to vibratory insults, these changes are nearly if not as impressive (14) in age- and sex-matched workers in heavy industries not exposed to vibratory insults. Furthermore, and emphatically, frank lunate collapse was not seen in any of these surveys. It is a rare event, too rare to be detected even in the nearly 1,000 workers at risk in these surveys. For that matter, no impressive or clinically important radiographic abnormality of the hand or wrist of heavy workers exposed to vibratory insult is established (15).

It is also important to realize that at least 24 electrodiagnostic surveys have been performed in populations of workers who experienced prolonged exposure to vibratory insults (2). Nearly all of these had reasonable sample size, ranging from 30 to 230 workers, were controlled, and were performed by experienced clinical electrophysiologists. The majority demonstrated no abnormality and, where minor abnormalities were detected, they did not involve a particular nerve and they proved inconsistent across series. If anything, these electrodiagnostic studies suggest damage to the digital sensory nerve endings rather than to the proximal nerve trunks. By way of transition to our next topic, the American concept of cumulative trauma disorder, it is worth emphasizing that multiple extensive studies of the arms and hands of workers who perform physically demanding tasks with vibrating tools demonstrate no consistent damage to the bones, joints, or nerves of the upper extremity! These workers are at risk for discomfort and for vascular lability.

USE-RELATED ARM PAIN

For reasons that are entirely unclear, NIOSH is restricting their rubric *cumulative trauma disorders* to use-related disorders of the upper extremity and no other anatomic region. Officers of NIOSH and the Occupational Safety and Health Administration are quoted in the lay press as claiming that more than 5 million workers, some 4% of the American work force, suffer "motion injuries" annually, with predictions that the figure will reach 50% by the year 2000 (16). Union health and safety officers are appropriately concerned and warning their constituents (17). In 1989 the Department of Labor reported over 30,000 cases of "repetitive motion disorders," contrasting with relatively few in prior years. The incidence of the diagnosis of carpal tunnel syndrome and the frequency of wrist surgery are escalating dramatically (18). OSHA thinks that underrecognition and underreporting account for the sparse earlier incidence and has targeted CTDs for a "national special emphasis program." OSHA is so convinced of the concept and so certain that damage is being suffered by American workers that many major employers have been issued citations under Section 5(a)(1), the "general duty clause," of the Occupational Health and Safety Act. This clause is designed to ensure that recognized workplace hazards not encompassed by specific standards are alleviated. OSHA is so wedded to the CTD concept that the agency is demanding that all arm symptoms in workers be elicited and recorded as injuries on OSHA logs, that an excess of such diagnoses impugns the safety of the tasks performed, and that the danger inherent in these tasks is so patent and of such magnitude that employers can be cited and fined for egregious practices even in the absence of ergonomic standards (19).

Today, the clinical diagnoses that are subsumed by CTDs are the entire array of terms to describe soft tissue disorders of the upper extremities from the tendinitides to the entrapment neuropathies (20). Not only are the conditions detailed in Chapters 8 and 10 included, but the complete cacophony of labels, from the antiquated to the undefinable, are bandied about. But the legal remedy offered by both the Occupational Health and Safety Act and the Workers' Compensation paradigm relates to damage, to disruption or distortion of anatomy! Neither legal construct is a remedy for discomfort. (There are exceptions in some Workers' Compensation jurisdictions.) Many of the soft tissue syndromes discussed in Chapter 8 would not qualify as damaging. A few, rare conditions would, such as the entrapment neuropathies detailed in Chapter 10. That was why the bureaucracy was appropriately attuned to the initial studies regarding the role of ergonomic factors in the pathophysiology of carpal tunnel syndrome.

Based on anatomic considerations, it was first postulated over a decade ago that ergonomically unsound upper extremity usage, particularly wrist flexion with power pinch, could result in the carpal tunnel syndrome (21). Shortly thereafter, this association was purported in a sample of workers who had received Workers' Compensation benefits for the diagnosis of carpal tunnel syndrome (22). The basis for this assertion was the difference in percentage of time utilizing power pinch when 18 female claimants with putative carpal tunnel syndrome were compared to 18 co-workers who also were sewing automobile seat covers but had not been labeled as having carpal tunnel syndrome. The magnitude of the greatest difference detected was 51.9% in power pinch for the claimants but only 43.9% for the nonclaimants. I cannot conceive of this being a meaningful or measurable difference. Furthermore, the statistic applied was inappropriate for the multiple comparisons studied. This study is fatally flawed. Even the authors no longer impugn a single motion, power pinch, in their writings. Clearly, the science that ushered in the American decade of CTD alarm was inauspicious. Nonetheless, the inference was presented as axiomatic to physicians in the early 1980s who were attending "miniresidencies" at the Universities of Michigan and Cincinnati, seeking the credential that would qualify them to sit for the board in Occupational Medicine. This cohort of physicians took the lesson of CTD back into their industrial settings. Just as "chance favors the prepared mind," misinformation can be persuasive to the mind in preparation.

Furthermore, once the paper was published the specter of carpal tunnel syndrome rapidly came to drive much of the research and health policy related to CTDs. Today carpal tunnel syndrome hangs like an imprecation over the American work force (23). A vast array of ergonomic stressors are impugned, based mainly on theory and conviction (24). Endemics of wrist surgery, underwritten by Workers' Compensation insurers, dot the landscape and even appear in the clinical literature (25). In fact, surgical division of the flexor retinaculum has rapidly risen to become the most frequent compensable surgical procedure in America.

At first blush, the recognition, prevention, and management of CTDs seems a triumph of occupational health sciences in the 1980s. We have come from theory to recognition of disease, to intervention, and even to targeted health policy in a decade. For one to have reservations, to raise questions, seems antilabor at least, un-American at worst. But I feel compelled to do so. I am concerned that this "triumph" is a sophistry. I have argued that CTD is an iatrogenic concept (26) promulgated in the face of a contrary body of informa-

TABLE 13.2. *Six discrete bodies of information supporting the premise that carpal tunnel syndrome does not qualify for the CTD construct*

Epidemiologic surveys in and out of industry
Clinical literature directly testing the hypothesis
The "RSI" experience in Australia
Perusal of the Ann Arbor industrial engineering studies
Multivariate studies of risk and studies of ergonomic intervention
My studies: Burlington Industries, Oscar Mayer, US West, Pepperidge Farms

tion (27,28). I am further convinced that the entire paralogism operates to the benefit of all involved except the worker whose arm hurts. That individual is not well served. For that reason, I am forced to the posture of an iconoclast but not without considerable ammunition. As was made clear in Chapter 10, carpal tunnel syndrome can be defined with considerable confidence. Furthermore, among the putative CTDs, carpal tunnel syndrome is the only entity associated with a damaging pathoanatomic outcome that has sufficient prevalence to be studied systematically. In the absence of damage, neither Workers' Compensation Insurance nor the execution of the Occupational Health and Safety statute need pertain. If carpal tunnel syndrome did not qualify as a CTD, the policy makers at NIOSH and OSHA would be at a loss to argue for the CTD concept; the principle argument reflects their willingness to extrapolate from their interpretation of the carpal tunnel syndrome data to all forms of arm discomfort. For that reason, I will target carpal tunnel syndrome in our assault on the CTD concept. Six discrete bodies of information provide the ammunition (Table 13.2).

THE EPIDEMIOLOGY OF CARPAL TUNNEL SYNDROME

One of the themes of this monograph is the distinctions among being a person with a predicament, a patient with an illness, and a claimant with an illness or an accident. These distinctions are nowhere more crucial than when trying to come to grips with the data that address the frequency of upper extremity disorders in general and carpal tunnel syndrome in particular.

The Predicament

At least 5% of us will experience discomfort in our neck and upper extremities every 6 wk (29). Although the discomfort often will last a week, it seldom gives us much pause. It is familiar, or we are reassured by the advice of a significant other, or OTC medications and the like provide sufficient palliation. Rarely do we consider recourse to our physician. However, experiencing this morbidity is so commonplace that some episodes are exceptional. Nearly 5% of us have experienced an episode of upper extremity morbidity distinctive in that it persisted for 1 mo of the past year and was memorable (30). Clearly, all of us have learned to process the experiences of regional musculoskeletal symptoms intellectually, each in our own way and usually with a successful outcome. Only occasionally do we need assistance and only occasionally do we find ourselves unable to circumvent functional compromise.

What drives us to seek medical care for a regional musculoskeletal illness of the upper extremity? Outside of the context of the workplace, there is little substantive information bearing on this crucial question. Clearly, becoming a patient with such morbidity is volitional and predicated on some preconceived notion of what is expected of the interaction with a physician. An episode that was unusually intense or just unfamiliar might drive us to patienthood. There is an implicit contract between patient and physician, a contract rooted in the past 200 yr of Western medicine. A person with a predicament of regional musculoskeletal symptoms of the upper extremity chooses to become a patient because of the expectation, if not promise, that the physician can find the cause of the illness and effect specific palliation, if not cure. No people are more wedded to this algorithm than the American people, and no group of practitioners is willing to hold to the precept with more unbridled zeal than the American physician (31,32). Sometimes the contract is rewarded by the establishment of a valid diagnosis that leads to a specific treatment, even cure. With regional musculoskeletal illness of the upper extremity, this is exceptional. However, the exceptions are noteworthy; sentinel among them is carpal tunnel syndrome.

The natural history of carpal tunnel syndrome has not been defined and may not be definable. After all, it is quite rare. Judging from the surveys of workers exposed to vibratory insult discussed above and from the household surveys, sizable populations followed for considerable intervals yield few if any sufferers of carpal tunnel syndrome. This turned out to be the case in Finland, where several surveys seeking upper extremity illness have been conducted in work sites (33–35). These surveys, in essence, are screening people for the predicament of upper extremity disorders; the people happen to be accessed at work. Teams of investigators entered various workplaces and examined workers. Their screening criteria (36) included the quest for carpal tunnel syndrome. Carpal tunnel syndrome was rarely detected (Table 13.3). Clearly the prevalence of carpal tunnel syndrome must be so low that a different approach is necessary to measure the prevalence with some accuracy.

The Medically Defined Illness

A different epidemiologic design is necessary to gain some insight into the incidence and prevalence of carpal tunnel syndrome. If we assume that all people with carpal tunnel syndrome, or with important carpal tunnel syndrome, will choose to be patients, then patient accrual rates reflect the inci-

TABLE 13.3. *Point prevalence of carpal tunnel syndrome among Finnish workers*

Worker description	Cases/number screened (average years on job)
Light mechanical industrial workers	0/93 (4)
Female food packers[a]	0/163 (6)
Female shop assistants	0/143 (13)
Slaughterhouse workers	1/113 (12)

From Kuorinka and Koskinen, ref. 33; Luopajarvi et al., ref. 34; and Viikari-Juntara, ref. 35.

[a] Although no carpal tunnel cases are tabulated in this paper, there is a cryptic statement on page 52 of ref. 34, "The carpal tunnel syndrome is probably combined more often with tenosynovitis of the flexors. Four separate cases were found among the packers and none among the shop assistants."

dence in the population at large. The Mayo Clinic is particularly suited to such an exercise; the clinic is essentially the sole provider of care for the population of the county in which it resides and has long kept records from that perspective. The incidence of presenting as a patient with an illness that Mayo clinicians diagnose as carpal tunnel syndrome is 99/100,000 person-years (37). In other words, if you follow a population of 1,000 people for 1 yr, 1 person will choose to be a patient with an illness that turns out to be carpal tunnel syndrome. The basis for diagnosis at the Mayo Clinic was a synthesis of signs, symptoms, and tests (Table 13.4). The clinicians felt the need to resort to electrodiagnostic confirmation in about half the patients and persisted in their diagnostic certainty in the 27% of those whose testing was interpreted as normal. Mayo clinicians are apparently comfortable with the uncertainties regarding the need for a classic presentation to diagnose carpal tunnel syndrome; some or all classic symptoms and signs were absent in many patients in their series. The salient point is that nocturnal dysesthesias, Phalen's and Tinel's signs, and other classic features contribute to diagnostic certainty. No single feature carries the day, and no single sign or symptom is adequate for screening purposes. Furthermore, not every patient with the diagnosis of carpal tunnel syndrome requires surgery; conservative therapy suffices for most (38). There are instances when clinical judgment holds that thenar atrophy is impending or that symptoms are intolerable in spite of conservative treatment. In these cases, surgical interruption of the tunnel is a reasonable option. It is common practice to seek diagnostic certainty before any carpal tunnel surgery. Unequivocal electrodiagnostic confirmation of the diagnosis is to be expected in the vast majority; leading centers of hand surgery document impressive abnormalities in nearly 90% of the patients taken to surgery (39). Given the uncertainties regarding symptoms and classic signs, adequate electrodiagnostic confirmation should be sought in any patient offered surgical decompression of the carpal tunnel. Furthermore,

TABLE 13.4. Clinical features of residents of
Olmstead County, MN, who chose to be patients
at the Mayo Clinic between 1961 and 1980
and were diagnosed with carpal tunnel syndrome

Parameter	Finding
Total number	1016
Female	798
Male	218
Unilateral (%)	42
Right (%)	29
Left (%)	13
Mean age at diagnosis (yr)	
Men	50
Women	51
Electrodiagnostic studies	
Number studied	505
% positive	73
Symptoms (%)	
Median paresthesias	100
Nocturnal paresthesias	71
Proximal radiation	38
Signs (%)	Right/Left
+ Tinel's	55/54
+ Phalen's	55/52
Decreased hand sensation	30/26
Thenar atrophy	20/15

From Stevens et al., ref. 37.

performance of the procedure in the face of normal studies requires justification and should be an exceptional happenstance.

The rationale for my dogmatism in this regard relates to the usefulness of the clinical criteria to diagnose carpal tunnel syndrome outside a referral center such as the Mayo Clinic or even in a referral center in recent times when the pattern of referral has been dramatically perturbed by the CTD hypothesis. The consensus is that unequivocal electrodiagnostic findings should be present in some 90% of patients with carpal tunnel syndrome. We will discuss shortly the difficulties with this technology and the greater difficulties of choosing appropriate "normals." However, let's accept the 90% sensitivity for the moment. If we use electrodiagnostic criteria to "make the diagnosis" and then see how useful the clinical criteria actually were, the exercise is sobering. The calculations in Table 13.5 are those of Katz (40) based on the data generated at Boston's Brigham and Women's Hospital (41). Even among patients referred to the Brigham's electrodiagnostic laboratory, where the prevalence of "true" carpal tunnel syndrome by electrodiagnostic criteria approached 40%, the utility of the classic signs was marginal. Only Tinel's sign and a drawing by the patient of discomfort that conformed to the distribution of the median nerve were useful. Clearly, the Mayo Clinic diagnosticians are capitalizing on the high prevalence

TABLE 13.5. *Utility of clinical signs and symptoms for the diagnosis of carpal tunnel syndrome, which is critically dependent on the prevalence of the condition*

		PPV/NPV[a] at prevalence of:	
Clinical finding	Sensitivity/specificity	40%	15%
Tinel's sign	0.60/0.67	.55/.72	.25/.91
Phalen's sign	0.75/0.47	.48/.74	.20/.91
Sensory loss	0.32/0.81	.54/.63	.23/.87
Pain drawing	0.61/0.71	.59/.73	.27/.91
Nocturnal symptoms	0.77/0.28	.42/.64	.16/.87
Bilateral symptoms	0.61/0.58	.49/.69	.20/.89

From Katz, ref. 40.
[a] PPV, positive predictive value; NPV, negative predictive value.

of the "true" condition once all selection pressures involved in referral had operated. But if these signs are used as a screening technique in populations with a lower prevalence, they become totally nonspecific. In Table 13.5 the calculation is given for a hypothetical population with a prevalence of 15% of electrodiagnostically confirmed carpal tunnel syndrome. In such a population, any of the classic signs are as likely to be associated with normal electrodiagnostic values as with truly positive patients. Realize that only one of the American endemics (25) approached even 15% prevalence (and we will have more to say about that endemic shortly). Using the "classic" signs and symptoms to screen a population of people, working or not, is an exercise doomed from the start.

Carpal Tunnel Syndrome as an Industrial Claim

The Mayo experience suggests that you would need to observe 1,000 people for a year before 1 would present to a physician with upper extremity symptoms that represented carpal tunnel syndrome (37). There is yet another way to gain insight into the incidence of carpal tunnel syndrome; if a worker reports arm symptoms that are thought to represent a consequence of work demands, the illness is considered an injury and is recorded as an incident on an OSHA 200 log and as a claim for Workers' Compensation Insurance purposes. Both data sets are readily accessible in larger companies. Although the literature is replete with such data masquerading as illness, it is important to realize that the process to the claimant status is very different from that to the patient status (42). Nonetheless, two surveys in Table 13.6 (43,44) demonstrate that the likelihood of becoming a claimant with carpal tunnel syndrome is less than one would predict if the claimant option were comparable to the patient option as revealed in the Mayo experience. The Pratt & Whitney analysis of claims data (44) is particularly striking and received considerable notoriety in the lay press. A

TABLE 13.6. *Epidemiology of claims for the "injury" of carpal tunnel syndrome in the American workplace*

Job/task description	Number of cases/workers at risk/years at risk
Microelectronics[a]	0/960/6
Aircraft engine manufacturing[b]	20/20,000/2

[a] From Hymovich and Lindholm, ref. 43.
[b] From Cannon et al., ref. 44.

review of claims data disclosed 20 cases of carpal tunnel syndrome over a 2-yr period. The claimants were women, many had undergone hysterectomies, and many had been employed in tasks requiring repetitive motion of the upper extremities. The widely disseminated interpretation of the authors was that women, particularly those who had undergone surgical menopause, were at risk for carpal tunnel syndrome if employed in repetitive tasks. However, the Mayo data would predict that there should have been 40 cases in this number (20,000) of workers over 2 yr. Perhaps repetitive motion is protective (not all that facetious a comment, as will become clear). It is also possible that patients with carpal tunnel syndrome were disallowed access to the roles of the injured simply because this illness was not indemnified in this fashion. However, based on the community, workplace, and patient epidemiology, it is difficult to argue for indemnification of carpal tunnel syndrome under the rubric of compensable injury. Recently, the judiciary of Florida, in a class-action case in Dade County, came to the same conclusion.

THE CLINICAL LITERATURE DIRECTLY TESTING THE HYPOTHESIS THAT CARPAL TUNNEL SYNDROME IS A CTD

One can find musings about the pathogenesis of idiopathic carpal tunnel syndrome in the clinical literature dating back decades. There is no doubt that forceful impact on the median nerve at or just distal to the wrist can produce the syndrome acutely (45). There is even reason to suggest that forceful usage might be damaging over time. After all, paraplegics who rely on their hand strength for transfer and mobility seem at special risk, and the risk increases with the passage of time from the onset of their paraplegia (46). It is also true that those individuals who have idiopathic carpal tunnel syndrome have measurably increased pressure in the tunnel, which increases further with flexion (47,48). So, for those already afflicted, usage may be an exacerbating influence. Interestingly, the symptoms are far more frequent at night than during usage. Nonetheless, usage cannot be discounted in those who already have the syndrome. But this does not mean that usage caused these individuals to develop the syndrome in the first place. A relevant analogy might be angina. Activity may provoke angina, but there is little reason to suggest that activity provokes the underlying atherosclerosis. To the contrary.

Anecdotal Experience

Based on clinical impression, the contributors to the literature on carpal tunnel syndrome are divided on whether ordinary or repetitive usage is a primary insult. "Clinical impression" may be useful to the particular practitioner when approaching a particular patient, and "clinical impression" may provide the investigator impetus to generate hypotheses. But clinical impression offers little to the policy maker and less to the process of litigation if either hopes to base judgment on "fact" or even probability. It is no surprise that, based on his uniquely extensive clinical experience as a pioneer in the surgery of carpal tunnel syndrome, George Phalen has the clinical impression that carpal tunnel syndrome is unrelated to occupation or usage (49). It is equally no surprise that other observers were impressed that nearly 80% of their 658 patients with carpal tunnel syndrome in Northamptonshire, England, were employed in work requiring light repetitive movements of the wrists and fingers (50). Perhaps the referral pattern to George Phalen in the Cleveland Clinic excluded manual workers. Perhaps the British physicians, whose referral base was a catchment area, were observing a pattern of employment that simply reflected the demographics of Northamptonshire. And there are innumerable other explanations that render these "clinical impressions" nothing more than guesses. No wonder the guesses can be diametrically opposed.

At least these guesses are based on "clinical impression" from experience with patients who in all likelihood actually had carpal tunnel syndrome. The same is true for the observation by Katz (40) in his elegant study of the sensitivity and specificity of the classic symptoms and signs of carpal tunnel syndrome; he pointed out that the true positive patients were not enriched for employment in tasks requiring repetitive motion. Unlike the thrust of the study, this gratuitous assertion is appealing but cannot be supported by the study as designed.

Flawed Epidemiology

There is another type of observation in the literature, one that is becoming disconcertingly more frequent. Perhaps such publications would have been excusable in decades past when we were more naive in terms of methodology and in terms of our understanding of the pathogenesis of arm complaints. These are publications that are masquerading as state-of-the-art epidemiology but are so patently flawed that they should be an embarrassment to the authors and a reproach to the editorial and peer review process. There are publications describing surveys performed with instruments that are neither standardized or validated (51). Other papers describe a cluster of complaints of arm pain which is ascribed to carpal tunnel syndrome (52). The authors fail to measure the specificity of any finding they use to support the diagnosis of carpal tunnel syndrome. Furthermore, the authors impugn the ergonomics of the task without adequate controls and without considering other influences that might lead to the spate of complaints. There is even a recent attempt at a case-control study where 34 men who had undergone carpal tunnel release between 1974 and 1980 were compared with other patients and with randomly selected men matched for age for putative risk factors (53). Some 60% of the patients had less than 1 yr of exposure to vibrating tools or to tasks with repetitive motion or heavy loading at the wrist. About 15% were exposed in this fashion for more than 20 yr. We are asked to accept that the small number of cases with prolonged exposure to vibration or repetition but not to force is more than would be expected based on the exposure history of the controls. However, case control studies are exquisitely sensitive to selection bias. Inferences based on such small numbers in only the artificial category of >20 yr of exposure are tenuous regardless of the statistic applied.

There is another form of epidemiology that has long provided the data for administrative decisions in government and in the insurance industry but rarely appears in the medical literature. However, one such paper was recently published. Industrial commissions and other insurers have ready access to claims data. After all, that is their function. If one is interested in surveillance for claims, there is no better source. However, the claims process, as we have discussed in Chapters 11 and 12, is highly convoluted. Individuals with legitimate claims may not consider themselves qualified or may not find ready access to the claims process. Or, as in the case of the current regulatory climate, any individual with an upper extremity symptom who approaches medical recognition is recorded on an OSHA 200 log and often becomes a Workers' Compensation claimant. The change in policy has dramatically perturbed the nosology, as well as the claims rate. Using claims data offers documentation of the claims rate—but offers little insight into the process that perturbed the rate. The recent analysis of the claims rate for carpal tunnel syndrome in Washington State (54) takes cognizance of the distinction between a claim for carpal tunnel syndrome and other venues for the experience of arm pain by labeling the claim "occupational carpal tunnel syndrome." The Washington administration that regulates Workers' Compensation is aware that the demographics of the "occupational" form of the syndrome differs from medical epidemiology in that it has nearly a twofold higher incidence and afflicts younger individuals with less female preponderance. It also seems to plague certain industries more than others. However, these data allow no insight into the pathogenesis of the claim, in terms of either motivation or pathologic condition at the arm.

Electrodiagnostic Surveys

Electrodiagnostic studies are easy to perform poorly. The instruments must be of high quality and standardized to achieve reproducibility. This renders field studies a challenge. Attention to ambient temperature is crucial. So is the temperature of the subject's limb; anxiety and a predisposition to vascular lability are well-documented and frequently encountered stumbling blocks to valid measurements. Young women in particular can experience vasoconstriction with anxiety or cold challenge to a degree that is not easily reversed by local warming maneuvers. One can monitor surface skin temperature with a thermistor, but monitoring of dermal vasoconstriction is not routine. Finally, calluses and other individual differences in the integument are important variables. All of these technical issues are well appreciated (55). It behooves any clinician to explore the accuracy with which electrodiagnostic studies are performed before relying on such data. When it comes to sensory conduction measurements or the interpretation of subtle motor abnormalities, documentation of accuracy is critical.

Equally critical is an appreciation of what is meant by "normal" values. Because of the vagaries of the testing, it is critical that each laboratory establish its own definition of normal individuals, including a statistical description of their limitations. But who should be the controls? Most laboratories choose normal volunteers, often from the technical staff. However, as will become clear, there are measurable differences in "normal" values for strata defined by age, sex, and weight. Seldom is a "normal" sample, chosen for convenience, matched to individuals in whom abnormality is suspected by even these demographic features. Particularly relevant to this chapter is the fact that normal values have not been established as a function of time of day, length of exposure to any hand motion or usage, or interval since usage stopped. I suspect that all of these biomechanical variables and others result in measurable changes in "normal" values.

Three groups of investigators with great experience in electrodiagnostic testing have performed surveys in industry. Feldman et al. (56) interpreted their study of workers in an electronic assembly plant as demonstrating progressive impairment of median nerve conduction after a year of performing tasks requiring repetitive motion. I am not convinced. They screened over 80 workers in the microelectronics industry on two occasions separated by a year. The workers were chosen because their tasks called for considerable hand usage and because they experienced frequent discomfort. Unfortunately, electrodiagnostic values obtained in nonaffected persons of the same age group were the standard for comparison, rather than studying co-workers whose tasks differed substantially in manual demands. Whether such normal values generalize to "high-risk" workers with measurably cooler fingertips is problematic. Far more problematic is the fact that these authors did not support their inferences with a statistical analysis of their data. On the first occasion, between 1.2% and 8.4% of the conduction velocities and latencies were beyond normal limits, consistent with a "normal distribution" of values. The distribution of median sensory latencies was normal and reproducible after a year of continued task performance. The distribution of median distal motor latencies shifted toward the abnormal on retest—a change that was not impressive and not shown to be statistically significant. The data are presented, and clearly there is no difference, no clinically meaningful difference and no statistically significant difference. This paper was published in the *Journal of Hand Surgery*, the highly reputable organ of the American Society of Surgery of the Hand—but it was published in a supplement that was not peer reviewed and that was underwritten by outside moneys.

I can offer no such scathing criticism of the paper published by Schottland et al. (57). Electrodiagnostic studies were performed on 93 randomly selected employees of a poultry processing plant and on 85 subjects who were applicants for these jobs. There was no description of the prior exposure of the applicants. The distribution of values for both the workers and the applicants conformed remarkably well to a normal distribution. The calculation for the power of this study, the ability of the study to detect a difference if one really existed, was adequate. Yet the only difference detected was a small impairment in the right median sensory latency for female workers that attenuated if the difference in age between female workers and applicants was taken into consideration. In other words, the employees in poultry processing are at no risk for median neuropathy! This does not mean that their job is comfortable, their wages are adequate, or their benefits and work environment are tolerable. It only speaks to carpal tunnel syndrome!

P. Nathan, a practicing hand surgeon in Oregon, and his colleagues also performed a series of electrodiagnostic surveys in industry. These investigators employed a technique that involves assessing median sensory conduction inch by inch along the course of the nerve, the Kimura technique (58). This is laborious. It is also uncomfortable—something that is true for most of the electrodiagnostic studies but is seldom emphasized. Using this technique they surveyed 471 industrial employees from 27 occupations in four industries (59); after age adjustment nearly 40% of employees had values that were outside the normal range. These "abnormal values" are probably not abnormal; rather the "normal range" is inappropriate to this population. More to the point, the slowing did not correlate with task demands at the upper extremity! Particularly for women, sensory slowing was a function of age, not of task (60). In fact, when these workers were restudied 5 yr later, the development of impaired sensory conduction correlated with weight and body mass index; task was not a determinant (61).

If we accept that electrodiagnostic criteria are the closest we can come to a gold standard for the diagnosis of carpal tunnel syndrome, there is no reason to postulate that carpal tunnel syndrome is a cumulative trauma disorder. To the contrary, it is clear that there is no measurable risk to the median nerve from performing repetitive tasks wherein the elements are customary and comfortable.

THE AUSTRALIAN EXPERIENCE WITH RSI

In the early 1980s a physiatrist in Melbourne (62) and a rheumatologist in Sydney (63) described a clinical experience that they thought was novel.

Women, employees in some of the "state of the art" industries involved in data entry and processing, were presenting with incapacitating arm pain. Their illness was remarkable because their symptoms defied the traditional nosology and because no dystrophic, atrophic, or neuropathic process was present. In particular, carpal tunnel syndrome was excluded. The condition was labeled *repetitive strain injuries,* a term that like CTDs lends itself to a facile acronym, RSI. The inescapable implications of this label include that this cluster of symptoms is a pathophysiologic entity, the workplace task is causal of "RS" and therefore the employer culpable, and the symptoms are a reflection of an underlying damaging process, the "I" of RSI. Furthermore, in the tradition of preventive medicine, it was argued that early symptoms, "Stage 1," portend more symptoms, "Stage 2," and even irreversible symptoms, "Stage 3." The latter was observed to occur in the absence of dystrophic or inflammatory signs. There followed in Australia over the next 5 yr a veritable epidemic of incapacitating arm pain (64); in some industries 30% of the workforce was off the job with disabling arm pain. It was at this juncture that I had the opportunity to study this epidemic, thanks to the sponsorship of the World Health Organization. That is why CTD is déjà vu. I offered my thoughts about the sociopolitical phenomenon that was manifest as RSI in lecture and in the Australian medical literature (65). Others reemphasized (66) and supported (67) the message in the press and in court so that today the epidemic has been put to rest (68). The Australian experience with RSI in its entirety, including the dearth of carpal tunnel syndrome and the proscription of surgery, is directly relevant to our considerations of CTD. Observers on the scene now also speak to the role of sociopolitical turmoil in promulgating the epidemic (69). And what is RSI really? The illness, which is pervasive and unremittent, shares many features of what is called by others *fibrositis* or *fibromyalgia* (70,71). It seems that the process outlined in Chapter 3 can take hold in epidemic form if anxiety about vincibility sweeps through the people, the medical profession is driven more by hubris and greed than reflection and circumspection, and the statutory sociopolitical substratum is nurturing.

THE UNIVERSITY OF MICHIGAN'S FORM OF ERGONOMETRICS

Based on clinical and legal precedents, it should have been difficult to consider carpal tunnel syndrome a CTD. In fact, it was difficult until the work of the single group of ergonomists at the University of Michigan discussed above (68–70). The senior members of this group remain at Ann Arbor, but their disciples are numerous and represent the majority of the voice that supports the CTD hypothesis.

The Ann Arbor investigators first became convinced that motion at the wrist (21), particularly wrist flexion with power pinch (22), was a prime factor in the pathogenesis of carpal tunnel syndrome. They based their assertion on biomechanic and histologic considerations and first tested the inference by performing an ergonometric analysis on 36 women employed in the fabrication of automobile seat covers, half of whom had presented to the company medical department with a "history of numbness or pain in the areas of the hand innervated by the median nerve or surgical decompression of the median nerve, or with a positive Phalen's test, or thenar atrophy" (22). They discerned multiple differences in the way the two groups performed their tasks; differences that were unimpressive in magnitude and would not reject a null hypothesis had an appropriate statistic for multiple comparisons been used. However, Armstrong and Chaffin were impressed and asserted that the difference in Table 13.7 had reached their level of confidence for meaningfulness. It has not reached mine! I am not convinced that the "diseased" workers actually had carpal tunnel syndrome or, for that matter, the controls did not; I am not convinced that an 8% difference in any element of a complex task performed in repetitive cycles can be discerned from inherent variability; I am convinced that the statistic applied was inappropriate and that this is a negative study designed with little statistical power. The authors were convinced that their observation was sound and meaningful; they proceeded to seek the sinister motion in a poultry processing plant, where it was readily discernible and forcefully decried (73). That the motion is present is not an issue; it is common to most hand usage. Their reasons for sounding the alarm are an issue. After all, an untoward clinical outcome, particularly a likelihood of carpal tunnel syndrome, consequent to this pattern of usage in the poultry plant was not discernible in the plant claims records (Table 13.8).

To their credit, the same group designed and performed a more appropriate test of their hypothesis regarding cumulative trauma disorders. In publishing their results, the authors have presented derivitized data and such statistical descriptors as odds ratios to make their points (74,75). However, analysis of the original data, found in the doctoral dissertation that underlies these publications (76), is far more edifying. The study involved approaching 20 manufacturing plants; 6 agreed to participate, of which 3 had previously participated in studies with this investigative team. In each plant the investigators identified those tasks that could be categorized as low repetitiveness/low force (LR/LF), low repetitiveness/high force, high repetitiveness/low force, and high repetitiveness/high force (HR/HF) based on the usage of the hands. This is a difficult exercise in ergonometrics that requires many assumptions to account for indi-

TABLE 13.7. *Data on which Armstrong and Chaffin base their imputation that usage is a cause of carpal tunnel syndrome*

Subjects	% of task cycle in "pinch"
Patients with putative carpal tunnel syndrome (n = 18)	51.9
Matched "controls" (N = 18)	43.9

From Armstrong and Chaffin, ref. 22.

TABLE 13.8. *Regional musculoskeletal illnesses of the upper extremities claimed by employees of a poultry processing plant according to medical department records*

Clinical outcome	Number afflicted
"Injury or illness of a nerve such as carpal tunnel syndrome"	2
"Inflammation, tearing or any other injury or illness of a tendon or tendon sheath"	3
"Nonspecific"	27

From Armstrong et al., ref. 73.
Exposure was >500,000 man-hours performing one of eight separate tasks.

vidual differences, handedness, variability in pattern and force in all tasks, etc. For the sake of our discussion, I will accept this categorization. I will further accept that, if a task is categorized as HF/HR at the hand, it must also require HF/HR at the proximal arm, and likewise with LF/LR. If a subject recalled "recurring difficulty in one or more parts of the upper extremity . . . in the previous two years," then a more detailed interview followed, probing the location, duration, onset, aggravating factors, and treatment. If the pain occurred more than once or lasted more than 1 wk, the volunteers were subjected to a standardized orthopedic examination of their upper extremities. Of 641 employed in the particular tasks in the six plants, 574 volunteered for the study. These workers averaged about 40 yr in age and had spent about 8 yr on their jobs. The results of this survey are presented in Table 13.9. The prevalence of

TABLE 13.9. *Prevalence of upper extremity musculoskeletal symptoms[a] and signs[b] in workers according to category of ergonometric exposure*

Task category	Number of cases				Total number (%)
	LF/LR[c]	HF/LR	LF/HR	HF/HR	
Total	136	153	143	142	574
Neck/shoulder					
Symptoms	13	25	29	29	96 (17)
Signs	7	18	15	13	53 (9)
Elbow/forearm					
Symptoms	9	7	12	13	41 (7)
Signs	2	3	4	7	16 (3)
Hand/wrist					
Symptoms	12	24	32	52	120 (21)
Signs	4	12	15	32	63 (11)

From Silverstein et al., ref. 76.

[a] Those who answered the questionnaire in the affirmative to the presence of symptoms since on the current job which lasted more than 1 week and/or occurred more than 20 times in the previous year.

[b] Those who were interviewed and examined and exhibited objective evidence of a pathologic condition.

[c] Tasks are categorized as low (L) or high (H) force (F) or repetitiveness (R).

recurrent and memorable symptoms of the neck, shoulder, elbow, and forearm is impressive; it is higher than one would have predicted based on the household surveys, suggesting that awareness and recall are enhanced in this population. However, neither symptoms nor signs at these regions correlated significantly with task category; all groups suffered. Recall of symptoms and the presence of signs at the hand/wrist were also greater for all categories than one would have expected. However, at this anatomic region there was a correlation with morbidity and task demand. The HF/HR workers had recalled more symptoms than the other groups, statistically significantly more, but had no more disease on examination!

And what is the clinical outcome at the hand/wrist? Osteoarthritis was detected frequently but was comparable across categories. The only difference detected was in two clinical categories, tendinitis and carpal tunnel syndrome (Table 13.10). However, the relationship between usage and carpal tunnel syndrome was only with the history of symptoms suggestive of that diagnosis, not even with signs of median entrapment neuropathy at the time of examination! Furthermore, we are dealing with only a marginal increment of workers recalling such symptoms; the entire data set supporting the idea that carpal tunnel syndrome is a CTD boils down to fewer than 10 of 574 workers who recalled compatible symptoms.

That is not the most disconcerting aspect of this line of investigation. The publications (74) and congressional testimony by these authors asserted that HF/HR imparted a >15-fold risk of the development of carpal tunnel syndrome. No statistic can be applied to Table 13.10 to generate such an odds ratio with a $p < .001$. To do so, the authors apply a factor termed *plant effect*. But "plant effect" was not defined in the thesis or subsequent publications, nor could Dr. Silverstein define or defend it when under oath (Secretary v. Pepperidge Farm, Inc. OSHRC Docket No. 89-0265). No legitimate statistical maneuver can be applied to the distribution of the scant numbers of afflicted workers

TABLE 13.10. *Distribution of the diagnoses of hand/wrist tendinitis and of carpal tunnel syndrome across task categories*

Task category	Number of cases				Total number (%)
	LF/LR	HF/LR	LF/HR	HF/HR	
Total	136	153	143	142	574
Tendinitis					
Symptoms	2	8	11	23	54 (9)
Signs	1	6	5	17[a]	29 (5)
Carpal tunnel syndrome					
Symptoms	2	2	4	15[a]	23 (4)
Signs	1	0	3	8	12 (2)

From Silverstein et al., ref. 75.
[a] These were the only two categories that reached statistical significance according to the published analysis.

in Table 13.10 to arrive at an assertion of a >15-fold odds ratio with any degree of certainty. Such an assertion is unconscionable, a sophistry, and indefensible.

"Plant effect" is a fudge factor that is trying to weigh the fact that many of the workers putatively afflicted with carpal tunnel syndrome were from a single plant, an "investment casting plant" that we will discuss in the next section. The outcome in Table 13.10 documents the fact that, in spite of the high prevalence of recalled hand and wrist discomfort (Table 13.9), this study lacks the power to detect objective differences in the hands at the time of examination. That may be because the method for detection was not precise; certainly, it falls short in that the electrodiagnostic gold standard was not sought. More likely, the study failed to detect a difference as a function of task because there is none to detect. That is more likely because the analysis failed to detect a correlation between outcome and duration of exposure; if the tasks were causing "cumulative trauma disorders," the outcome should accumulate with prolongation of exposure, and it did not. Furthermore, symptoms in the HF/HR correlated more with the forcefulness than with the repetitiveness of the tasks; again, somewhat counterintuitive for a putative "cumulative trauma disorder." And, finally, female employees were not at increased risk for putative carpal tunnel syndrome, an observation that runs counter to all of the epidemiologic studies discussed above.

This is not to impugn the reliability of or belittle the intensity of the symptoms experienced by these workers. To the contrary. They had symptoms and many had some element of soreness. However, neither the symptoms nor the soreness correlated with ergonomic categories of exposure. And I am not certain that any suffered carpal tunnel syndrome. The specificity of the symptoms and signs employed in this study is inadequate for screening (Table 13.5) when the number putatively afflicted with carpal tunnel syndrome is no more than 12 of 574 at risk; the false positives will overwhelm the result. An electrodiagnostic definition of carpal tunnel syndrome is a far more appealing criterion in terms of reproducibility and specificity, assuming that the studies are well done—but there was no electrodiagnostic assessment in this study.

One should realize that these data do not entirely exclude usage/motion from the pathogenesis of carpal tunnel syndrome. Carpal tunnel syndrome is a well-defined and important entity (77). However, it is too rare and the impugned variable, motion, too ubiquitous to test such a hypothesis effectively. If we are to consider carpal tunnel syndrome a work-related injury when there is no uncomfortable or unusual precipitant, we do so in the absence of substantive supporting data; we do so in the absence of data suggesting that carpal tunnel syndrome is increased in frequency or prevalence in workers performing comfortable and customary tasks; we do so in the absence of data demonstrating that carpal tunnel syndrome occurs in more than 1/1,000 workers/year in any of the industries mentioned. To declare carpal tunnel syndrome an injury or an occupational disease is not science. It is policy, and we need to query who is served by such policy.

Are there any CTDs? That carpal tunnel syndrome is an unappealing candidate for such a rubric does not exclude other clinical entities. The most obvious is patent in the Silverstein data (Table 13.10); how about tendinitis? The Ann Arbor investigators found more signs of tendinitis in the HF/HR workers in the absence of an excess of symptomatic recall! Tendinitis is an abused term (see Chapter 8). There are individuals who experience frank inflammation—swelling and erythema and warmth and induration—in tendons, but these are extraordinarily rare presentations, many of which have been awarded eponymic distinction. They are rare events in the industrial surveys as well; all that is being described in these many surveys is tenderness, soreness, and discomfort with particular motions. There are no signs of frank inflammation, nor can one demonstrate specific pathologic conditions by state-of-the-art imaging techniques or by histology. Yet the term *tendinitis* is bandied about to raise the specter that these subtle conditions are the forme fruste of the more dramatic exceptions. There are no supporting data for this postulate or for the fear it engenders. In fact, Table 13.10 documents the discrepancy between soreness to palpation and symptomatic recall.

MULTIVARIATE STUDIES OF RISK AND STUDIES OF ERGONOMIC INTERVENTION

If ergonomic variables were the, or even a, major cause of arm symptoms in the workplace, then ergonomic remedies should be possible. One of the six plants that participated in the University of Michigan study was an investment casting plant. In fact, this plant contributed 152 of the original 574 subjects and 4 of the 12 diagnosed with so-called carpal tunnel syndrome (Table 13.10). Ergonomic modification was introduced as a result of the original survey. However, when Silverstein and her colleagues returned to the plant 3 yr later, there was no discernible change in the incidence of arm symptoms recorded as cumulative trauma disorders (78). There are two obvious explanations; either the ergonomic interventions were irrelevant or their effect was thwarted by noncompliance. The authors offer only the second possibility as explanation.

There is no controlled trial of ergonomic modification, but there are four other published descriptions of the effect of ergonomically modifying the workplace, in addition to the experience in the investment casting plant. Adjustable work stations offered little palliation to keyboard operators (79). In an Australian office complex, the prevalence of RSI did not correlate with work station design but with work volume and duration. Readjusting schedules and similar "policies for prevention" led to an increased incidence of complaints, although they were less severe and were managed with alternative work rather than resulting in absenteeism (80). There are also two reports from Scandinavia, where aggressive programs of instruction and workplace redesign in two companies led to a decrease in upper extremity complaints and consequent absenteeism

(81,82). To be fair, the authors who reported little to no effect of their ergonomic intervention impugned the compliance and insight of the work force along with the state of ergonomic science to explain their failure. At least they have some cognizance of the complex nature of the CTD outcome.

CTD is an acronym that is designed to indicate tissue damage. As was the case for RSI in Australia, it is a frightening term causing anxiety among workers who experience any discomfort and calling for redress at many levels. Furthermore, it embroils workers in a maelstrom that serves them poorly while serving so many interested parties well. Neither the theory nor the data suggest that repetitive usage where the elements are themselves customary and comfortable will cause any damage! CTD is a malapropism.

This does not mean that repetitive usage can't lead to soreness at the end of the day. Furthermore, since we will all suffer more than one regional musculoskeletal illness of the upper extremity as the years go by, usage, repetitive or not, can confound our predicament by exacerbating the symptoms. The issue is not damage, but how do we minimize such morbidity, particularly in the workplace. The answer that is offered by NIOSH is "ergonomics," and to some extent it is reasonable. Workplaces should be designed with comfort in mind and must be designed with safety in mind. However, it is naive to think that ergonomic adjustments can abrogate the experience of regional upper extremity symptoms or obviate the need to seek help as a consequence.

The science of ergonomics is still in its infancy; there is no consensus for standards for upper extremity usage, let alone studies validating such standards. But even the most ergonomically sound workplace will not spare one from upper extremity regional musculoskeletal illness and will not dissuade one from proclaiming morbidity in the company medical department. That process is far more multivariate.

If we divorce ourselves from the simplistic notions of task design, it is possible to investigate how individuals with regional musculoskeletal symptoms of the upper extremity cope in the workplace. Clearly, task design cannot be ignored. However, the worker's perceptions of the implications of the discomfort, personal resources on and off the job, job flexibility and alternatives, and personal satisfactions on and off the job are potential confounders of the experience of any illness. Our arm discomfort is real, but the quality of the experience can be perturbed by these and other confounders. Three studies of the complaint of arm pain in the workplace have considered aspects of the work environment in addition to task demands. In data processing and secretarial jobs (83,84), the psychosocial variables were shown to overwhelm the task demands as correlates with arm symptoms. In the third study, in heavy industry, psychosocial variables were less critical, though discernibly important (85).

The realization that work environment and other psychosocial factors are critical to understanding the pathogenesis of CTDs is long overdue (86). In fact, it is disconcerting that any debate rages. First, there is the precedent of backache in industry, which we discussed in Chapter 12. But there is also a wealth of directly relevant experience that derives from the press of studies regarding the health of video display terminal (VDT) workers. Realize that these tasks are high on the list of tasks demanding repetitive usage of the upper extremity. Our understanding of the health and safety issues faced by such workers has been summarized in a recent report of a consensus meeting sponsored by the World Health Organization (87). The inferences of this group of scientists are relevant to our conclusions.

In the past, the health debate has tended to focus more on the technology (the physical manifestations and possible hazardous processes within the device) than the information-handling requirements of the task and the related information-processing limitations of the user, as well as wider organizational aspects. This would seem to be a reflection of perception of risk on the part of users rather than an objective assessment of its size. More recently, however, information-processing aspects, cognitive demands in VDT work, and wider organizational considerations have received greater scrutiny.

And they put ergonomic issues into perspective.

When the operator's job consists of a variety of tasks, only some of which may be related to VDT operation, minor faults in the ergonomics of the equipment may not be critical. Conversely, when intense and continuous operation is required, the need for optimum workplace and screen characteristics becomes crucial. However, solutions based entirely upon attention to ergonomic factors are not a panacea for low motivation and poor morale; work design and organizational factors are likely to be more important in determining the operator's overall acceptability of the computer.

A SAMPLING OF MY OWN INVESTIGATIONS INTO DISORDERS OF THE UPPER EXTREMITY IN INDUSTRY

When I first conceptualized "Industrial Rheumatology" as an investigative discipline some 17 yr ago (88), it was clear that industry offered a setting in which the pattern of musculoskeletal usage could be isolated and studied as an independent variable. It was also clear that the upper extremity could be studied unfettered by major psychosocial issues. The American backache was already so embroiled, but the American arm had engendered little notoriety. As investigators we were blessed with an opportunity to study an issue that was fascinating but still not important.

The first study we undertook was to examine the hypothesis that repetitive motion of the upper extremity led to no discernible alteration in structure or function. We identified three groups of women in a single knitting mill operated by Burlington Industries in rural Virginia. Each group had performed a distinctive, highly repetitive, and stereotyped task for a minimum of 20 yr. All the volunteers were examined by rheumatologists to exclude neuropathies and systemic rheumatic disease; we detected no instance of carpal tunnel syndrome or other neuropathy and one instance of rheumatoid arthritis among the 67 volunteers. By radiographic and clinical criteria we could discern differences in the structure of the hand and wrist in the 64 workers who qualified, and these changes correlated with their pattern of usage (8). We could not account for individuals who were no longer in this cohort of workers and might have left because of illness. However, the "survivors" were successful production workers. Extrapolating from community-based epidemiology, even though the groups were distinguishable, we had reason to presume that no group had greater impairment than the population at large matched for age and sex (as discussed in Chapter 8).

Now studies of the upper extremity in the workplace must take into consideration the sociopolitical confounders that render studies of the industrial backache so challenging. In recent years, I have had the opportunity to study groups of workers who were embroiled in considerable medical and sociopolitical turmoil regarding their arm structure and comfort. In such populations, studies designed to examine a single variable, such as our Burlington study, would be naive. I came to this realization when I had the opportunity to examine the Australian RSI epidemic discussed above. I have chosen three of the more dramatic American endemics of putative carpal tunnel syndrome to illustrate the fashion in which a simple concept, that of CTDs, when introduced into the American form of recourse for workplace injury, can engender outcomes that benefit many—but seldom the worker who is hurting and who is at risk for being harmed not by the task but by the recourse.

The Oscar Meyer Endemic

For years Oscar Meyer, Inc., operated a pork processing plant in Beardstown, Illinois. Before 1978, an occasional employee had been subjected to carpal tunnel release. Then the surgical rate began to escalate so that between 1978 and 1983 there were 213 separate carpal tunnel releases in a work force of 788. This means that 20% of the 55 women employees and 15% of the male employees had at least one release. A report of these events was published by hand surgeons (25), some of whom were involved in performing the surgery. It was also an endemic that generated a wealth of documentation that I had the opportunity to study after the fact. The publication offers an accurate data set, although the authors are wedded to supporting the surgery as appropriate for carpal tunnel syndrome of "industrial cause." As the authors are aware, this experience is extraordinary because of the incidence figure of 15%, the male predominance, and the relative youth of the afflicted. They ascribe the endemic to an increase in overtime hours for the meat cutters between 1978 and 1983, since little else about the task description had changed in decades.

The authors mentioned in their discussion several aspects of the endemic that should have shaken their confidence in their pathogenetic inference after the fact and in their diagnosis and management during the endemic. Not only was its onset discrete, but also it terminated abruptly in 1984. At its peak, in 1983, when there were 68 releases in Beardstown, there were only 3 at a sister plant in Iowa with a similar work force. As did the authors, I reviewed a sample of the electrodiagnostic studies performed on the work force during the endemic; these were exhaustive and expensive studies performed by one of several neurologists. About 15% of the studies were impressively beyond normal limits for the particular laboratory. However, Oscar Meyer had initiated an electrodiagnostic preemployment screening program; about 15% of candidates were beyond these normal limits. Therefore, the electrodiagnostic studies of employees were no different than what one would expect in that community.

When I first examined this documentation, it was my impression that the basis for the diagnosis of carpal tunnel syndrome was unconvincing and the surgery was unwarranted. Similar to my arguments earlier in this chapter, I believed even then that the theoretical underpinnings of the CTD concept were anything but solid. I felt that labor-management turmoil that was rife at the time of the endemic rendered the work force susceptible to empirical interventions offered by the local surgical community. I argued these impressions before OSHA, after which OSHA withdrew its general duty clause citation. However, the withdrawal was contingent on Oscar Meyer's contracting with Armstrong and Silverstein from the University of Michigan (for some $50,000) to perform a study of the effectiveness of ergonomic measures in the Beardstown plant. The contracted study was not designed in an experimental fashion and, as predicted, offered no information when completed, since there was no longer a case accrual rate to diminish. The citation was ill-founded. However, demanding that the company contract such flawed investigations is a reproach to the regulatory process that benefits only the coffers of the investigators.

The US West Experience

The Version II console, manufactured by Computer Consoles, Inc. (CCI), is specifically designed for use in the directory assistance operation of telephone companies. By 1983 11 telecommunication entities, both independent companies and subsidiaries of ATT, had purchased over 8,500 units and converted to their use.

By early 1984, what had been the Mountain Bell subsidiary of ATT (before divestiture created US West Communications, Inc.) had also replaced their IBM hardware with CCI terminals. The Version II machine was introduced into the directory assistance operations based in Salt Lake City, in Phoenix, and in Denver. A newer model, the Version III, was introduced into the Phoenix center in 1986. This seemingly minor event passed relatively without incident only in Salt Lake City. In both Denver and Phoenix there are some 500 directory assistance operator positions. Shortly after the equipment change, the corporate medical departments serving each city were faced with a spate of complaints of arm and hand pain by directory assistance operators. However, here the similarity ends. In Denver events unfolded, resulting in a sizable population of workers who suffer incapacitating illness, many of whom have been subjected to multiple surgical procedures. In Phoenix the illness was transient and comparatively benign.

The turmoil surrounding the directory assistance operators employed in Denver is anything but private. It has been the subject of mass media reporting on numerous occasions, including investigative reporting by a team from National Public Radio. However, the details became a matter of record as a result of a class action product liability suit brought by 30 of the directory assistance operators against CCI. The suit alleged that the hand and arm pain was a consequence of flaws in the design of the Version II keyboard which constrained usage to motions that induced pain and tissue damage and which required aggressive medical intervention. The fact that the pain was recalcitrant to such intervention and that the disability was irremediable was further testimony to the severity of the tissue damage incurred in operating the Version II computer keyboard. Although scheduled for hearing in federal court, the claims were settled out of court. Nonetheless, a veritable mountain of clinical and ergonomic data was assembled, along with volumes of sworn testimony. These documents and this documentation were the basis for the current analysis. Data of this nature have disadvantages in that their reliability and validity must be taken at face value. However, these are the same data that fuel litigation and drive policy. If they are good enough for the policy makers, then their analysis is worth our while.

The Incidence of CTDs in the US West Work Force

As I pointed out in Chapter 11, in 1970 Congress enacted the Occupational Health and Safety Act (89). The intent was prophylactic; employers were to provide safe and healthful work environments. One provision was that larger employers were to maintain a register, the OSHA 200 log, of all workplace injuries. For example, backache (even in the absence of traumatic precipitation) reported at work is generally considered a workplace injury (90) and therefore is recorded on OSHA 200 logs. Similarly, use-related arm and hand pain may have been recorded on OSHA 200 logs. In 1986, for consideration as policy, the National Institute for Occupational Safety and Health declared that such use-related arm pain reflects the injurious consequence of microtrauma; the rubric "cumulative trauma disorders" was offered as the appropriate clinical label (1). After this declaration, the Occupational Safety and Health Administration mandated the recording of use-related arm pain on OSHA 200 logs (19). Figure 13.1 is the annual incidence of recorded CTDs among all US West employees broken down into the three geographic areas formerly served by the ATT subsidiaries: Mountain Bell, Northwestern Bell, and Pacific Northwest

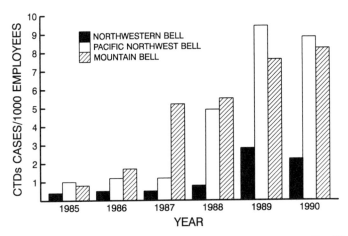

FIG. 13.1. The CTD case rate as reflected by the OSHA 200 logs maintained by US West. The work force is broken down into the three regions served by the former ATT subsidiaries that were merged to form US West Communications. The former Northwestern Bell has a total work force of approximately 15,000 and serves the states of North Dakota, South Dakota, Nebraska, Minnesota, and Iowa. The former Mountain Bell has a work force of approximately 28,000 and serves Arizona, New Mexico, Utah, Colorado, Wyoming, Montana, and most of Idaho. The former Pacific Northwest Bell has a work force of approximately 15,000 and serves Washington, Oregon, and the panhandle of Idaho. The incidence rate for 1990 is extrapolated from the data for the first quarter.

Bell. It is clear that the incidence of recordings of CTDs starts to increase in 1986 in the Mountain Bell work force. There is a lag of about a year before the Pacific Northwest Bell work force is similarly afflicted. The work force of Northwestern Bell seems relatively spared.

The average age of US West workers afflicted and recorded with CTDs was 36 yr. Their average length of service was 11 yr, and the ratio of female to male sufferers was 4.4. However, it is clear from Fig. 13.1 that the likelihood of suffering from recorded CTDs was not uniform by region or time. It is also not restricted to the directory assistance task category; nearly as many cases emerge from other task categories in the company. However, the incidence among directory assistance operators is about tenfold greater than that in the general work force and accounts for most of the increments in incidence demonstrated in Fig. 13.1.

Figure 13.2 is the CTD incidence rate for three of the Mountain Bell states where CCI equipment was introduced in the mid-1980s. The Version II keyboard was introduced in the Salt Lake City and Denver centers and initially in the Phoenix center, yet the incidence rates for CTDs are dramatically different in the states served. The Arizona rate even exceeds that in Colorado, although it was for the Phoenix/Tempe center that the newer Version III keyboard was procured in 1986.

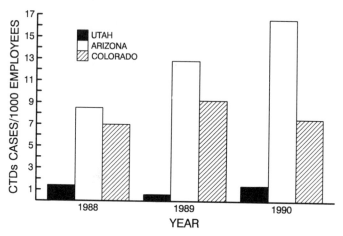

FIG. 13.2. The annual incidence rate of CTDs as recorded by US West on OSHA 200 logs for their work force in Utah, Arizona, and Colorado. The US West work force in each state is approximately 3,000, 7,000, and 12,000, respectively. The rate for 1990 is extrapolated from the data for the first quarter. CCI Version II keyboards were used in the directory assistance centers in these states. In 1986, the Version III was introduced into the Arizona center. (From Hadler, ref. 93, with permission.)

In addition to the three centers illustrated in Fig. 13.2, the directory assistance operators in 9 of the 11 other states served by US West were provided with CCI Version II consoles. For these 9 states, CTDs remained a relatively infrequent event according to the OSHA 200 logs. However, in Oregon and Washington CTDs increased in frequency, accounting for the increase noted in Fig. 13.1 in the Pacific Northwest Bell region. Paradoxically, in Oregon and Washington the directory assistance operators persisted in using the IBM hardware that had been in place for some years. Figure 13.3 details the incidence of CTDs in Oregon and Washington in contrast with Minnesota, which is representative of states with lower rates using the CCI Version II.

Considerable insight into the phenomenon represented by these disparate incidence rates is forthcoming from a dissection of the course of events in Denver and Phoenix. The incidence of CTDs recorded for directory assistance operators in the Denver and Phoenix/Tempe centers accounts for much of the incidence reflected in the data for the respective geographic regions in Figs. 13.1 and 13.2.

The CTDs Endemic in Denver

The physicians and nurses staffing the US West Medical Department in Denver were receptive to the complaints of arm pain. The initial presumption was that these workers were suffering from some form of soft tissue problem,

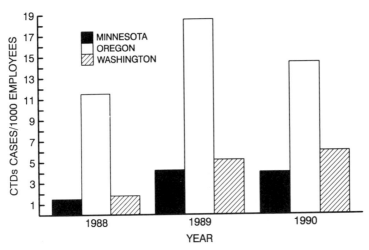

FIG. 13.3. The annual incidence rate of CTDs as recorded by US West on OSHA 200 logs for the work force in the states of Minnesota, Oregon, and Washington. The work force in each state numbers approximately 6,500, 4,500, and 9,500, respectively. The rate for 1990 is extrapolated from the data for the first quarter. Directory assistance operators in Oregon and Washington did not switch to CCI equipment but persisted in the use of IBM equipment. Minnesota utilized the Version II CCI console. (From Hadler, ref. 93, with permission.)

often labeled "tendinitis" or the like. Conservative therapy including antiinflammatory drugs, splinting, and proscription of hand activities was employed. Sessions of physical therapy under the direction of a staff therapist and necessitating further work proscription became a mainstay of intervention. Workers who did not respond were referred to one of a small number of surgeons, often with the possibility of carpal tunnel syndrome in mind. Since the referents were considered injured workers by the US West medical staff, they were entitled to coverage under their Workers' Compensation Insurance program (91). For all of the interval in question, US West was "self-insured"; the task of monitoring care fell back on the Medical Department making the referral. Prior approval was prerequisite if the cost of outside care was to be covered. This requirement forced the consultants to defend their judgments in writing, accounting for the completeness of the records upon which this analysis is based.

In spite of these best of intentions, the results were disappointing. By June 1986 many cases were becoming chronic and new cases were presenting. The corporate industrial hygienist and a consultant ergonomist recommended alterations in the work station, which were followed with some decrease in the case accrual rate. But this was short lived. By early 1987 educational sessions for the workers were conducted by physicians on staff, the staff physical therapist, and one of the cadre of consulting hand surgeons. These sessions involved describing the concept of cumulative trauma disorders and the consequences of not adhering to ergonomic recommendations at the work station. Committees met throughout 1987 with input from directory assistance managers, corporate labor relations and legal officers, and union representatives. All to no avail. At the beginning of 1987, 40 directory assistance operators had been treated for arm pain. By the end of 1987, 147 operators had been treated but only 80 had returned to their prior work, and most of the remainder had persisting restrictions. Furthermore, the clinical records of the Medical Department are rife with demonstrations of the contentious nature of the clinical interactions. For example, workers were often accompanied during their clinic appointments by union representatives attempting to assure that complaints were met with due consideration.

The Occupational Health and Safety Act (89) provides for workers to report perceived hazards to OSHA in a privileged fashion. In response to such complaints, the two principle Denver work sites were inspected in 1987. On January 4, 1988, the company was cited for violations of the act and penalties were proposed. The basis for the citation is the so-called "general duty clause" of the Act of 1970; Section 5(a)(1) obligates the employer to "furnish each of his employees employment and a place of employment which are free from recognized hazards that are causing or likely to cause death or serious physical harm." The intent of this clause is to empower OSHA to enforce safety expeditiously should the agency encounter a hazard that is so patently harmful to justify forgoing the usual setting of standards and rules (92). US West was cited (OSHRC Docket Nos. 88-0308 and 88-0309) for exposing directory assistance operators to "undue repetitive motion trauma . . . due to repeated hand and wrist exertions causing, aggravating, or precipitating Carpal Tunnel Syndrome, Tendinitis, Tenosynovitis, numbness of hands and elbows, strains of hands and elbows, ganglionic cysts, or epicondylitis." The citations further accused US West of ignoring a known "hazard of serious injury" that "could have been eliminated or materially reduced . . . by educating and training its employees as to what Carpal Tunnel Syndrome is . . . by installing adjustable, ergonomically designed work chairs, and by replacing the keyboards currently in use." US West settled with OSHA on August 25, 1988, agreeing to institute a program of ergonomic reforms rapidly, including modification of equipment, educational programs, and management restructuring.

By early 1988 a phasing out of the inculpated keyboard commenced, replacing it with CCI's Version III already in use in the Phoenix/Tempe center. Yet new cases of use-related arm pain presented to the Medical Department at nearly the same pace as in 1987. By the end of 1989, 190 of the directory assistance operators had reported to the medical department, were considered to have suffered a work-related injury qualifying for benefits under their Workers' Compensation Insurance, were recorded on the OSHA 200 log, and were treated (Table 13.11). The majority, 63%, of these claimants were labeled by the Medical Department as suffering from "overuse syndrome" and were treated in-house with work restriction and conservative modalities. Eventually, over 90% of those treated exclusively in-house could return to work without

TABLE 13.11. *Descriptive statistics for the epidemic of hand/arm pain experienced by directory assistance operators employed by US West in Denver from early 1986 through 1989*

Parameter	Finding
Total number of claimants	190
Female/male ratio	2.8
Length of service (range in yr)	6–10
Total number subjected to surgery	29
Number of procedures	41
Number managed "in-house"	119
Given a single diagnosis	105
Resolved without restrictions	113
Number given multiple diagnoses	56
Subjected to surgery	25
Resolved without restrictions	16
Instances each diagnosis was listed on insurance forms	
Epicondylitis	8
Ganglion	5
Fibromyositis/tendinitis	52
Overuse syndrome	121
Thoracic outlet syndrome	18
Reflex sympathetic dystrophy	2
deQuervain's tenosynovitis	8
Carpal tunnel syndrome	26
Other	35

restrictions and often on the same equipment. However, such was not the fate of the 37% for whom outside consultation was either recommended by the Medical Department or demanded by the claimant. It is in this group that the 30 claimants who pursued the product liability suit against CCI can be found.

Table 13.12 presents the descriptive statistics on these 30 litigants, including the diagnoses that led to their multiple surgical procedures. Nearly all were evaluated by more than one consultant, usually by referral from the first consultant but often and also at the request of the Medical Department. There was considerable variability in the symptoms elicited by each consultant and even wider variability in the signs interpreted as indicative of particular soft tissue diseases. It was typical for diagnoses to range from single to multiple soft tissue syndromes and from neuropathic disease to "fibrositis" in each claimant as he or she made the rounds. No patient was ever described as having any consistent atrophic, dystrophic, or overtly inflammatory manifestation of disease. Nearly every litigant was subjected to routine laboratory and radiographic studies that were, without exception, normal. More inventive diagnostic studies were performed in at least 11 instances, ranging from bone scans to arteriograms, without revealing a pathologic condition. These 30 individuals were subjected to electrodiagnostic testing on 46 separate occasions; nearly always the studies were exhaustive, including assessment of sensory and motor conduction in the median and ulnar nerves of both arms, along with electromyograms of multiple hand muscles. In every instance, these studies were entirely normal and, in almost every instance, they were interpreted as well within normal limits by the consulting neurologists who performed the tests.

The small cadre of hand, thoracic, and vascular surgeons involved as the principal consultants took no issue with the negative electrodiagnostic interpretations, and neither did they find the result compelling. They were not dissuaded by the widely divergent diagnostic impressions they generated or by the circumspect and tentative opinions of consultants outside this cadre. To the contrary, they simply postulated that these claimants were suffering from multiple discrete soft tissue and neuropathic processes simultaneously in both arms. Several relied on clinical signs of their own invention; signs interpreted as diagnostic of thoracic outlet syndrome or various entrapment neuropathies. Driven by their clinical impression, they discounted the softness and variability of symptoms and signs and they discounted the total dearth of supporting laboratory, imaging, and electrodiagnostic findings in developing their plan of intervention. They behaved as if cure must be accomplished at all cost and at any

TABLE 13.12. *Descriptive statistics (from early 1986 through early 1990) for the 30 US West employees in Denver who were the plaintiffs in the product liability suit brought against CCI from the design of its Version II console*

Parameter	Finding
Age at onset of symptoms	
Mean	31.3
Range	21–44
Female/male ratio	26/4
Instances of specialized diagnostic testing	
Electrodiagnostic testing	46
Invasive testing (arteriogram,	
arthrogram, bone scan)	11
Number of claimants spared surgery	9
Invasive/surgical procedures performed	70
For entrapment neuropathy	
Carpal tunnel release	18
Radial tunnel release	1
Ulnar nerve release	1
Re-do for median entrapment	2
For reflex sympathetic dystrophy	
Series of stellate blocks	12
Series of Bier blocks	6
Stellate ganglionectomy	1
Brachial artery stripping	3
For thoracic outlet syndrome	
Supra/infraclavicular approach	9
Transaxillary approach	1
For soft tissue diseases	
Of tendons	14
Ganglionectomy	1
Scar revision	1

risk/benefit ratio given the desperate straits of their patients. They behaved as if more than a job was at risk; limb was at risk, if not life itself. They behaved in this fashion in spite of the absence of clinical precedent in their own practices. The relevant literature was never cited. Rather, the group of surgeons plied each other with pathogenetic hypotheses, and they convinced each other that they were at the forefront of insight into a new industrial disease. When one procedure was unsuccessful or only transiently successful, a new diagnosis rose to the fore and a new intervention was proposed to the claimant and usually accepted. And all of their intellectual and therapeutic machinations were met with "prior approval" by the Medical Department; their bills were paid promptly by the telephone company. The direct cost to compensate for the lost wages and to pay for the medical care of these 30 litigants exceeded $1.5 million.

In this fashion a small cadre of surgeons, consulting among themselves, found the temerity to undertake 70 separate invasive procedures on 21 of the 30 litigants. All 21 submitted to surgical procedures for putative entrapment neuropathies, 22 designed for peripheral releases and 10 for thoracic outlet syndrome. In addition, these same 21 claimants were subjected to 16 separate surgical procedures offered as remedies for such putative soft tissue diseases as various forms of the tendinitides. Even the 21 procedures designed as remedies for various manifestations of putative reflex sympathetic dystrophy were performed in the absence of demonstrable cutaneous or osseous dystrophy. Yet the interventionalist zeal was intransigent.

The CTDs Endemic in Phoenix

The incidence of CTDs reflected by the OSHA 200 log in Phoenix outstripped even that in Denver (Fig. 13.2). The Phoenix medical staff also initiated on-site programs designed to render the entire work force more knowledgeable regarding the conservative management of arm pain, including the roles for biomechanics, physical medicine, and ergonomics. Workers were encouraged to report any arm discomfort. Such complaints led to one-on-one consultations with the staff physical therapist at the worker's work station. Labor/management committees were formed to address the issue of CTDs, and work station modification commenced.

Much of this also occurred in Denver. However, the clinical consequences are dramatically divergent. The majority of the workers, again mainly directory assistance operators, felt no need to make a second visit to the Medical Department. The working diagnoses recorded in the Phoenix Medical Department were similar to those in Denver (Table 13.1). Of the first 165 workers with CTDs, 129 were back at work full-time without restrictions by early 1990. In Phoenix, as in Denver, referrals to outside physicians were common, also to a small cadre of surgeons. However, a recommendation for surgery was seldom the result, and multiple procedures were never undertaken. In fact, less than 20 procedures were performed on this population. About half were designed for a putative entrapment neuropathy, including a single case of surgery for putative thoracic outlet syndrome. Some procedures were performed in Phoenix but not Denver, such as several wrist arthroscopies and a shortening of the radius in a patient whose symptoms were ascribed to radiographic Kienböck's disease. The majority of the workers who underwent these procedures were well enough to return to work. Even an OSHA inspection did not result in a citation.

The Ergonomics of the CCI Keyboard

The Version II keyboard is just that, a keyboard (Fig. 13.4). At first blush, nothing could appear more innocuous. In fact, it was designed with the comfort and efficiency of the operator in mind and successfully marketed for that reason. It is a "Dvorak" keyboard, meaning that the keys are positioned with a view toward the biomechanics of usage rather than the traditional "QWERTY" configuration. This also means that practice is necessary to overcome unfamiliarity with this array. As part of the product liability suit, the plaintiffs hired five specialists in ergonomics and human factors to opine on the pathogenetic potential of this keyboard. One after another concurred with the first assessment; the design of the Version II keyboard was faulted because the user receives no tactile, visual, or auditory feedback when depressing the key. It was asserted that without such feedback as a "click" or "breakaway," the user is at risk of exerting excess force and therefore of incurring CTDs. In addition, it was opined that the keyboard casing is shaped so that a "sharp edge" awaits the resting wrist. Since usage by directory assistance operators is intermittent, resting their wrists on the edge might similarly induce CTDs. The frequency of keying or any other motion was not considered an issue.

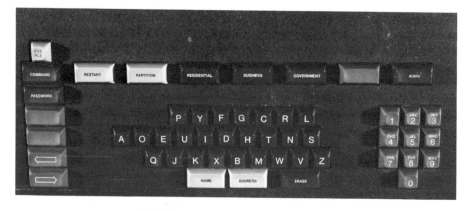

FIG. 13.4. The Version II CCI keyboard.

It is noteworthy that the CCI Version III was sanctioned for substitution in Denver as part of the OSHA settlement with US West. The Version III also passed muster at the OSHA inspection in Phoenix. The Version III keyboard has a different design to take advantage of technologically advanced low-profile switches. The casing is less deep, there are more keys, and they are arrayed in the QWERTY configuration. The Version III keying characteristic is the same as that of the Version II.

The Object Lesson

Is this a saga of omission? Could it be that the arm pain of the directory assistance operators in Minnesota or Utah is being ignored? Are the CTDs of the workers in Arizona undertreated by the local surgical community? Could it be that the Denver experience should be our "gold standard"? I think not. The literature relevant to these questions is overwhelmingly in support of the refutation. Furthermore, close inspection of the experience of the US West directory assistance operators provides an object lesson in the human costs of prematurely basing workplace health and safety policy on as tenuous a concept as CTDs. This small area analysis (93) leaves several questions unanswered. However, it tests two of the inferences that are critical to the CTD hypothesis: ergonomic causality and the damaging outcome. Since the clinical outcome is unrelated to the ergonomics of the task, holding the ergonomics of the keyboard at fault is untenable. Since the clinical outcome varies from predicaments to illnesses that lead to mutilating surgery, one must question the validity of the latter clinical diagnoses and the wisdom of the intervention.

The Pepperidge Farm Experience

Pepperidge Farm is another employer that was cited by OSHA under the general duty clause at two of its facilities, Downingtown, Pennsylvania, and Downers Grove, Illinois. The Downingtown plant has some 1,500 employees. However, the citation followed an inspection in response to complaints from workers on only a few of the tasks at the facility. Not only had workers solicited an OSHA inspection, but also many were experiencing arm pain that had been recorded by the plant's medical department. The task that was considered most egregious involved the manufacture of Milano cookies. Almost the entire process is automated until one cookie has to be manually placed on top of another to create a sandwich. Minimal force is involved; otherwise, the cookie would crumble. The task is more highly repetitive than any involved in the other endemics we have discussed.

However, the clinical outcomes were tragic. Downingtown never reached the unconscionable outcomes that befell the Denver directory assistance operators. However, these women met a fate similar to the Beardstown butchers even though their only exposure was to maneuvering cookies. Sixty-eight workers received 190 separate diagnostic labels as they progressed from the plant physician to the consultant chosen by the plant physician. Forty workers underwent 60 exhaustive electrodiagnostic tests; only 2 were clearly abnormal. And 28 workers underwent 42 separate surgical procedures, of which 33 were carpal tunnel releases. The complaint rate at the Downers Grove facility was similar. However, the outcomes were far less drastic. In particular, few workers underwent empirical surgical procedures.

Pepperidge Farm appealed the two citations. The Downingtown appeal (OSHRC Docket No. 89-0265) was brought before the federal judiciary. An opinion is pending. The Downers Grove appeal was also brought before the federal judiciary (OSHRC Docket No. 90-1236), but action proved unnecessary as OSHA withdrew the citation.

SUMMARY

CTDs are an inappropriate rallying cry for workplace safety. The legislated redress for worker health and safety is designed to prevent trauma and to provide redress for tissue damage. If we use discomfort as a surrogate for damage, the legislated redress can backfire: The worker who hurts is drawn into the contest of causation. The pain becomes the evidence for hazard, and the persistence of pain is necessary to carry forth the argument. Likewise, when pain is the cause of disability, persistence of pain is necessary to carry forth the argument. In either contest, the hurting worker is poorly served; no one can get well if he or she has to prove illness! To the contrary, the patients are at risk for getting sicker. They can become angry, beleaguered, desperate claimants willing to grasp at any straw, even multiple, unproven surgical interventions, in defense of their claim (see Chapter 5). This is the vortex that was precipitated by the RSI hypothesis in Australia, that (as we saw in Chapter 12) has enveloped the industrial backache for decades (94), and that now threatens to confound our predicaments of arm pain even to the extreme seen in the US West directory assistance operators in Denver. This vortex is the topic of Chapter 15. It is one of the major pitfalls of the format for disability determination that all of the West inherited from the Prussian statutes of 100 yr ago (95). Other countries have experimented with alternatives (96). But compassionate, major reform is long overdue to provide more efficient redress for the illness of work incapacity, whether a consequence of damage or of discomfort.

Regional musculoskeletal illness of the upper extremity or axial skeleton is an important target for improved worker comfort and workplace healthfulness. These predicaments, like stress and unhappiness, color all of our lives at some time, both in and out of the workplace. But it is in the workplace where salutary reform is feasible. We need to be able complain when our own coping mechanisms are exhausted. Interpersonal relationships, fiscal and other rewards, information and misinformation, personal psychosocial confounders, and, yes, even ergonomics are relevant variables. Compassionate micromanagement should be the response to our plea—not contests, gauntlets, and ill-conceived medical and ergonomic interventions. The rallying cry is for enlightenment of labor, management, and the individual worker.

REFERENCES

1. Association of Schools of Public Health/National Institute for Occupational Safety and Health. *Proposed National Strategies for the Prevention of Leading Work-related Diseases and Injuries: Part 1.* Washington, DC, Association of Schools of Public Health, 1986:19.
2. Brammer A, Pyykkö I. Vibration-induced neuropathy: detection by nerve conduction measurements. *Scand J Work Environ Health* 1987;13:317–22.
3. Schumacher HR, Agudelo C, Labowitz R. Jackhammer arthropathy. *J Occup Med* 1972;14:563–4.
4. Miyashita K, Shiomi S, Itoh N, Kasamatsu T, Iwata H. Epidemiological study of vibration syndrome in response to total hand-tool operating time. *Br J Ind Med* 1983;40:92–8.
5. National Institute of Occupational Safety and Health. Vibration syndrome in chipping and grinding workers. *J Occup Med* 1984;26[Suppl]:766–88.
6. Taylor W. Hand-arm vibration syndrome: a new clinical classification and an updated British standard guide for hand transmitted vibration. *Br J Ind Med* 1988;45:281–2.
7. Vibration syndrome. *Current Intelligence Bulletin 38.* March 29, 1983. US Public Health Service, Centers for Disease Control. DHHS(NIOSH) Publication No. 83-110.
8. Hadler NM, Gillings DB, Imbus HR, Levitin PM, Makuc D, Utsinger PD, Yount WJ, Slusser D, Moskovitz N. Hand structure and function in an industrial setting: influence of three patterns of stereotyped, repetitive usage. *Arthritis Rheum* 1978;21:210–20.
9. Douglas G, Rang M. The role of trauma in the pathogenesis of the osteochondroses. *Clin Orthop* 1981;158:28–32.
10. Meilá I, Braborscu E, Meilá D. Aseptic necrosis of the lunate bone caused by repeated microtrauma in the mining and metallurgic industry. *Oncol Radiol* 1963;II:89–93.
11. Beckenbaugh RD, Shives TC, Dobyns JH, Linscheid RL. Kienböck's disease: the natural history of Kienböck's disease and consideration of lunate fractures. *Clin Orthop* 1980;149:98–106.
12. Kumlin R, Wiikeri M, Sumari P. Radiological changes in carpal and metacarpal bones and phalanges caused by chain saw vibration. *Br J Ind Med* 1973;30:71–3.
13. Suzuki K, Takahashi S, Nakagawa T. Radiological studies of the wrist joint among chain saw operating lumberjacks in Japan. *Acta Orthop Scand* 1978;49:464–8.
14. Bovenzi M, Florito A, Volpe C. Bone and joint disorders in the upper extremities of chipping and grinding operators. *Int Arch Occup Environ Health* 1987;59:189–98.
15. Gemne G, Saraste H. Bone and joint pathology in workers using hand-held vibrating tools. *Scand J Work Environ Health* 1987;13:290–300.
16. Mallory M, Bradford H. An invisible workplace hazard gets harder to ignore. *Business Week* 1989;January 30:92–3.
17. LeGrande D. Carpal tunnel syndrome: it hurts, it cripples. *CWA News* 1989;48:6–7.
18. Occupational disease surveillance: carpal tunnel syndrome. *MMWR Morb Mortal Wkly Rep* 1989;38:485–9.
19. Freeman RS. Going around and around with CTDs: a look at the legal issues. *Occup Safety Health Rep* 1990;June 13:63–7.
20. Armstrong TJ, Silverstein BA. Upper-extremity pain in the workplace—role of usage in causality. In: Hadler NM (ed.) *Clinical Concepts in Regional Musculoskeletal Illness.* Orlando, Grune & Stratton, 1987:333–54.
21. Armstrong TJ, Chaffin DB. Some biomechanical aspects of the carpal tunnel. *J Biomech* 1979;12:567–70.
22. Armstrong TJ, Chaffin DB. Carpal tunnel syndrome and selected personal attributes. *J Occup Med* 1979;21:481–6.

23. Baker EL, Ehrenberg RL. Preventing the work-related carpal tunnel syndrome: physician reporting and diagnostic criteria. *Ann Intern Med* 1990;112:317–9.
24. Armstrong TJ. Ergonomics and cumulative trauma disorders. *Hand Clin* 1986;2:553–65.
25. Masear V, Hayes J, Hyde A. An industrial cause of carpal tunnel syndrome. *J Hand Surg* 1986;64:271–301.
26. Hadler NM. Cumulative trauma disorders: an iatrogenic concept. *J Occup Med* 1990;32:38–41.
27. Hadler NM. The roles of work and of working in disorders of the upper extremity. *Baillieres Clin Rheumatol* 1989;3:121–41.
28. Hadler NM. Work-related disorders of the upper extremity. In: Hadler NM, Bunn WB (eds.) *Occupational Problems in Medical Practice*. New York, DellaCorte, 1990:219–48.
29. Verbrugge LM, Ascione FJ. Exploring the iceberg: common symptoms and how people care for them. *Med Care* 1987;25:539–69.
30. Cunningham LS, Kelsey JL. Epidemiology of musculoskeletal impairments and associated disability. *Am J Public Health* 1984;74:574–9.
31. Hadler NM. The language of diagnosis. In: Hadler NM (ed.) *Clinical Concepts in Regional Musculoskeletal Disease*. Orlando, Grune & Stratton, 1987:3–6.
32. Payer L. *Medicine & Culture*. New York, Holt, 1988:1–204.
33. Kuorinka I, Koskinen P. Occupational rheumatic diseases and upper limb strain in manual jobs in a light mechanical industry. *Scand J Work Environ Health* 1979;5[Suppl 3]:39–47.
34. Luopajarvi T, Kuorinka I, Virolainen M. Prevalence of tenosynovitis and other injuries of the upper extremities in repetitive work. *Scand J Work Environ Health* 1979;5[Suppl 3]:48–55.
35. Viikari-Juntara E. Neck and upper limb disorders among slaughterhouse workers. *Scand J Work Environ Health* 1983;9:283–90.
36. Waris P, Kuorinka I, Kurppa K, Luopajarvi T, Virolainen M, Pesonen K, Nummi J, Kukkonnen R. Epidemiologic screening for occupational nick and upper limb disorders: methods and criteria. *Scand J Work Environ Health* 1979;5[Suppl 3]:25–38.
37. Stevens JC, Sun S, Beard CM, O'Fallon WM, Kurland LT. Carpal tunnel syndrome in Rochester, Minnesota, 1961–1980. *Neurology* 1988;38:134–8.
38. Pfeffer GB, Gelberman RH. The carpal tunnel syndrome. In: Hadler NM (ed.) *Clinical Concepts in Regional Musculoskeletal Illness*. Orlando, Grune & Stratton, 1987:201–16.
39. Louis DS, Hankin FM. Symptomatic relief following carpal tunnel decompression with normal electroneuromyographic studies. *Orthopedics* 1987;10:434–6.
40. Katz JN. Carpal tunnel syndrome and other workplace-related upper extremity pain disorders. In: *Postgraduate Advances in Rheumatology IV-XI*. Berryville, Virginia, Forum Medicum, 1991:3.
41. Katz JN, Larson MG, Sabra A, Krarup C, Stirrat CR, Sethi R, Eaton HM, Fossel AH, Liang MH. The carpal tunnel syndrome: diagnostic utility of the history and physical examination findings. *Ann Intern Med* 1990;112:321–7.
42. Hadler NM. To be a patient or a claimant with a musculoskeletal illness. In: Hadler NM (ed.) *Clinical Concepts in Regional Musculoskeletal Illness*. Orlando, Grune & Stratton, 1987:7–23.
43. Hymovich L, Lindholm M. Hand, wrist and forearm injuries: the result of repetitive motions. *J Occup Med* 1966;8:573–7.
44. Cannon LJ, Bernacki EJ, Walter SD. Personal and occupational factors associated with carpal tunnel syndrome. *J Occup Med* 1981;23:255–8.
45. Ford DJ, Ali MS. Acute carpal tunnel syndrome. *J Bone Joint Surg [Br]* 1986;68B:758–9.
46. Gellman H, Chandler DR, Petrasek J, Sie I, Adkins R, Waters RL. Carpal tunnel syndrome in paraplegic patients. *J Bone Joint Surg [Am]* 1988;70A:517–9.
47. Gelberman RH, Rydevik BL, Pess GM, Szabo RM, Lundborg G. Carpal tunnel syndrome: a scientific basis for clinical care. *Orthop Clin North Am* 1988;19:115–24.
48. Okutsu I, Ninomiya S, Hamanaka I, Kuroshima N, Inanami H. Measurement of pressure in the carpal canal before and after endoscopic management of carpal tunnel syndrome. *J Bone Joint Surg [Am]* 1989;71A:679–83.
49. Phalen GS, Kendrick JL. Compression neuropathy of the median nerve in the carpal tunnel. *JAMA* 1957;164:524–30.
50. Birbeck MQ, Beer TC. Occupation in relation to the carpal tunnel syndrome. *Rheum Rehabil* 1975;14:218–21.
51. Margolis W, Kraus JF. The prevalence of carpal tunnel syndrome symptoms in female supermarket checkers. *J Occup Med* 1987;29:953–6.

52. Barnhart S, Rosenstock L. Carpal tunnel syndrome in grocery checkers: a cluster of work-related illness. *West J Med* 1987;147:37–40.
53. Wieslander G, Norbäck D, Göthe C-J, Juhlin L. Carpal tunnel syndrome (CTS) and exposure to vibration, repetitive wrist movements, and heavy manual work: a case-referent study. *Br J Ind Med* 1989;46:43–7.
54. Franklin GM, Haug J, Heyer N, Checkoway H, Peck N. Occupational carpal tunnel syndrome in Washington State 1984–1988. *Am J Public Health* 1991;81:741–6.
55. Feldman RG, Jabre JF. Electrodiagnostic aspects of the carpal tunnel syndrome. In: Hadler NM (ed.) *Clinical Concepts in Regional Musculoskeletal Illness.* Orlando, Grune & Stratton, 1987:217–26.
56. Feldman RG, Travers PH, Chirico-Post J, Keyserling WM. Risk assessment in electronic assembly workers: carpal tunnel syndrome. *J Hand Surg [Am]* 1987;12A(2 Pt 2):849–55.
57. Schottland JR, Kirschberg GJ, Fillingim R, Davis VP, Hogg F. Median nerve latencies in poultry processing workers: an approach to resolving the role of industrial "cumulative trauma" in the development of the carpal tunnel syndrome. *J Occup Med* 1991;33:627–31.
58. Nathan PA, Meadows KD, Doyle LS. Sensory segmental latency values of the median nerve for a population of normal individuals. *Arch Phys Med Rehabil* 1988;69:499–501.
59. Nathan PA, Meadows KD, Doyle LS. Occupation as a risk factor for impaired sensory conduction of the median nerve at the carpal tunnel. *J Hand Surg [Br]* 1988;13B:167–70.
60. Nathan PA, Meadows KD, Doyle LS. Relationship of age and sex to sensory conduction of the median nerve at the carpal tunnel and association of slowed conduction with symptoms. *Muscle Nerve* 1988;11:1149–53.
61. Nathan PA, Keniston RC, Myers LD, Meadows KD. Obesity as a risk factor for slowing of sensory conduction of the median nerve in industry. *J Occup Med* 1992;34:379–83.
62. Stone WE. Repetitive strain injuries. *Med J Aust* 1983;2:616–8.
63. Browne CD, Nolan BM, Faithfull DK. Occupational repetition strain injuries: guidelines for diagnosis and management. *Med J Aust* 1984;140:329–32.
64. Ferguson D. The "new" industrial epidemic. *Med J Aust* 1984;140:318–9.
65. Hadler NM. Industrial rheumatology: the Australian and New Zealand experiences with arm pain and backache in the workplace. *Med J Aust* 1986;144:191–5.
66. Cleland LG. "RSI": a model of social iatrogenesis. *Med J Aust* 1987;147:236–9.
67. Hocking B. Epidemiological aspects of "repetition strain injury" in Telecom Australia. *Med J Aust* 1987:147:318–322.
68. Ferguson DA. "RSI": putting the epidemic to rest. *Med J Aust* 1987;147:213–4.
69. Reilly PA, Travers R, Littlejohn GO. Epidemiology of soft tissue rheumatism: the influence of the law. *J Rheumatol* 1991;18:10–1.
70. Simms RW, Goldenberg DL. Symptoms mimicking neurologic disorders in fibromyalgia syndrome. *J Rheumatol* 1988;15:1271–3.
71. Miller MH, Topliss DJ. Chronic upper limb pain syndrome (repetitive strain injury) in the Australian workforce: a systematic cross sectional rheumatological study of 229 patients. *J Rheumatol* 1988;15:1705–12.
72. Armstrong TJ, Castelli WA, Evans FG, Diaz-Perez R. Some histological changes in the carpal tunnel contents and their biomechanical implications. *J Occup Med* 1984;26:197–201.
73. Armstrong TJ, Foulke JA, Joseph BS, Goldstein SA. Investigation of cumulative trauma disorders in a poultry processing plant. *Am Ind Hyg Assoc J* 1982;43:103–16.
74. Silverstein BA, Fine LJ, Armstrong TJ. Hand-wrist cumulative trauma disorders in industry. *Br J Ind Med* 1986;43:779–84.
75. Silverstein BA, Fine LJ, Armstrong TJ. Occupational factors and carpal tunnel syndrome. *Am J Ind Med* 1987;11:343–58.
76. Silverstein BA. *The Prevalence of Upper Extremity Cumulative Trauma Disorders in Industry.* [Dissertation]. Ann Arbor, Michigan, University of Michigan, 1985:1–262.
77. Hadler NM. Entrapment neuropathies. In: McCarty DJ (ed.) *Arthritis and Allied Conditions.* Philadelphia, Lea & Febiger, 1989:1485–91.
78. Silverstein B, Fine L, Stetson D. Hand-wrist disorders among investment casting plant workers. *J Hand Surg [Am]* 1987;12A:838–44.
79. Green RA, Briggs CA. Effect of overuse injury and the importance of training on the use of adjustable workstations by keyboard operators. *J Occup Med* 1989;31:557–62.
80. Oxenburgh MS, Rowe SA, Douglas DB. Repetition strain injury in keyboard operators. *J Occup Health Safety Aust NZ* 1985;1:106–12.

81. Westgaard RH, Aaras A. The effect of improved workplace design on the development of the work-related musculoskeletal illnesses. *Appl Ergonomics* 1985;16:91–7.
82. Parenmark G, Engvall B, Malmkvist A-K. Ergonomic on-the-job training of assembly workers. *Appl Ergonomics* 1988;19:143–6.
83. Ryan GA, Bampton M. Comparison of data process operators with and without upper limb symptoms. *Community Health Studies* 1988;12:63–8.
84. Linton SJ, Kamwendo K. Risk factors in the psychosocial work environment for neck and shoulder pain in secretaries. *J Occup Med* 1989;31:609–13.
85. Dimberg L, Olafsson A, Stefansson E, Aagaard H, Odén A, Andersson GBJ, Hansson T, Hagert C-G. The correlation between work environment and the occurrence of cervicobrachial symptoms. *J Occup Med* 1989;31:447–53.
86. Smith MJ, Sainfort PC. A balance theory of job design for stress reduction. *Int J Ind Ergonomics* 1989;4:67–79.
87. World Health Organization. Work with visual display terminals: psychosocial aspects and health. *J Occup Med* 1989;31:957–68.
88. Hadler NM. Industrial rheumatology: clinical investigations into the influence of pattern of usage on pattern of regional musculoskeletal disease. *Arthritis Rheum* 1977;20:1019–25.
89. Occupational Health and Safety Act of 1970. 29 U.S.C. 651 et seq.
90. Hadler NM. Regional musculoskeletal diseases of the low back: cumulative trauma versus single incident. *Clin Orthop* 1987;221:33–41.
91. Hadler NM. Occupational illness: the issue of causality. *J Occup Med* 1984;26:587–93.
92. Stillman NG, Wheeler JR. The expansion of occupational safety and health law. *Notre Dame Law Rev* 1987;62:969–1009.
93. Hadler NM. Arm pain in the workplace: a small area analysis. *J Occup Med* 1992;34:113–9.
94. Hadler NM. The vortex of disability determination: the object lesson of impairment rating for axial pain. In: Hadler NM, Bunn WB (eds.) *Occupational Problems in Medical Practice.* New York, DellaCorte, 1990:261–6.
95. Hadler NM. Criteria for screening workers for the establishment of disability. *J Occup Med* 1986;28:940–5.
96. Hadler NM. Disabling backache in France, Switzerland, and the Netherlands: contrasting sociopolitical constraints on clinical judgment. *J Occup Med* 1989;31:823–31.

14

Social Security

The Process of Pensioning the Invalid

Are there still worthy poor? Are there individuals among us who, in spite of their best efforts and because of circumstances they cannot control, are particularly deserving of empathy and fiscal support? This question is woven into the fabric of Western society.

Codification of the need to care for the worthy poor can be dated to Elizabethan England. Before that, these individuals had to plead their desperation to merit the charity of family and religious orders. But the government of Elizabeth I came to their assistance in the form of a series of statutes called the "Poor Laws" (1). These statutes placed the onus of asylum care of the crippled on the fiscally competent. Well into the 18th century, the gentry were charged with assessing work capacity; charity was tendered to those deemed deserving. In fact, on the great estates of the time in England, asylum care was provided in terms of housing and food for the needy.

The Poor Laws offer a window into Western ambivalence regarding such magnanimousness. Helping the worthy is an incontrovertible tenet—even if it is ignored. But the idea that someone less deserving might benefit from this largess has always seemed, to most, to be intolerable. That's why all Poor Laws included some consideration of the unworthy poor. These are individuals that request assistance but do not deserve it. The same gentry who meted out beneficence were required to identify the unworthy poor, who were entitled to punishment, even corporal punishment. The unworthy poor included "those whose defects make them an abomination." The Poor Laws crossed the Atlantic into the American colonies. In colonial America a destitute individual surviving as a beggar, even physically disabled but still judged unworthy, could be "warned out of town" and punished upon returning, "36 lashes on the bare back if a man, 25 if a women." They added sexism to injury!

Paranoia about rewarding the unworthy poor has driven the thinking of Western politicians and philosophers up to the present. There are exceptions.

Henry Mayhew was a Victorian editorialist with an extraordinary social conscience. His essays are collected in a multivolume work entitled *London Labour and the London Poor*, in which he championed the "street people" whom he saw as driven to desperation by the callousness of society. Mayhew argued that the "effects of uncertain labour drive the labourers to improvidence, recklessness, and pauperism." However, unlike most liberal thinkers, Mayhew championed the street people, regardless of the cause of their desperation, "those that will work, those that cannot work, and those that will not work" (2). The traditional sociopolitical imperative is not that indiscriminate; Western society is willing to spend a fortune making a distinction between the categories of "will work" but unemployed, "cannot work" from disability, and, the most dreaded of all, those who "will not work" even though they can. To most Westerners, the prospect of rewarding those whose plight reflects a degree of volition is anathema. That explains the violent underbelly of the Poor Laws in demanding that the gentry exclude the unworthy from benefits and punish them for their impertinence. It also explains the extraordinary lengths to which society has gone and the moneys it has expended to ferret out the unworthy poor. This exercise of designing and operating the perfect mouse trap is the exercise of disability determination, which we will dissect in Chapter 15.

The Poor Laws were active statutes in Great Britain into this century. They were superseded by the social insurance acts of 1911, which were Prussian in precedent and were shepherded through the Edwardian parliament by David Lloyd George. His description of the operation of the Poor Laws, in a speech delivered on June 11, 1911, at the Birmingham Town Hall, will stand forever as the condemnation of noblesse oblige (3).

> You may say there is the Poor Law. Ah! Let me say this to the honour of the workers of this country, the last thing they pawn is their pride. There is no greater heroism in history as you find in the humble annals of those who fight through life against odds to maintain their self-respect and independence. They will suffer the last privation before they pin the badge of pauperism over their hearts, and certainly before they will put it on the breast of their children.

One can identify some laudatory features, even ethic, in the Poor Laws, but that ethic was distorted by the often arbitrary nature of the assessment of worthiness and the stigma attached to the charity. What remained of the ethic could not cope with the advent of the industrial revolution, when large numbers of citizens opted to enter the workplace as employees. That dialectic led to the formulation of the Prussian reforms in social legislation at the turn of the century. As discussed in Chapter 12, these statutes created the distinction between those who were worthy but not necessarily poor as a consequence of injury incurred in the workplace and those who were worthy and poor as a consequence of catastrophe that was not work related. The largesse not only was greater for the former, but also was the only form of disability insurance to be introduced into the United States in the early decades of the 20th century.

THE HISTORY OF THE U.S. PROGRAM FOR
GLOBAL DISABILITY INSURANCE

America found itself dealing with the precepts of Workers' Compensation Insurance by 1911. The time should have been ripe for further social reform. Theodore Roosevelt ran for president in 1912 under the Progressive Party banner. His platform, with the support of the American Medical Association, included national health insurance. He made an impact on the election; he garnered sufficient votes to enable Woodrow Wilson to become president. Reformers such as Professor Henry Seager of Columbia University, Isaac M. Rubinow, Louis Brandeis (the Boston attorney who would later join the Supreme Court), and many in the labor movement all called for social reform. But the American voter, still imbued with the 19th century spirit of rugged individualism, turned a deaf ear to the cries of the unemployed, whether from physical incapacity or age. With the Great Depression, the American sense of invincibility crumbled.

Franklin D. Roosevelt stood before Congress on June 9, 1934, and changed the course of American humanism. FDR demanded "some safeguard against misfortunes which cannot be wholly eliminated in this man-made world of ours. . . . I am looking for a sound means which I can recommend to provide at once security against several of the great disturbing factors in life—especially those related to unemployment and old age." Roosevelt brought the Wisconsin economist, Edwin E. Witte, to Washington to provide the "sound means" (4). The Witte Committee probably had the talent to address the entire scope of the human predicament, with such members as Dorothy Perkins, Frank Porter Graham, and others. The machinations of the committee are recorded in Witte's diary and are awe inspiring (5). The product of their work was the Social Security Act of 1935. The act provided the old-age pension program Roosevelt sought, funding the plan by assessing wages and requiring employer contribution. But political exigencies blocked any consideration of disability or health insurance. The AMA had withdrawn its support shortly after the last Theodore Roosevelt campaign and even coined the descriptor *socialized medicine* for national health insurance to play on American fears of "socialism"—the term is used as an implicit aspersion even today.

Disability insurance did not regain a place on the national agenda until the 1950s, a half-century after nearly every European power had developed its programs. These were the Eisenhower years—the decade of American empire. Nonetheless, empire did not guarantee social awareness; the return of disability insurance to political consciousness was somewhat insidious. In 1951 it was decided that contributions to the Old Age Pension Fund could be waived without jeopardizing benefits if the worker was incapacitated and unable to continue his contributions. This legislation provided the daylight for broader disability legislation. Spearheaded by Witte's disciple, Wilbur Cohen, Social

Security Disability Insurance was passed into law in 1954 and became operational in 1956. As with Old Age Insurance, wages were assessed, employers contributed, and the moneys accumulated in a separate fund that was meant to be restricted for the payment of disability benefits. To qualify for a disability pension, the claimant had to be over 50 yr of age, have worked for at least half of the previous 10 yr, and demonstrate an impairment of "long continued and indefinite duration." In 1960 the age limitation was eliminated, and in 1967 the duration of incapacity was reduced to a minimum of 12 mo.

In its first decade of operation (1957–1967) the annual cost of the SSDI program climbed from $59 million to $2,089 million. The number of disabled workers rose from 149,850 to 1,193,120. The number of dependent beneficiaries (spouses and children of disabled workers and the like who also receive benefits) reached 1 million. These figures and those which follow are culled from a report prepared by the U.S. Senate Finance Committee in September 1983 (6). The second decade saw a dramatic increase in the number of disabled workers and in the cost of the program. Two acts of Congress were responsible for this expansion: the Black Lung Benefits Act and Title XVI of the Social Security Act.

The Black Lung Benefits Act

In 1969 Congress passed the Black Lung Benefits Act (30 USC 901 et seq.). This act is the product, heralded as the culmination, of some 50 yr of labor-management acrimony. It was to be the vindication and the salve for generations of downtrodden, exploited coal miners. It has proven a Pyrrhic victory.

In the aftermath of World War II, John L. Lewis, the president of the United Mine Workers, turned his attention to the plight of injured and disabled miners. In 1946 mine operators agreed to utilize some percentage of coal-tonnage royalties to underwrite a Welfare and Retirement Fund. Public health nurses and physicians were sent into the hollows of Appalachia to locate paralyzed miners and transport them to rehabilitation centers. Lewis also pressured the federal government to bolster the funding of state vocational rehabilitation agencies. And he added the voice of the United Mine Workers to that of others calling for the establishment of SSDI in the 1950s. But by 1960, only the most catastrophically impaired of the miners had recourse.

Their cause was taken up by two champions: Ralph Nader, the consumer advocate, and I. E. Buff, a physician practicing in West Virginia. Buff decried conditions in the mines and coined the term *black lung*. With Nader he argued that external force injury was only the most patent of the perils of the mine; the scourge was pneumoconiosis. Neither the United Mine Workers Union nor Congress felt compelled to action until November 20, 1968, when another in a long line of mining calamities occurred; an explosion at the Consolidation Coal

Company mine in Farmington, West Virginia, entombed 78 miners. Press coverage was extensive, and the country was enraged. The coal mines of Appalachia can be found in seven states: Pennsylvania, Virginia, West Virginia, Kentucky, Ohio, Illinois, and Alabama. Driven by national outrage and spearheaded by seven congressional delegations, legislation was soon to follow in the form of the Coal Mine Health and Safety Act of 1969. Appended to the act was coverage for an occupational disease, black lung disease. There was precedent for coverage of occupational disease in the Federal Workers' Compensation system, which indemnified longshoremen, railroad workers, and federal employees. Covering miners for black lung seemed reasonable. However, the Black Lung Program was distinctive for the federal administration—and an administrative Trojan horse for the Social Security Administration, under whose aegis it fell until 1973, when the Department of Labor assumed responsibility for new claims.

Congress' intent was that black lung would be handled by the Social Security Administration just like any other claim. As we shall discuss shortly, the critical criterion for a disability award is the inability to maintain any substantial gainful employment. Applying this standard of rather global disability dictated an overwhelming likelihood of denial for any miner who filed a claim. The United Mine Workers and other lobbying groups brought pressure on Congress so that the Black Lung Benefits Act of 1972 and the Black Lung Benefits Reform Act of 1977 were forthcoming. No longer did one have to demonstrate severe pulmonary impairment and argue successfully that the impairment was a consequence of mining and not, for example, of smoking. Duration of exposure, even if continuing to work in the mine, was to be accepted as a surrogate for impairment. The moneys to underwrite the program were derived from a tax on coal tonnage and from wage assessment to create an exclusive Disability Trust Fund. The annual cost of the program escalated from some $100 million in 1970 to nearly $1 billion in 1980, where it has leveled off.

From my perspective, the magnitude of moneys is not an issue, nor is the number on the roles if they perceive themselves as disabled (7). The issue is the quality of life of those on the roles and the quality of life of those who will qualify with the passage of time. The assumption was that, after a decade of exposure, there was a high likelihood of a disabling pneumoconiosis qualifying for benefits. Predictably, most miners stopped mining after a decade and retired on tax-free benefits (8). Between 1970 and 1980 the federal government, in effect, was providing Appalachia with a form of social insurance. However, it was not a pension, in that it was not a reward for onerous service performed well. Nor was it designed as an instrument to be used to seek a better quality of life. It was in the form of compensation for work-related lung damage with the understanding that the recipient was sentenced to a life of the illness of work incapacity.

The law and its administration have changed the sociology of Appalachia. No one could defend the quality of life before these reforms. But few would declare the trade-off an improvement. Appalachia has become a disabled society. As Horton stated (9), "disability is not experienced as it would be in general middle class United States, as a sharp insulting surprise. Disability is not only inevitable, but it inevitably accompanied age . . . it is not a matter of 'if' you'll be crippled, only 'when.'. . . Even fit, healthy, hardworking young males are resigned to being 'past it' by their 30th birthday." Instead of being sentenced to the drudgery and danger their fathers knew, the young men of Appalachia have been sentenced to disability, to a lifetime of the illness of work incapacity. Rather than retirement or vocational retraining, Appalachia added "a surfeit of illness behavior, all superimposed on passive, dependent individuals with borderline normal intelligence and exposed to profound sociocultural deprivation" (10).

Mining communities, whether in Appalachia, Wales, or Woolongong, have a history of subjugation and exploitation of miners. The communities are usually remote, poor, undereducated, and vulnerable to abuse from mine operators, who are the sole employers and whose greed too often overwhelmed their sense of justice. The miners are also at some risk from union bosses, whose anger and desperation became an end rather than a means. Today, mining communities are further decimated by an epidemic of illness behavior legislated from 1970 to 1980 by the federal government.

In response to these events, the Black Lung Benefits Amendments of 1981 returned the format to one similar to that for Workers' Compensation. The Department of Labor is responsible for monitoring the program, which is administered by each state (see Chapter 12). Most states employ a guide that sets the standards for the provision of health care. The guide, MINER (an acronym for Miner's Instrument for Entitled Reimbursement), was contracted by the National Council on Compensation Insurance (a private-sector research and econometrics resource for Workers' Compensation insurers) in 1985. The level and cost of medical care are based on the degree of pulmonary impairment which, in turn, is based on radiographs, hypoxemia, and symptoms; pulmonary function testing is deemphasized. MINER has proven highly efficient from the perspective of insurers in controlling medical costs and rendering them predictable. It has probably also spared the claimants from the egregiously unnecessary medical interventions that have plagued others under Workers' Compensation. MINER is not used for disability determination. The approach to disability determination for lung disease is to attempt to measure functional capacity (11). The shortcomings of this approach will be considered in the next chapter. Measuring hypoxemia has the appeal of accuracy; but it correlates poorly with disability (12).

Appalachia remains a disabled society today. Furthermore, the contests of Workers' Compensation that were to have been eliminated by the black lung legislation have returned, to the benefit of those who operate the system. The miners remain the exploited (13).

Title XVI of the Social Security Act

SSDI is funded by moneys tithed from wages and supplemented by employer contributions. What happens if the disabled individual has little or no work experience? Before 1972, the recourse was to the uneven and parsimonious state welfare programs. Title XVI was passed in 1972 and became operational in 1974 as the Supplemental Security Income (SSI) program. Under this act, disabled state welfare recipients could turn to the Social Security Administration for benefits. This program is funded by general revenues rather than the Disability Trust Fund, but its administration is identical to that of SSDI. The Social Security Administration is in the Department of Health and Human Services. The disability programs, however, are contracted to the states for administration, with close monitoring and regulation by the Social Security Administration. Some 75,000 Americans are employed by the Social Security Administration!

Between 1972 and 1974, the Social Security Administration prepared for the additional burden anticipated because of the SSI legislation. Nonetheless, the administration was overwhelmed by the increase in applications, particularly from applicants whose medical documentation was less readily retrievable. By 1977 the annual cost of SSDI/SSI had risen to $11,946 million and by 1983 to $17,852 million. The number of disabled workers receiving benefits escalated from 1,193,120 in 1967 to 2,837,432 a decade later, with an equivalent increment in dependent beneficiaries. Since then, the number of beneficiaries has somewhat stabilized, as has the number of applicants at some 1.5 million annually. But the costs of administration and of benefits continue to escalate. On June 9, 1980, President Carter signed the Social Security Disability Amendments (PL 96-265) into law. The statute required the Social Security Administration periodically to review all beneficiaries and to rereview 65% of allowances to assure that the process was reliable. The amendment also provided major incentives to return to work without placing benefits at risk if the attempt was unsuccessful.

The Carter administration placed the incentives into play. It took the Reagan administration to leap to the challenge of purging the roles of the unworthy. What was soon discovered was that the traditional standards had been relaxed by the Social Security Administration when faced with the flood of applicants for SSDI and SSI when the latter program was established in the mid-1970s. Many of those who received awards between 1974 and 1980 would be denied today and therefore were vulnerable to the purge. However, most who applied considered themselves disabled. In fact, most who are denied never return to work (14). What cruelty to deprive anyone whose sole support might be a SSDI/SSI pension (monthly payments average nearly $600 for a disabled worker and $165 for a dependent spouse or child) and who depends on SSDI/SSI for health insurance. And what was to come of them? The Reagan purge was met with outcry and with litigation. Multiple class-action suits arrived in federal courtrooms. In April 1992, as part of a settlement of one such case, the federal government agreed to reopen the files on some 200,000 residents of New York State who had been purged from the roles. SSDI/SSI is a moving target.

THE SSDI/SSI ENTITLEMENT

Wilbur Cohen took on not only the noble task of constructing a broad Social Security safety net for America, but also the political challenge of creating a safety net to be available exclusively for the most worthy (15,16). Defining the elderly was arbitrary but straightforward. Defining the disabled was also arbitrary but seemingly as straightforward. You are disabled if you are unable to engage in any "substantial gainful activity." Following is the definition of disability as stipulated in 20 Code of Federal Regulations 404.1501.

Inability to engage in any substantial gainful activity by reason of any medically determinable physical or mental impairment or impairments which can be expected to result in death or which have lasted, or can be expected to last, for a continuous period of not less than 12 months.

The operational definition of "substantial gainful employment" today is the inability to earn $300 per month in any job anywhere. In other words, you must be so disabled that even earning minimum wage is impossible. If you're an accountant capable of only a few hours of work per month, you wouldn't be disabled. It follows that, to apply, one can no longer be working. An application based on the argument that you are having difficulty and probably can't continue is doomed.

If you qualify, you receive a monthly stipend, as may your dependents. The stipends are based on contributions for SSDI and vary considerably from state to state for SSI. Furthermore, if you qualify your medical care is indemnified by the Medicare program for SSDI beneficiaries and the Medicaid program for SSI beneficiaries. By definition, those with disabilities who qualify have considerable medical needs. However, there is considerable delay before SSDI applicants become eligible for Medicare coverage. If they have no other coverage than from their employer and they must cease working to apply, they incur considerable personal risk in coping with a disabling disease without insurance. This risk is yet another feature of the application process that renders it a gauntlet.

THE ADMINISTRATION OF SSDI/SSI

The algorithm for the administration of SSDI/SSI is diagrammed in Fig. 14.1. A treating, personal physician who is knowledgeable about the algorithm can do little to perturb its inexorableness but can do much to alleviate anxiety and avoid anger on the part of the claimant simply by demystifying the experience. If nothing else, it is predictable.

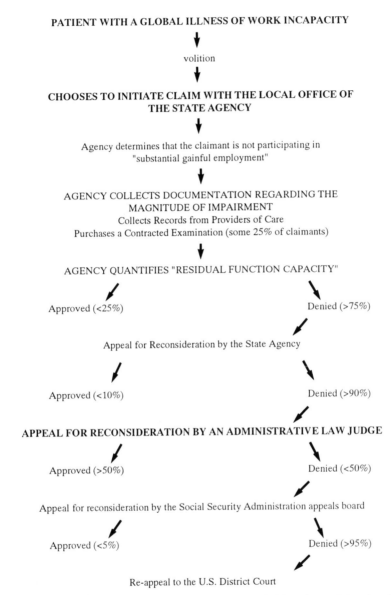

FIG. 14.1. The algorithm operated by the Social Security Administration to determine eligibility for an award under SSDI/SSI. The process is defined by a single statute. However, the rules that apply to the three levels of federal disability determination are distinctive. The levels are first at the state agency, then appellate options within the Social Security Administration [first to an administrative law judge (ALJ) and then to an appeals board], and final recourse in U.S. District Court.

Disability Determination at the Agency Level

Some 1.5 million Americans choose to apply for benefits under SSDI/SSI each year. To do so, each must approach an intake clerk at a branch of the state agency that administers the program for the Department of Health and Human Services. This interview is designed to establish sources of information regarding current and past employment and current and past medical care. Although reforms are under way, the program is designed so that the agency has no need to interview the claimant regarding any personal aspect of his or her predicament such as symptoms, suitability and availability of employment, and the like; decisions are to be based on material retrieved from medical providers to quantify the claimant's impairment. "Impairment" and the role of impairment in disability determination at the agency level are stipulated by the 20 Code of Federal Regulations 404.1501; this is the basis upon which the state agency can eschew interviewing the claimant. Only "objective" data are sought.

A physical or mental impairment is an impairment that results from anatomical, physiological, or psychological abnormalities which are demonstrable by medically acceptable clinical and laboratory diagnostic techniques. Statements by the applicant, including his own description of his impairment (symptoms) are, alone, insufficient to establish the presence of a physical or mental impairment.

The definition of disability determination (20 Code of Federal Regulations; 404.1502) charges the state agency to operate a purely impairment-based system.

Primary consideration is given to the severity of the individual's impairment . . . age, education and work experience. Medical considerations alone (including the physiological and psychological manifestations of aging) can . . . justify a finding that the individual is under a disability where his impairment is one that meets the duration requirement and is listed.

In Chapter 6, I discussed the history of the concept of differential diagnosis. The basic tenet of scientific medicine, established by Thomas Syndenham at the turn of the 18th century, is that people should choose to be patients with the expectation that the cause of their symptoms can be deduced. The exercise can be rewarding; the patient complains of sputum production and fever, and the physician defines the pathogen causing the pneumonia and prescribes specific and effective therapy. Such syllogisms are the reason the scientific physician struts the Western world. The process is not always successful. It can even be iatrogenic (Chapter 3). But the process and its successes are the pride and joy of contemporary medicine and have been so for nearly 200 yr, even deservedly so since World War II. This syllogism—from symptoms we deduce disease, for disease we effect cure—permeates Western concepts of the role of the physician. No wonder the converse seemed so rational. If you name the disease, the physician can predict the symptoms. If you have sufficient disease, work incapacity will be one of your symptoms. With disease of great magnitude, the work incapacity will be so global as to render one incapable of earning even minimum wage. If the reader substitutes the word "impairment" for disease in this seemingly corollary syllogism, you will be reading the definition of impairment-based disability determination. This is the definition with which the Social Security Administration is saddled. It is the reason that the state agency can eschew probing the claimant's symptoms. It is also the reason that the agency can ignore any other subjective input regarding the claimant's plight, including that of the claimant's treating physician. The precept of impairment-based disability determination holds that no subjective input is necessary. Even the impressions of the treating physician can be ignored. The agency can rely solely on objective data (20 Code of Federal Regulations 404.1526).

> The function of deciding whether or not an individual is under a disability is the responsibility of the Secretary. A statement by a physician . . . shall not be determinative. . . . The weight to be given such a physician's statement depends on the extent to which it is supported by specific and complete clinical findings and is consistent with other evidences as to the severity and probable duration.

This stipulation is a snare just waiting for the naive physician who writes the typical letter to the agency, "I have known Mrs. X for years and she can no longer perform her job." Such a letter is to be ignored and, when the claimant is denied, will result in anger toward the agency by the physician and toward the physician by the patient/claimant. For reasons that seem diabolic and certainly are contrary to the Code of Federal Regulations, many of the forms sent to physicians by Social Security ask for an impression as to the claimant's disability—usually a gratuitous question appended to questions probing impairment. I urge physicians to ignore this question.

Each claimant's file is assigned to two reviewers on the agency staff. One is a physician generally in full-time employment, and the other has a background in vocational rehabilitation or a related field. The file thickens with the data documenting the claimant's impairment, work history, age, and education. The decision process pivots on the assessment of "inability to maintain substantial gainful employment." Thus, the exercise undertaken by the agency is an attempt to quantify whether the claimant has "sufficient function" to earn minimum wage. Since individual variation is so great, no single set of criteria could encompass the combinations and permutations of medical, vocational, and educational variables. Rather, there is an attempt to integrate this information by determining the applicant's "residual functional capacity." The physician or the vocational specialist derives this composite score by integrating estimates of how much the applicant can lift, how long he or she can sit, etc. There is some leniency for the older and less educated claimant. The "residual functional capacity" score is then compared with listings of occupations to determine if appropriate jobs exist anywhere in the national economy. Whether the jobs are available or desirable to the applicant is not determinative.

The critical variable in the integration, and the one that is most contentious, is impairment. When a treating physician or another of the claimant's health-care providers receives a request from the agency for information regarding the patient, the patient is best served by a response that addresses the issue of impairment in the same frame of reference as is employed by the agency.

The Listings in the Handbook

Guiding the agency in its determination of impairment is a pamphlet last updated by the Social Security Administration in 1986. The pamphlet is enti-tled "Disability Evaluation Under Social Security" and is generally referred to as the "Handbook." The Handbook was widely distributed to the medical com-munity in the hopes that treating physicians would respond to the agency's request by providing prerequisite clinical information when one of their pa-tients chose to be a claimant. The information deemed to be critical is "listed" in the Handbook. The listing relevant to musculoskeletal diseases, both sys-temic and regional, is presented as Appendix 1. The fallacious reasoning that led to the promulgation of these listings is obvious to any experienced rheumatologist.

1. All systemic rheumatic diseases are treated as similar to rheumatoid arthri-tis. However, systemic lupus erythematosus, scleroderma, and others can be catastrophic without any joint involvement. This shortcoming of the listing has recently been remedied so that systemic rheumatic diseases are treated as dis-tinct entities (17).

2. Listing 1.02 will exclude most patients who do not have rheumatoid arthri-tis. Listing 1.05 will exclude most patients who do not have a backache. How-ever, both listings will also exclude most with the respective illness.

3. The severity of impairment is not quantified.

4. Sections 1.03 and 1.04 list failed surgery on one major lower extremity joint or major joint damage in the upper extremity, respectively. In the setting of rheumatoid arthritis, one joint is not listed. Sections 1.03 and 1.04 reflect a historical surgical agenda. That agenda was still operating when the Reagan Administration established a "Musculoskeletal Panel" to consider revisions of the Handbook. The panel was divided into medical and surgical subsections over my objections (as a panel member representing the American College of Physicians), and considerations of disabling backache, monarticular disease, and surgical failure were delegated to the surgical subcommittee. The revisions have yet to be enacted.

5. Sections 1.11 and 1.12 are for nonunion fractures. Again, surgical failure is deemed a greater impairment than a more global disease.

6. Section 1.13 is most disconcerting, as it demands a series of surgical proce-dures for "soft tissue injuries" of a single extremity. Such a listing presupposes the surgical indication; the initial thinking probably encompassed congenital anomalies, catastrophic diseases (such as sarcomas), or violent trauma outside

of the workplace context. But, in effect, Social Security is indemnifying the impairment even if it is iatrogenic. Given the climate in the United States today, which promulgates the "cumulative trauma disorder" hypothesis in the workplace with occasionally devastating outcomes (Chapter 13), the existence of Section 1.13 is disconcerting, to say the least.

The Contracted Examination

Usually, particularly for the applicant under SSDI, the agency can collect sufficient documentation to feel secure regarding impairment and therefore go on to determine residual functional capacity. Sometimes the data are inadequate. More often, the documentation does not apply to the Handbook listing. The Social Security Administration has explicit instructions as to how to remedy these deficits. The definition of an unlisted impairment is also the rationale for the contracted examination (20 Code of Federal Regulations 404.1505).

> An impairment . . . shall be determined to be medically the equivalent of an impairment listed . . . only if the medical findings with respect thereto are at least equivalent in severity and duration to the listed findings. . . . A decision . . . shall be based on medical evidence demonstrated by medically acceptable clinical and laboratory diagnostic techniques.

Adequate objective data are to be purchased so that the claimant's impairment can be compared directly to the relevant listing for similarity or comparability. To this end, the Social Security Administration purchases over 250,000 "contracted examinations" annually. There are physicians who do little else, so-called "mass providers," an activity that has been sanctioned by Congress (18). Until a decade ago, many agencies employed a physician as a "physician recruiter" to identify and induce practitioners to perform contracted examinations. Such is no longer necessary; practitioners seem to have both time and interest.

I will expand on the role of physicians in disability determination in the next chapter. However, two studies are worth noting at this juncture: One study was performed by our group at the University of North Carolina (19). A group of physicians who had performed three to ten contracted examinations participated. They were given a stack of clinical vignettes and asked to address their certainty that the SSDI/SSI claimant with low back pain we described was or was not disabled. The vignettes varied only in the description of four measures of impairment and one of pain. The four measures of impairment proved influential in the way these physicians thought; pain was irrelevant. Behaving in this fashion is consonant with the Code of Federal Regulations but inconsonant with their role as physicians. They were thinking as agents of the state. Even Thomas Sydenham is turning in his grave.

The other study compared the impressions of the agency with those of experienced rheumatologists for patients with rheumatoid arthritis (20). Both groups came to similar scores for residual functional capacity. Furthermore, the scores are valid; if the estimate was that the applicant was capable of a 20-pound lift, that turned out to be the case. The paper does not address two critical issues: Are residual functional capacity determinations comparably reliable, let alone comparably valid, for diseases other than rheumatoid arthritis? And, even for rheumatoid arthritis, is the score speaking to the aspect of the illness that is disabling? The answer to both questions, as will be discussed in Chapter 15 in depth, is NO! For example, there are data in rheumatoid arthritis to support the contention that aspects of the applicant's task description are far more determinative of disability than any variable encompassed by the residual functional capacity score (21).

MOVING ON TO THE ADMINISTRATIVE LAW JUDGE

Nearly 80% of applicants are found to have sufficient residual functional capacity to earn $300 per month and therefore are denied any pension. Unlike Workers' Compensation programs (Chapter 13), there are no temporary awards of any magnitude and no permanent partial awards. The disappointed applicant can request rereview by the agency with little inconvenience. Their folder is assessed by another team of evaluators. Seldom is the agency's decision reversed.

However, that is not as likely to be the outcome at the next level of appeal, before the administrative law judge (ALJ). The state agency employs 20 or so individuals, most with law degrees, to hear the next level of appeal. The stipulations of the Code of Federal Regulation quoted above do not pertain to the function of the ALJ. The ALJ can truly "hear" the predicament of the claimant, including the claimant's symptoms. Claimants appear before the ALJ to describe their predicament and plead their case. Furthermore, the ALJ has access to and may take advantage of insights from treating physicians, clergy, and others who are considered relevant. In fact, the federal judiciary has determined that the opinion of the treating physician at this level of appeal offers more "substantial evidence" than the conclusions of a government physician.

The guideline to be followed by the ALJ in determining disability is less stringent than that stipulated for the agency. The ALJ is to determine whether the impairment renders the applicant unable "to do basic work activities"; the agency requires that the same "impairment will not be considered to be severe even though it may prevent the individual from doing a highly selective group of jobs, including work that the individual has done in the past." The upshot is that the ALJ is asked to deduce the fashion in which the illness, much more broadly defined, might operate in the workplace. No wonder the ALJs of America reverse some 50% of agency denials. This is particularly true if the claimant is represented by counsel (22).

BEYOND THE ADMINISTRATIVE LAW JUDGE

Appeals before the Social Security Administration appeals board and further to the U.S. District Court had been infrequent. That is no longer the case. Occasionally, individuals plead their case. However, class-action suits are re-shaping the program. I mentioned earlier how the federal judiciary has recently demanded reconsideration of all who were purged from the roles when *ex post facto* review was mandated by Congress in 1980. The protestation and appeal was spearheaded by class-action suits brought by individuals whose initial claim for disability was based either on mental impairment or on illnesses where pain or fatigue were the predominant features. These categories of illness are associated with the least objective data, in the traditional sense, and the highest rate of denial at the agency level. The clinical diagnoses most relevant to the topic of this monograph (and highly relevant to the operation of SSDI/SSI) include back pain (Chapter 7) and fibrositis (Chapter 3). In 1984 Congress mandated that the Secretary of the Department of Health and Human Services appoint a commission to study the issue of pain evaluation as it relates to SSDI/SSI (23). The report of the commission appeared in 1987 (24); the treatise is a comprehensive discussion of the issues. However, as is true for too many commission reports, it consumed considerable resources, postponed the need to make a difficult decision, rehashed information that was already in the literature, and offered no new insight—only the predictable cry for more research.

The federal judiciary has no similar way out. Clearly, the nation also is going to be forced to come to grips with the validity of impairment-based disability determination. Any argument for the validity of impairment-based disability determination has to contend with defending the gauntlet it fosters and the simple fact that even those denied SSDI/SSI seldom return to work (25). If impairment-based determination is as invalid for those who are awarded as for those who are denied, there must be a better approach. One answer is to pursue investigations that might provide a technological solution: a serologic correlate of pain, an electrodiagnostic correlate of fatigue, or, the Holy Grail of disability determination, a serologic measure of veracity. I, obviously, think the pursuit is worse than futile. While commissions meet and scientists do science, more and more claimants are being measured by the standards of impairment rating and are inexorably drawn into a vortex of disability determination that renders them more ill as well as more disabled.

It is noteworthy that the European programs that serve the needs of those disabled by illness are often called "Invalid Pensions." It is equally noteworthy that the word *invalid* can mean either infirm or not valid. Its use in the context of disability determination is not just irony; it is a statement of society's ambivalence about helping those who perceive the need. How many of the disabled have been relegated to a disabled society, as has happened in Appalachia, but one that is dispersed and hidden among us? That question will be rejoined in the next chapter.

ON LEAVING THE WORK FORCE

Mayhew (2) considered the unemployed in the context of "street people," those who can, cannot, or will not work. We had, until recently, made progress during this century so that many of the unemployed, but far from all, are not street people. Furthermore, we have created a new form of the "will not work"; if you are unemployed and you are not seeking employment, labor statisticians consider you out of the work force. For some, being out of the work force is considered a positive event; those with a working spouse and those with pensions may have chosen this station and may be content.

Maintaining gainful employment through life, losing employment, and relinquishing employment are stations in life that have very complex interactions (Fig. 14.2). The ability to choose when to leave the work force is a privilege enjoyed by too few. Some of us will want to and be able to stay employed until the day we die. Some of us will choose to quit because we have other options including pensions to fall back on. Others will lose their job; either the employee will be terminated or the employment will cease. Those who persist in the quest for employment are counted as among the unemployed members of the work force. And still others will leave the work force because they find themselves incapable of continuing. Only the minority are out of the work force because of incapacity (Table 14.1). However, this minority represents an impressive number of Americans.

It is a reflection of contemporary American society that most individuals

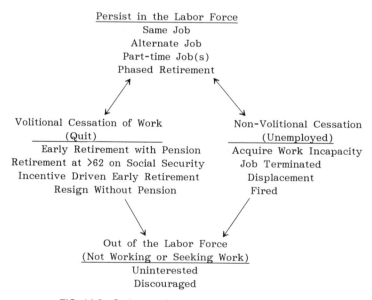

FIG. 14.2. Options and transitions for the aging worker.

TABLE 14.1. Demographics of the illness of work incapacity in the United States in 1989

| Age (yr) | Sex | Percentage of the total population not in the work force | |
		For any reason	For incapacity
35–44	Total	15.5	1.6
	Men	5.4	1.9
	Women	23.2	1.1
55–64	Total	43.6	3.5
	Men	31.7	5.4
	Women	53.3	2.5

From ref. 30.

who are out of the work force are not incapacitated. The younger women are likely to be engaged in child rearing; the older men and women have savings, pensions, and the income of a spouse as an option. Predictably, most leave the work force after age 55 when pensions, including the Social Security Old Age Pension, become available. That our society has evolved to permit so many to leave the work force and not fear joining the ranks of the "street people" is a tribute to FDR and to our collective ethic.

In this chapter we have been concerned with those who acquire the illness of work incapacity and are forced to leave the work force. SSDI/SSI was designed to provide for such individuals with the stipulation that those who "will not work" will be barred access to the dole. In particular, it was feared that Americans would seek the benefits of SSDI/SSI rather than persist in the quest for a job in times of unemployment or persist in the performance of a job that was unappealing. "Unappealing" would also encompass the possibility that SSDI/SSI would function as a form of early retirement pension. The percentage who are out of the work force because of incapacity does not parallel those who leave for other reasons. In fact, it seems to be a linear function of aging (Fig. 14.3). But that doesn't mean that SSDI/SSI is not serving as a form of early retirement.

As has been suggested and as will be reemphasized in the next chapter, the context in which one suffers illness is more determinative of work incapacity than the actual disease itself (26). Those who qualify for SSDI/SSI after age 50 represent over half the new beneficiaries. Furthermore, they qualify by criteria that seldom would lead to the awarding of a pension to a younger applicant. As I mentioned earlier, the concept of "residual functional capacity" is inversely dependent on age. It is also inversely dependent on education, and the older applicant is less likely to be educated. In addition, older applicants seldom meet any single Handbook listing. Rather, they tend to present with milder illness inferred to represent impairment in more than one organ system—usually including some component of musculoskeletal symptoms (27)—which in aggregate are considered to be comparable to any single listing (26). Many such

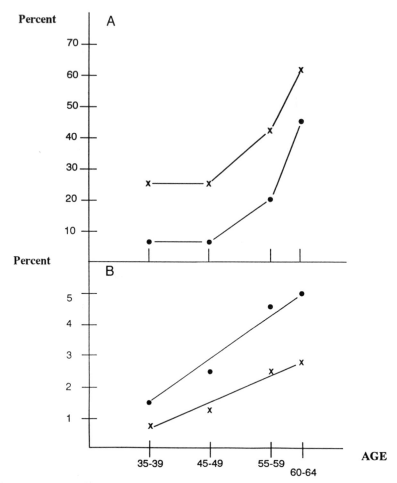

FIG. 14.3. Top: Percentage of the total labor force not working for any reason as a function of age. *Closed circles*, men; *crosses,* women. The data are for 1989 (30). Clearly, women are far more likely to be out of the work force at all ages. Clearly, as well, both sexes leave the work force at an impressive rate after age 55. The reasons for this exit are many: difficulties with reentry, displacement, lack of availability of higher-paying jobs, and increasing availability of pensions (31) **Bottom:** Percentage of the total work force that leaves because of incapacity. Clearly, this is not an explanation for the impressive increase in egress from the labor force observed after age 55.

individuals are forced to negotiate the SSDI/SSI gauntlet to the ALJ level to receive their award. However, this is not to say that the ALJ can be more readily duped than the agency process. Rather, the ALJ may have sufficient humanity to be empathic with the trials and tribulations of an unskilled laborer attempting to persist in manual labor into the sixth decade of life. Furthermore, even the clinical insights of the ALJ seem to be valid. Those who leave the work force because of incapacity, whether they are denied or allowed benefits under SSDI/SSI, are at greater risk of dying within 2 yr than age-matched workers (29). These claimants have sufficient illness, beyond the scope of impairment rating, to warrant assistance. Furthermore, their plight is begging for far more investigation than has been undertaken to date and far more assistance than even the benefits of SSDI/SSI.

Clearly, SSDI/SSI is in need of radical reform in its process. Just as clearly, it embodies a precious ethic. There is no evidence that it is egregiously abused (Fig. 14.3) as currently constituted. There is room to render the program more humane without having to be taken to task by those who fear rewarding the unworthy.

REFERENCES

1. Wright GN. The history of rehabilitation. In: *Total Rehabilitation.* Boston, Little Brown, 1980.
2. Mayhew H. *London Labour and the London Poor.* Volumes 1–4. London, Dover Press, 1983.
3. Grigg J. *Lloyd George: The People's Champion, 1902–1911.* London, Eyre Methuen, 1978.
4. Schlabach TF. *Edwin E. Witte, Cautious Reformer.* Madison, State Historical Society of Wisconsin, 1969.
5. Witte EE. *The Development of the Social Security Act.* Madison, University of Wisconsin Press, 1963.
6. Dole RJ, Committee of Finance, United States Senate. Staff data and materials related to the Social Security Act disability programs. Washington, US Government Printing Office, 1983; S. Prt. 98-93.
7. Hadler NM. Lessons from the Black Lung Compensation program. In: Hadler NM, Bunn WB (eds.) *Occupational Problems in Medical Practice.* New York, DellaCorte, 1990:163–6.
8. Erlenborn JN. *An Examination of Federal Workers Compensation Programs: Workers Compensation and Workplace Liability.* Washington, DC, National Legal Center for Public Interest, 1981:173–7.
9. Horton C. Women have headaches, men have backaches: patterns of illness in an Appalachian community. *Soc Sci Med* 1984;19:647–54.
10. Ludwig AM. "Nerves": a sociomedical diagnosis . . . of sorts. *Am J Psychother* 1982;36: 350–7.
11. Boehlecke B. Pulmonary diseases and work capacity. In: Hadler NM, Bunn WB (eds.) *Occupational Problems in Medical Practice.* New York, DellaCorte, 1990:149–62.
12. Morgan WKC, Zaldivar GL. Blood gas analysis as a determinant of occupationally related disability. *J Occup Med* 1990;32:440–4.
13. Barth PS. *The Tragedy of Black Lung: Federal Compensation for Occupational Disease.* Kalamazoo, Michigan, WE Upjohn Institute for Employment Research, 1987.
14. US General Accounting Office Report to Congressional Requesters. Social Security disability: denied applicants' health and financial status compared with beneficiaries'. Washington, DC, General Accounting Office, 1989; GAO/HRD-90-2:1–78.
15. Cohen WJ. *Retirement Policies Under Social Security.* Berkeley, University of California Press, 1957:43–68.
16. Haber W, Cohen WJ. *Social Security: programs, problems and policies.* Homewood, Illinois, Irwin, 1960.

17. Department of Health and Human Services. Social Security Administration 20 CFR Part 404. *Federal Register* 1991;56:65705–6.
18. US House of Representatives, 97th Congress, 1st Session, Subcommittee on Social Security and Subcommittee on Oversight on the Committee on Ways and Means. Volume providers of medical exams for SSA, hearings 18 September 1981. Washington, US Government Printing Office, 1982; Serial No. 4-12. [Y4.W36:97-27].
19. Carey TS, Hadler NM, Gillings D, Wallsten T. Medical disability assessment of the back pain patient for the Social Security Administration: the weighting of presenting clinical features. *J Clin Epidemiol* 1988;41:691–7.
20. Liang MH, Daltroy LH, Larson MG, et al. Evaluation of Social Security disability in claimants with rheumatic disease. *Ann Intern Med* 1991;115:26–31.
21. Yelin E, Meenan R, Nevitt M, Epstein W. Work disability in rheumatoid arthritis: effects of disease, social, and work factors. *Ann Intern Med* 1980;93:551–6.
22. The Bellmon report. *Soc Secur Bull* 1982;45:3–27.
23. US House of Representatives, 98th Congress, 2nd Session. House Resolution 3755, Social Security disability benefits reform act of 1984. Washington, US Government Printing Office, 1984 [Y1.1/8:98-618].
24. Osterweis M, Kleinman A, Mechanic D (eds.) *Pain and Disability.* Washington, DC, National Academy Press, 1987:1–306.
25. Bound J. The health and earnings of rejected disability insurance applicants. *Am Economic Rev* 1989;79:482–503.
26. Hadler NM. Work disability and musculoskeletal disease. *Arthritis Rheum* 1986;29:1410–1.
27. Yelin EH, Henke CJ, Epstein WV. Work disability among persons with musculoskeletal conditions. *Arthritis Rheum* 1986;29:1322–33.
28. US General Accounting Office. Briefing report to congressional requesters: Social Security disability. Demographic and economic characteristics of new beneficiaries. Washington, US Government Printing Office, January 1988; HRD-88-35BR.
29. Boaz RF, Muller CF. The validity of health limitations as a reason for deciding to retire. *Health Serv Res* 1990;25:361–86.
30. US Department of Labor Statistics. *Employment and Earnings*, 1990;37:1–241.
31. McLaughlin A. Labor Market Problems of Older Workers. Report of the Secretary of Labor in response to Labor Department Appropriations Act in Public Law 100–202. Office of Current Employment Analysis, Division of Labor Force Statistics, Bureau of Labor Statistics, 1989.

APPENDIX 1: "HANDBOOK" LISTING FOR CATEGORY OF IMPAIRMENTS, MUSCULOSKELETAL

1.02 *Active rheumatoid arthritis and other inflammatory arthritis:* With both A and B.

A. History of persistent joint pain, swelling, and tenderness involving multiple major joints (see 1.00D) and with signs of joint inflammation (swelling and tenderness) on current physical examination despite prescribed therapy for at least 3 months, resulting in significant restriction of function of the affected joints, and clinical activity expected to last at least 12 months; and

B. Corroboration of diagnosis at some point in time by either

1. Positive serologic test for rheumatoid factor; or
2. Antinuclear antibodies; or
3. Elevated sedimentation rate; or
4. Characteristic histologic changes in biopsy of synovial membrane or subcutaneous nodule (obtained independent of Social Security disability evaluation).

1.03 *Arthritis of a major weight-bearing joint (due to any cause):*
With history of persistent joint pain and stiffness with signs of marked limitation of motion or abnormal motion of the affected joint on current physical examination. With:

A. Gross anatomical deformity of hip or knee (e.g., subluxation, contracture, bony or fibrous ankylosis, instability) supported by X-ray evidence of either significant joint space narrowing or significant bony destructive and markedly limited ability to walk and stand; or

B. Reconstructive surgery or surgical arthrodesis of a major weight-bearing joint and return to full weight-bearing status did not occur, or is not expected to occur, within 12 months of onset.

1.04. *Arthritis of one major joint in each of the upper extremities (due to any cause):*
With history of persistent joint pain and stiffness, signs of marked limitation of motion of the affected joints on current physical examination, and X-ray evidence of either significant joint space narrowing or significant bony destruction. With:

A. Abduction and forward flexion (elevation) of both arms at the shoulders, including scapular motion, restricted to less than 90 degrees; or

B. Gross anatomical deformity (e.g., subluxation, contracture, bony or fibrous ankylosis, instability, ulnar deviation) and enlargement or effusion of the affected joints.

1.05 *Disorder of the spine:*
A. Arthritis manifested by ankylosis or fixation of the cervical or dorsolumbar spine at 30° or more of flexion measured from the neutral position, with X-ray evidence of:

1. Calcification of the anterior and lateral ligaments; or
2. Bilateral ankylosis of the sacroiliac joints with abnormal apophyseal articulations; or

B. Osteoporosis, generalized (established by X-ray) manifested by pain and limitation of back motion and paravertebral muscle spasm with X-ray evidence of either:

1. Compression fracture of a vertebral body with loss of at least 50 percent of the estimated height of the vertebral body prior to the compression fracture, with no intervening direct traumatic episode; or
2. Multiple fractures of vertebrae with no intervening direct traumatic episode; or

C. Other vertebrogenic disorders (e.g., herniated nucleus pulposus, spinal stenosis) with the following persisting for at least 3 months despite prescribed therapy and expected to last 12 months. With both 1 and 2:

1. Pain, muscle spasm, and significant limitation of motion in the spine; and
2. Appropriate radicular distribution of significant motor loss with muscle weakness and sensory and reflex loss.

1.12 *Fractures of an upper extremity* with non-union of a fracture of the shaft of the humerus, radius, or ulna under continuing surgical management directed toward restoration of functional use of the extremity and such function was not restored or expected to be restored within 12 months after onset.

1.13 *Soft tissue injuries of an upper or lower extremity* requiring a series of staged surgical procedures within 12 months after onset for salvage and/or restoration of major function of the extremity, and such major function was not restored or expected to be restored within 12 months after onset.

15

Disability Determination in America

The following is an excerpt from *The Trial,* written by Franz Kafka in the winter of 1916–1917. Imagine Joseph K., who has appeared before a tribunal where he was required to prove his innocence when the charge against him was not stated. There is no decision yet. But Mr. K. has an opportunity to discuss the course of events with one knowledgeable in the proceedings. I have taken one liberty with the translation (1); I have substituted the words in brackets for "superstition" or "superstitious" in the original.

"Apparently you don't know the people there yet and you might take it up wrongly. You must remember that in these proceedings things are always coming up for discussion that are simply beyond reason, people are too tired and distracted to think and so they take refuge in [supposition and preconception]. I'm as bad as anyone myself. And one of the [suppositions] is that you're supposed to tell from a man's face, especially the line of his lips, how his case is going to turn out. Well, people declared that judging from the expression of your lips you would be found guilty, and in the near future too. I tell you, it's a silly [supposition], and in most cases completely belied by the facts, but if you live among these people, it's difficult to escape the prevailing opinion. You can't imagine what a strong effect such [suppositions] have. You spoke to a man up there, didn't you? And he could hardly utter a word in answer. Of course there's many a reason for being bewildered up there, but one of the reasons why he couldn't bring out an answer was the shock he got from looking at your lips. He said afterwards that he saw on your lips the sign of his own condemnation."

"How [arbitrary and capricious] these people are!" cried K. . . . "Do they meet each other so frequently, then, and exchange all these ideas?"

"As a rule they don't mix much . . . it would be hardly possible, there are too many of them. Besides, they have few interests in common. Occasionally a group believes it has found a common interest, but it soon finds out its a mistake. Combined action against the Court is impossible. Each case is judged on its own merits, the Court is very conscientious about that, and so common action is out of the question. An individual here and there may score a point in secret, but no one hears it until afterwards, no one knows how it has been done. So, there's no real community, people come across each other in the lobbies, but there's not much

249

conversation. The [preconceived notions and] beliefs are an old tradition and increase automatically."

Joseph K is driven mad by the process.

THE BIRTH OF CONTEMPORARY DISABILITY DETERMINATION

Franz Kafka was born in Prague, Czechoslovakia, in 1883 into a German-Jewish-Bohemian family. He received his doctorate in jurisprudence from the German University Karls-Ferdinand in Prague in June 1906. From 1908 until his death he was employed as a governmental bureaucrat. The position exempted him from military service during World War I and provided him with a comfortable living and short hours. During his lifetime he published only a few short stories, beginning with "Observations" in 1913. He worked on *The Trial* during the winter of 1916–1917 and on *The Castle* in 1918, but these novels, together with *Amerika*, other short stories, and his letters, were not published until after his death from tuberculosis on June 3, 1924, at age 41.

Kafka's short life was insular, even withdrawn. For our knowledge we owe much to his great friendship with Max Brod. Even more importantly, the world will forever be indebted to Brod for enabling Kafka to leave his mark indelibly on the Western conscience. Kafka was reclusive and, in spite of a consuming passion for writing, he seldom arrived at a sufficient sense of accomplishment, of completion, to agree to publication. His doubts about the value of his work caused him to instruct Brod in writing, on his death bed with "pulmonary fever," to destroy his manuscripts after his death. They should "be burned unread." Fortunately, Brod could search his conscience and the memories of his interactions with Kafka to find the will to offer these great works to posterity.

The story of Joseph K. has achieved the status of a modern myth. This is what is meant by "Kafka-esque." Scholars have attributed Kafka's ability to conjure up such an image to a combination of his childhood experiences and his legal background. I disagree—and so does Max Brod. As I said above, Kafka spent his professional life as a bureaucrat. That is true. From 1908 to 1913 he worked in the Workers' Accident Insurance Institute for the Kingdom of Bohemia in Prague. I am convinced that Kafka could never have imagined Joseph K. unless he witnessed disability determination. In the following excerpt from his biography of Kafka, Brod explained the torment Kafka internalized by virtue of his vocation (2).

> It is clear that Kafka derived a great amount of his knowledge of the world and of life, as well as his skeptical pessimism, from his experiences in the office, from coming into contact with workmen suffering under injustice, and from having to deal with the long-drawn-out process of official work, and from the stagnating life of files. Whole chapters of the novels *The Trial* and *The Castle* derive their outer

covers, their realistic wrappings, from the atmosphere Kafka breathed in the Workers' Accident Institute. Compare too the sketch "New Lamps," and an entry in the diary dated July 2, 1913: "Wept over the account of the trial of twenty-three-year-old Marie Abraham, who, through want and hunger, strangled her almost nine-months' old child with a tie which she was using as a garter and which she unwound for the purpose. A thoroughly typical story." Compare also the following scheme for reform, which is almost unique in Kafka's work, drawn up towards the end of his life, the plan of a workers' collective, voluntary of course, almost monastic.

Can it be that, within a decade of the establishment of the Prussian precedent for legislated worker health and safety, it could have gone so wrong as to become Kafka-esque? Or was it designed to go so wrong? Out of naivete?

SOCIAL LEGISLATION AND THE WORKPLACE: BENEFICENCE VERSUS SOPHISM

Workers' compensation insurance is a century-old watershed in social legislation. However, it was never meant to serve the worker. It serves the collective guilt of an industrialized capitalism. It is this specter that FDR evoked before Congress on June 8, 1934, in pleading for Social Security as a "safeguard against misfortunes which cannot be wholly eliminated in the man-made world of ours." Workers' Compensation Insurance acknowledges that some among us enjoy advantages because others toil in conditions that are onerous if not hazardous; at the very least, any laborer who must also suffer the consequences of an injury on the job is entitled to special consideration. How special the consideration relates to how much guilt each generation of leaders and policy makers is able to tolerate or suppress. The Prussian leadership that first formulated workers' compensation legislation had a high tolerance for such guilt. Franz Kafka bore witness. That Bismarck did not foster a kinder and gentler Prussia is no surprise. But are we doing much better? I appreciate that the question is anathema, if not heresy. After all, we are expending ever-increasing proportions of our wealth to assuage our guilt, proportions that Bismarck would have found inconceivable. But I ask again. Are we serving our workers? Or is much of this expenditure the exercise of a sophistry; under the banner of collective guilt, we have cultivated a system of self-service.

THE DISCRETE TRAUMATIC EVENT

The administration of workers' compensation programs pivots on three clinical issues: causation, consolidation, and consequence. For a discrete injury, one that involves a clear-cut traumatic event such as a laceration or amputation, the issues are straightforward. The cause is clear. Medical and surgical algorithms and prognosis are established and lend themselves to scientific validation. One can establish, even predict with some certainty, when the worker will be as well as possible—a station of health variously labeled *fixed and stable, maximal medical improvement,* or *consolidation,* the last term common in Europe. Since the consequence is a scar or a blinded eye or the like, any discussion of the magnitude of handicap is anchored in a concrete and incontrovertible pathologic outcome, an impairment. Finally, rehabilitation is in the best interest of all.

Given this algorithm, injurious events can be monitored and hazards eliminated. Why, then, do discrete injuries still represent the vast majority of workers' compensation claims? True, their processing is efficient in the sense that they represent a small percentage of the cost of the system. But such events should become vanishingly rare in a sophisticated society so that their indemnification would justify an ever-shrinking insurance enterprise underwriting less and less surgical care. Every discrete traumatic workplace injury is a reproach to our collective guilt.

The workers' compensation algorithm to offer redress for discrete traumatic workplace injuries is readily explicable. The logic that fostered the application of the same algorithm to clinical outcomes with uncertain or multivariate pathogenesis is recondite at best. Let's again couch our considerations in the context of regional backache.

EXPANDING THE APPLICABILITY OF THE INJURY LABEL

Before 1934, you could only "injure" your back as a consequence of discrete and major trauma. Since World War II, "I injured my back" has become a comfortable descriptive for every American. Every one of us wonders what we did to cause the illness. Often, no explanation is apparent. Even if there is a coincident event, seldom is it a unique event; similar experiences in the past and in the future will pass without consequence. We are joined in our puzzlement by our physicians, who find it irresistible to inquire, "What were you doing when it started?" Why this need to ascribe a backache to an external influence? None of us would feel comfortable describing our headache or angina as a head injury or heart injury.

The answer is that the workers' compensation paradigm has permeated the very fabric of society. In 1934 backache was first commonly ascribed to a "ruptured disc" (3). Given the specter of such catastrophic damage, adjudicators in the workers' compensation system still consider any worker's backache diagnosed as a ruptured disc to be a compensable injury (4). The American regional backache has never been the same (5). The experience, itself, of backache is confounded by a perception of damage, of injury. For the American Workers' Compensation system, this was a Rubicon.

Consider the challenge of forcing the regional backache into the workers' compensation paradigm, which pivots on causation, consolidation, and consequence.

Causation

Enough has been written on causation (3,6). It is important to realize that no aspect of anthropomorphics including lifting strength (7), of demographics, of clinimetrics, or of ergonomics will alter the likelihood of experiencing a backache or of deciding to launch a claim for a compensable back injury. The last is far more a function of the psychosocial context in which the backache is suffered (8). For 50 yr workers' compensation has underwritten the contest of causation, enjoined by "expert" ergonomists and physicians, as well as regulators and bureaucrats. To what end? Great sums of money benefit many of the perpetrators of this paralogism—these moneys do not service our collective guilt nor the worker with a regional backache.

Consolidation

Enter the medical entitlement, the most nefarious aspect of this algorithm. To choose the role of workers' compensation claimant with a backache is to find oneself in a gauntlet. The choice is often driven by job dissatisfactions (8) so that one starts out at a psychologic disadvantage in terms of making personal decisions. Then one has to negotiate the contest of causation—What were you doing when it started? And then you are entitled to medical care to try to put things right. It should be clear from Section II that nearly the entire diagnostic and therapeutic armamentarium for backache has been subjected to scientific testing and found to be woefully lacking, if not bogus. Nonetheless, under the banner of "standard of care" or "defensive medicine," the entire armamentarium has become a booming, egregiously profitable enterprise. If, however, the claimant refuses a study or an intervention, the veracity of the claimant is questioned rather than the intelligence, motivation, or ethic of the prescriber. No wonder the claimant with a back "injury" is so much more likely to be subjected to imaging, physical modalities, and surgery than the patient with a backache! If the claimant refuses, the claim is compromised. "Consolidation" or "fixed and stable" or "maximum medical improvement" is not a station of health; it is the station wherein all modalities have been exhausted. It is disconcerting but far from surprising that Workers' Compensation is willing to underwrite invasive procedures in the absence of data suggesting benefit—or even data suggesting decreased cost (9).

Consequence

Enter disability determination. This is the exercise where a hurting human being has to stand before experts and prove the hurting. This is the image of Joseph K. Furthermore, in this exercise, all petitioners for assistance in coping with the illness of work incapacity face the same nemesis. For a century, trust in the veracity of the petitioner has held little sway; surrogate measures have been sought, generally forms of impairment rating. All to no avail (10,11). People are disabled because of the quagmire their life has become. Forcing them to prove that they are ill causes them to be more ill. No wonder claimants in disability determination acquire illness behaviors. No wonder worker's compensation claimants with back pain compose a goodly portion of the sad and ill individuals who populate America's pain, work hardening, and similar clinics. To the escalating costs of unprovable remedies, we have added the escalating costs of causing and treating the illness that results from disability determination. Almost none of these moneys benefits the ill worker as much as the establishment designed to prove that the worker is less ill than claimed. It is more than unconscionable; it is Kafka-esque.

IMPAIRMENT RATING

Nonetheless, society is still advised, often by the medical community, to persevere. Somewhere, somehow, there will be a reliable and valid standard for measuring disability. To this end, most wave the banner of impairment rating: It should be possible to quantify impairment reliably and then base any award for disability on the magnitude of impairment. The syllogism is based on the assumption that impairment (disease or pathoanatomic derangement) correlates in some predictable fashion with disability. However, even Waddell (12), who is an intransigent proponent of impairment rating, admits to the enormous difficulties inherent in this assertion (13). Despite the admission, Waddell is convinced that the difficulties with impairment rating are surmountable and that the approach has too many redeeming features to consider alternatives.

I, on the other hand, am equally convinced that the notion of impairment rating is fatally flawed and should be discarded. The illness of work incapacity is a necessary consequence only of global disease, such as terminal heart or lung processes, a massive stroke, and other overt horrors. Short of such catastrophes, the illness of work incapacity is multivariate in precipitation and perpetuation. The pioneering work of Magora (14) 20 yr ago has been confirmed by more recent studies (8,15), rendering this conclusion inescapable for low back pain. Psychologic and sociopolitical confounders overwhelm both disease and ergonomic factors in predicting the illness of work incapacity.

Nonetheless, impairment rating is the business of the state agency assigned the task of determining the merits of disability claims for the Social Security Administration (see Chapter 14). American Workers' Compensation jurisdictions have abandoned impairment "schedules" for low back pain, but not reliance on impairment ratings in determining the degree of disability that is a consequence of injury in the workplace. Many jurisdictions persevere in spite of the disappointing reliability of purchased evaluations (16), even by experienced orthopedists and neurosurgeons (17,18). In other countries, impairment rating is downplayed; it is at most ancillary information to be considered along with psychosocial information by panels of educated citizens who are charged with determining disability (19). In America, we hold tenaciously to the precepts of impairment rating in the quest for a totally objective and quantifiable measure of disability. Some Workers' Compensation jurisdictions even rely exclusively on the AMA "Guides" for their gold standard in measuring impairment; others, like Texas, are attempting to legislate the usage of the Guides.

THE AMA GUIDES—AN OBJECT LESSON

The American Medical Association publishes the "Guides to the Evaluation of Permanent Impairment," a remarkable document with 20 yr of staying power. In 1988 the AMA published the third edition, which went into its second printing within the year. The stated intent of the Guides is to promulgate a standardized physical examination. The invited panel of experts who revise the Guides disclaim their usage for disability determination even though the AMA is aware that such is the principal reason for the impressive sales of the document. In fact, the AMA instructs the reader of the Guides on how to weight any measure of impairment so its influence on the function of the "whole person" can be deduced. For that reason impairment of the thumb is held to be more valuable than impairment of any other digit, the hand is the most valuable part of the arm, and the arm is more valuable than the leg. Therefore, loss of an arm is considered to diminish the "whole person" by 60%, whereas loss of the leg diminishes the person by 40%. Weighting of impairment in this fashion is a form of disability determination. The authors of the Guides are aware of the fallacy inherent in such calculations and state so quite explicitly in their introductory chapters. There is no consensus "whole person." The loss of a leg might result in a minimal disability for most physicians and surgeons and, with a good prosthesis, minimal handicap. The relative weighting of impairments is arguable; the absolute weighting is a fantasy.

In terms of the musculoskeletal system, the methods suggested for the extremities can be reliable if the examiners are patient and practiced (20). However, even for the extremities, the validity is easily subjected to question. Take the example of an amputation of the fifth finger. Quantifying the impairment is trivial. Inferring the disability is not. For most of us there would be little disability—but not for the flutist, pianist, and others for whom exquisite dexterity is critical.

Quantifying impairment of the axial skeleton is not so straightforward. The Guides go to great lengths to quantify the range of motion of spinal segments. The method suggested is held to be an improvement on the Schöber technique (Fig. 15.1). This technique suffers from wide standard errors on normal values with aging, from difficulties with skin landmarks, and from considerable interobserver error (21). The Guides call for abandoning tape measures and substi-

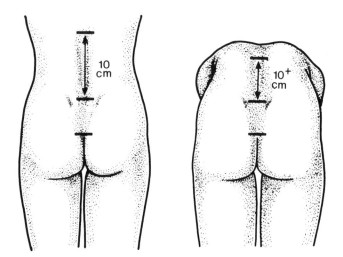

FIG. 15.1. The classic Schöber's Index is based on measuring the distraction of two points drawn on the back when the subject flexes. In the illustration, the marks are drawn 10 cm apart with the subject erect and are measured again when the subject flexes. A teen-ager is expected to distract the marks to 15 cm at least. With aging, we all lose suppleness but to varying degrees, so that the range of normal is too wide to render the test meaningful. In fact, in my hands, the only utility is in the presence of low back pain; if the distraction is maintained, one should wonder if the low back pain is referred from other than a musculoskeletal structure. In addition to the variability in mobility of the lumbosacral spine, the measurement is confounded by geometric consider-ations. Skin mobility, particularly obesity, and rotatory scoliosis are among these confounders.

tuting the use of inclinometers to measure spinal range of motion. The inclino-meter is a device with a straight-edge base that is placed on the skin, attached to which is a pendulum indicating degrees of deviation from the vertical as the subject flexes or extends. If the subject is free of "spasm" and the measurements are reproducible to 5°, the inclinometer provides a measure that, according to the AMA's panel of experts, correlates with radiographic range of motion as a "gold standard." That may be the opinion of the panel; it certainly is the pub-lished opinion of the only orthopedist to sit on the panel (22). But not all observers are convinced. In fact, careful analysis demonstrates that the incli-nometer offers little more reliability or discriminant validity than the tradi-tional Schöber technique (23).

For the axial skeleton, the measurement of impairment is problematic. Weighting the impairment is more than problematic. In a fashion reminiscent of the Handbook used by the state agency in disability determination for SSDI/SSI (as I pointed out in Chapter 14), the AMA Guides weights the impairment following surgery as greater than similar impairment without surgery. The im-plication is that if surgery failed, a priori, the underlying disease must be more severe. Of course, based on our analysis in Chapter 7 of the effectiveness of surgical intervention, a more defensible statement is that failed surgery is a

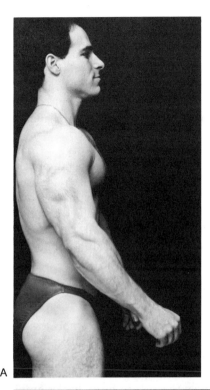

A

FIG. 15.2. In the classic Schöber measurement or in the traditional examination of the spine, the subject is asked to stand erect (**A**). The normal lumbar lordosis is apparent in this subject. With flexion (**B**), the lumbar curve normally reverses, becoming a kyphosis, and the spine distracts. In this subject, the lumbosacral segment can do no more than flatten. This is an impairment. The subject actually has ankylosing spondylitis. However, in spite of the impairment, this subject is not disabled. He is a competition body builder, excellent physician, and successful husband. So much for impairment rating.

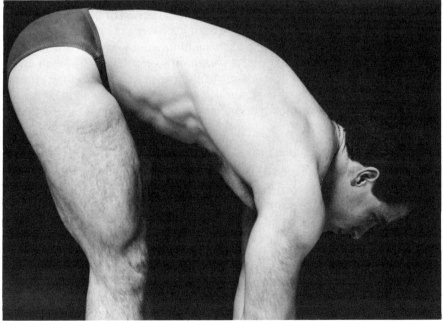

B

failure of surgical judgment and that, if there is greater impairment, it is iatrogenic. The Guides are a cover-up.

That the "Guides" for impairment rating for the axial skeleton has marginal reliability is no surprise. Experienced clinicians have long known that the history and physical examination are only one component of a therapeutic patient/physician relationship. Figure 15.2 is an example. The elements of the history and physical examination themselves are quite variable in reliability; most are of limited reliability and validity and cannot substitute for a more global interaction (24,25). For that reason, even the majority of Workers' Compensation jurisdictions eschew reliance on the AMA Guides. In fact, more are turning away from traditional impairment rating, hoping to devise rating systems that rely on combinations of traditional measures (16) or more novel behavioral measures (26,27). No one, yet, is making the leap to the realization that, just as impairment does not predict who will choose to be a claimant, impairment does not determine which claimant is disabled or to what degree.

THE VORTEX OF DISABILITY DETERMINATION

The vortex of disability determination draws the claimant inexorably toward a destiny with a pain clinic or work hardening program. When the claimant has submitted to all proffered interventions and still has the illness of work incapacity, the undercurrent of the entire gauntlet comes to the fore—disability determination. Is this worker really unable to return to work, to his or her prior job for Workers' Compensation or to any job for SSDI/SSI? The decision is administrative, even though the data used are clinical. Worker's Compensation insurers are faced with considerable financial outlay if a worker is declared partially or totally disabled. That cost is passed on to employers, who balk when they can no longer readily pass it on to the consumer. The Social Security Administration is subjected to political pressures to exercise fiscal constraint whenever the size and configuration of government programs targeted toward the disabled receive lesser priority, usually because of times of economic constraint (28). That is why both systems will grasp at any straw: any proffered cure, any way to deny an award. The Workers' Compensation system, in particular, has the money and prerogative to postpone the more costly granting of a permanent total or a permanent partial award under the guise of "rehabilitation." Rehabilitation programs underwritten by Workers' Compensation have a glorious tradition when it comes to workers who suffer external force trauma; these programs have broken ground in reconstructive surgery, physical medicine, and orthotics. However, for regional musculoskeletal illness, particularly for backache and recently for arm pain, the programs are laudable in intent but tragic in outcome.

The reader should be aware that most of the "patients" with chronic back or arm pain who populate the nation's pain clinics and work hardening programs are actually Workers' Compensation claimants. The settlement of their claims has been postponed contingent on their performance in rehabilitation. It is argued that, if they improve, they will be better off and the insurer will have less fiscal outlay in the long run. This is a seductive argument. However, there is a wealth of data to suggest that the programs are ineffective, if not harmful, and the approach needs to be reconsidered.

The claimants arrive in the pain clinic after negotiating the contest of causation and the gauntlet of consolidation discussed above. The process lasts for many months, if not years. The work of Bigos et al. (8,29) suggests that inherent psychologic abnormalities do not predispose to becoming a claimant with a back injury. The work of Crown (30), more importantly and in desperate need of confirmation, suggests that psychologic aberration is acquired as a consequence of negotiating the gauntlet. In any event, by the time they arrive in the pain clinic, these individuals are changed human beings. Many bear literal scars and even bear the blame for the unsuccessful surgery by carrying the label of "failed back" (31) or even the "back loser." They limp into the pain clinics with altered somatic perceptions (32,33). Many suffer socioeconomic deprivation (34), often confounded by psychosocial disenfranchisement, which correlates directly with the chronicity of their back pain (the time spent in the gauntlet) and inversely with their prognosis (35,36). All of these sad claimants have spent months to years in the gauntlet, trying to prove how ill they are to physicians and administrators who sit in judgment and can seldom be swayed in the absence of sufficient impairment. These claimants are Kafka's Joseph K.

The most diabolic aspect of the pain clinic and work hardening or "function restoration" programs is that they overturn all the rules by which the gauntlet operates. All of a sudden, impairment is irrelevant. All of a sudden, the proscription of function by treating physicians, employers, and insurers is thrown out. The bewildered claimant is no longer advised to "listen to your body," "don't perform if it exacerbates pain," "record all symptoms," consume all variety of analgesics, and the like. Rather, the pain is to be ignored, pills to be discarded, and performance demanded in spite of the pain. However, all of this advice falls on an altered human being whose very existence is validated by the persistence of pain and incapacity and who seeks the disability award as his ultimate validation and as a triumph over a system that has pursued him relentlessly—as relentlessly as another system pursued Joseph K. No wonder pain clinics and the like have such dismal track records. If the claimants complied with the program, they would be stripped of more than their disability, they would be stripped of their raison d'être and lose their pension to boot.

For inscrutable, if not perverse reasons, the response of the medical community involved and the Workers' Compensation industry is to take cognizance of this evolution in rehabilitation and spend even more money attempting to redress the illness behaviors that are a barrier to functional improvement. (Maybe the driving force is that some of these programs generate considerable income for their purveyors—if I might be allowed a fleeting moment of cynicism.) Some programs demand, and procure, well over $15,000 in fees from the insurer to house a single claimant for several weeks. Most centers immerse their clients in programs of physical medicine, behavioral therapy, and pain modulation (37–39). The published success rate is dismal; some claimants do increase their capacity to meet biomechanical demands, but a minority return to work. From my own observations in several countries, a minority of those who are finally pensioned are rewarded with a quality of life that they had hoped for or any of us would wish for them. They were disabled the moment they perceived themselves disabled. However, instead of comfort, compassion, and a path to a better future, society's provision is Sisyphean.

QUO VADIS

The American approach to providing for the disabled with regional musculo-skeletal illness is indefensible. Almost all of this money is expended in rendering the claimant with backache more ill. What is even more horrifying is that we do not seem to be able to learn the lesson of the compensable backache; we are repeating these sins with arm pain, so-called cumulative trauma disorders (Chapter 13), and with stress. I cannot believe that we are doing this out of ignorance. There must be driving elements of self-interest on the parts of the purveyors of health "care," of ergonomics, of advocacy, and of indemnity. There must also be some explanation for the intransigence of organized labor in realizing that entitlements such as Workers' Compensation are double-edged swords; discrete injuries receive state-of-the-art treatment but not state-of-the-art prevention, and atraumatic "injuries" fuel iatrogenic clinical algorithms. Reforms might offer a solution. No reform is a match for the power and wealth of the vested interests. The Quebec Workers' Health and Safety Commission found that out the hard way; their elegant risk/benefit analysis (40) of the treatment of regional spine "injuries" could never be implemented. The vested interests must be recognized and bridled first.

Reformers must reconsider some of the basic tenets of our approach to caring for the disabled.

Do we need to perpetuate the distinction between the ill invalid seeking an SSDI/SSI pension and the injured worker seeking help under Workers' Compensation?

Isn't it time to abandon the myth of impairment rating?

If we wish to maintain a distinct program to indemnify for workplace injuries, how can we countenance placing such predicaments of daily life as regional musculoskeletal symptoms under the umbrella? The precedent is overwhelmingly iatrogenic!

The burgeoning disability determination enterprise captures extraordinary wealth for the parties that operate the gauntlet and very little for the claimant who considers himself disabled. This must be decried. Furthermore, reform must disallow repetition of this unconscionable aspect of the American programs.

Other countries operate disability schemes that are far less convoluted and expensive and far more compassionate than ours (19,28,41). I am not suggesting that the United States borrow another's program. We are too heterogeneous, we have our own traditions, and we serve a peculiar national ethic. It would be naive to suggest that what works in Switzerland, or Sweden, or New Zealand would transpose easily. These other systems demonstrate only that alternatives exist. Our approach is not etched in stone. To the contrary, it is plastic and it is stained with the tears of all the disabled who limp through its gauntlet and mill about our pain clinics.

REFERENCES

1. Kafka F. *The Trial.* New York, Knopf, 1956:217–20.
2. Brod M. *Franz Kafka: a Biography.* New York, Schockian, 1947:84.
3. Hadler NM. Regional musculoskeletal diseases of the low back: cumulative trauma versus single incident. *Clin Orthop* 1987;221:33–41.
4. Hadler NM. Legal ramifications of the medical definition of back disease. *Ann Intern Med* 1978;89:992–9.
5. Hadler NM. Regional back pain. *N Engl J Med* 1986;315:1090–2.
6. Hadler NM. Occupational illness: the issue of causality. *J Occup Med* 1984;26:587–93.
7. Mostardi RA, Noe DA, Kovacik MW, Proterfield JA. Isokinetic lifting strength and occupational injury. *Spine* 1992;17:189–93.
8. Bigos SJ, Battié MC, Spengler DM, Fisher LD, Fordyce WE, Hansson TH, Nachemson AL, Wortley MD. A prospective study of work perceptions and psychosocial factors affecting the report of back injury. *Spine* 1991;16:1–6.
9. Shvartzman L, Weingarten E, Sherry H, Levin S, Persaud A. Cost-effectiveness analysis of extended conservative therapy versus surgical intervention in the management of herniated lumbar intervertebral disc. *Spine* 1992;17:177–82.
10. Hadler NM. Impairment rating in disability determination for low back pain: placing the AMA Guides and the Quebec Institute Report into perspective. *John Burton's Workers' Compensation Monitor* 1990;3:4–8.
11. Hadler NM. Backache and humanism. In: Frymoyer JW, Ducker TB, Hadler NM, Kostuik JP, Weinstein JN, Whitecloud TS III (eds.) *The Adult Spine: Principles and Practice.* New York, Raven Press, 1991:55–60.
12. Waddell G. Occupational low-back pain, illness behavior, and disability. *Spine* 1991;16:683–4.
13. Wadell G, Main CJ, Morris EW, et al. Chronic low-back pain, psychologic distress, and illness behavior. *Spine* 1984;9:209–13.
14. Magora A. Investigation of the relation between low back pain and occupation. V. Psychological aspects. *Scand J Rehabil Med* 1973;5:191–6.
15. Deyo RA, Diehl AK. Psychosocial predictors of disability in patients with low back pain. *J Rheumatol* 1988;15:1557–64.
16. Clark WL, Haldeman S, Johnson P, Morris J, Schulenberger C, Trauner D, White A. Back impairment and disability determination: another attempt at objective, reliable rating. *Spine* 1988;13:332–41.
17. Brand RA, Lehman TR. Low-back impairment rating practices of orthopaedic surgeons. *Spine* 1983;8:75–8.
18. Greenwood JG. Low-back impairment-rating practices of orthopaedic surgeons and neurosurgeons in West Virginia. *Spine* 1985;10:773–6.
19. Hadler NM. Disabling backache in France, Switzerland, and the Netherlands: contrasting sociopolitical constraints on clinical judgment. *J Occup Med* 1989;31:823–31.

20. Gloss DS, Wardle MG. Reliability and validity of the American Medical Association's Guide to ratings of permanent impairment. *JAMA* 1982;248:2292–6.
21. Miller SA, Mayer T, Cox R, Gatchel RJ. Reliability problems associated with the modified Schöber technique for true lumbar flexion measurement. *Spine* 1992;17:345–8.
22. Mayer TG, Tencer AF, Kristoferson S, Mooney V. Use of non-invasive techniques for quantification of spinal range-of-motion in normal subjects and chronic low-back dysfunction patients. *Spine* 1984;9:588–95.
23. Boline PD, Keating JC, Haas M, Anderson AV. Interexaminer reliability and discriminant validity of inclinometric measurement of lumbar rotation in chronic low-back pain patients and subjects without low-back pain. *Spine* 1992;17:335–8.
24. Nelson MA, Allen P, Clamp SE, de Dombal FT. Reliability and reproducibility of clinical findings in low-back pain. *Spine* 1979;4:97–101.
25. McCombe PF, Fairbank JCT, Cockersole BC, Pynsent PB. Reproducibility of physical signs in low-back pain. *Spine* 1989;14:908–18.
26. Spratt KF, Lehmann TR, Weinstein JN, Sayre HA. A new approach to the low-back physical examination: behavioral assessment of mechanical signs. *Spine* 1990;15:96–102.
27. Ahern DK, Hannon DJ, Goreczny AJ, Follick MJ, Parziale JR. Correlation of chronic low-back pain behavior and muscle function examination of the flexion-relaxation response. *Spine* 1990;15:92–5.
28. Burkhauser RV, Hirvonen P. United States disability policy in a time of economic crisis: a comparison with Sweden and the Federal Republic of Germany. *Milbank Q* 1989;67[Suppl 2 Pt 1]:166–93.
29. Bigos SJ, Spengler DM, Martin NA, et al. Back injuries in industry: a retrospective study. III. Employee-related factors. *Spine* 1986;11:252–6.
30. Crown S. Psychological aspects of low back pain. *Rheumatol Rehabil* 1978;17:114–24.
31. North RB, Ewend MG, Lawton MT, Kidd DH, Piantadosi S. Failed back surgery syndrome: 5-year follow-up after spinal cord stimulator implantation. *Neurosurgery* 1991;28:692–9.
32. Wesley AL, Gatchel RJ, Polatin PB, Kinney RK, Mayer TG. Differentiation between somatic and cognitive/affective components in commonly used measurements of depression in patients with chronic low-back pain. *Spine* 1991;16:S213–5.
33. Deyo RA, Walsh NE, Schoenfeld LS, Ramamurthy S. Studies of the modified somatic perceptions questionnaire (MSPQ) in patients with back pain. *Spine* 1989;14:507–10.
34. Volinn E, Koevering DV, Loeser JD. Back sprain in industry: the role of socioeconomic factors in chronicity. *Spine* 1991;16:542–8.
35. Polatin PB, Gatchel RJ, Barnes D, Mayer H, Arens C, Mayer TG. A psychosociomedical prediction model of response to treatment by chronically disabled workers with low-back pain. *Spine* 1989;14:956–61.
36. Barnes D, Smith D, Gatchel RJ, Mayer TG. Psychosocioeconomic predictors of treatment success/failure in chronic low-back pain patients. *Spine* 1989;14:426–30.
37. Moffett JAK, Chase SM, Protek I, Ennis JR. A controlled, prospective study to evaluate the effectiveness of a back school in the relief of chronic low back pain. *Spine* 1986;11:120–2.
38. Turner JA, Clancy S, McQuade KJ, Cardenas DD. Effectiveness of behavioral therapy for chronic low back pain: a component analysis. *J Consult Clin Psychol* 1990;58:573–9.
39. Oland G, Tveiten G. A trial of modern rehabilitation for chronic low-back pain and disability. *Spine* 1991;16:457–9.
40. Quebec Task Force on Spinal Disorders. Scientific approach to the assessment and management of activity-related spinal disorders. *Spine* 1987;12[Suppl 1]:S1–S59.
41. Carron H, DeGood DE, Tait R. A comparison of low back pain patients in the United States and New Zealand: psychosocial and economic factors affecting severity of disability. *Pain* 1985;21:77–89.

Subject Index